# Contents

D0505847

# Acknowledgements

**Elizabeth Haworth** would like to thank her husband Mike and her children Emma and Ben for their continued love and support throughout the writing process. She would also like to thank her parents, Dorothy and Trevor, and also her sisters Anne and Pamela, her stepdaughters Rachel and Sarah, and their respective husbands, Alec, Paul, Mike and Emmanuel, for their encouragement. Finally she would like to thank her brother Glynne, who is never far from her thoughts.

**Beth Allen** would like to thank all of those who supported her during her writing period, both on a professional and personal level. Special thanks to Juliet Mozley for her patience, Pen Gresford for her encouragement and enthusiasm, Natasha Mills for sharing her GP practice knowledge and her daughters Olivia and Yasmin and husband Rob for their love, encouragement, patience and support.

**Carol Forshaw** would like to thank Nigel Hudson, Crime Reduction Officer, Anti-Social Behaviour Strategy, Bolton Council for his assistance in the writing of Unit 6. She would also like to thank her husband Ellis, sisters Gillian and Christine, and friend Pat for their continual support during the writing of Units 6 and 7.

**Denise Nicol** would like to thank John for his patience during the writing; her children, Emma and James for their love, support and encouragement and her mum for having faith in her. She would also like to thank her colleagues at Fernwood School, for putting up with her during some busy times.

**Anne Vollbracht** would like to thank her colleague and friend, Valerie Knowles, for her constructive criticism and comment while she was working on Unit 5.

## Photographs

© Alamy: page 8 (Nick Gregory), page 30 (Kitt Cooper-Smith), page 39 (Kuttig – People), page 42 (Richard Sheppard), page 51 (eurekaimages.com), page 56 (Frank Chmura), page 90 (Janine Wiedel Photolibrary), page 142 (Simon Clay), page 144 (Sue Thraves), page 154 (David Chilvers), page 178 (Picture Partners), page 214 (David Hoffman), page 233 (Rob Wilkinson), page 237 (Ian Miles-Flashpoint Pictures), page 245 (Jeff Greenberg)

© Bananastock: page 6

© Corbis: page x (Ed Murray), page 2 (Rick Gomez), page 18 (Gideon Mendel), page 80 (Kim Kulish), pages 88, 92, page 104 (Fred de Noyelle/Godong), page 132, page 198 (Roy Morsch), page 212, page 226 (Richard Hutchings)

© Creatas: page 182

© Digital Stock: pages 160, 174

© Digital Vision: pages 164, 180 (Rob van Petten)

© Getty: page vi (Graeme Robertson), page 41 (Hans Neleman), page 157 (Stuart McClymont)

© Image100: page 192

© iStockphoto: page 32 (Angelika Schwarz, eb33), page 148 (Anthony Baggett)

© Pearson Education Ltd: pages vi, vii, 46, 168, 206, 210, 221, 223, 228 (Jules Selmes) / pages 23, 73 (Richard Smith) / pages 48, 194 (Mind Studio) / page 52 (Chris Parker) / page 132 (Martin Sookias) / pages 164, 176 (Tudor Photography) / page 172 (Gareth Boden)

© PhotoDisc: page viii (Duncan Smith), page 32 (x 2), page 96 (Jim Wehtje), page 132 (C Squared Studios), page 203

© PA Photos: page 146 (Barry Batchelor/PA Archive), page 219 (Joe Giddens/EMPICS Sport)

© RCN Publishing company: page 27

© Rex Features: page 4 (Stuart Clarke), page 112 (Clive Dixon), page 150 (Peter MacDiarmid)

© SPL: page vi (John Cole), page 205 (Samuel Ashfield)

## About the diploma

Welcome to the Society, Health and Development Diploma. The diploma is an exciting qualification that allows you to explore and develop your knowledge, skills and understanding of the health, social care, community justice and Children and Young People's sectors. It will enable you to work across a wide range of disciplines and get a real feel for the sectors.

### Health, social care, community justice and Children and Young People's sectors

The Diploma covers the four main care sectors: health, social care, community justice and children and young people. Each sector covers a large variety of disciplines; throughout your course, you will learn about these and the roles and responsibilities of each discipline. Some of the types of organisation involved in each sector are listed below, and the relevant sector skills councils (SSCs) are indicated.

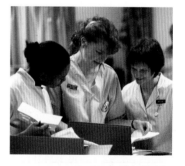

**Health (SSC = Skills for Health)**

* NHS primary care trusts; GPs; health centres; pharmacists; opticians, etc.
* NHS trust hospitals
* Voluntary organisations (e.g. Diabetes UK)
* Private providers; hospitals; hospices

**Social care (SSC = Skills for Care and Development), e.g.**

* Care homes
* Day centres
* Assessment and support services
* Housing associations

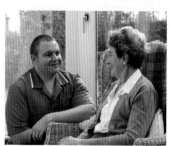

**Community justice (SSC = Skills for Justice)**

* Community safety and crime and disorder reduction partnerships; agencies working in local communities to reduce offending behaviour, including the probation service
* Voluntary organisations (e.g. Crime Concern, NACRO, SOVA, Rainer)
* Drug and alcohol services; National Treatment Agency for Substance Misuse; Phoenix House
* Providers of residential services in the community for offenders (hostels and housing associations)
* Groups working with victims, survivors and witnesses (e.g. Victim Support, Rape Crisis, Women's Aid)
* Youth justice services; youth offending teams (YOTs)

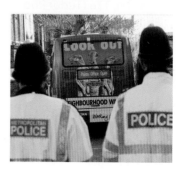

**Children and Young People (SSC = SkillsActive and Children's Workforce Development Council)**

* Education services, e.g. primary and secondary schools
* Private nurseries; local authority nurseries; nurseries based within schools and employer organisations
* Crèches and playgroups
* Mother and child groups

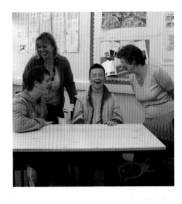

## What you will cover

Your diploma is made up of three elements and you will have to pass all three elements to achieve your qualification.

* **Principal learning** – this is the main part of the qualification and is organised into the units shown in the table on the right. The work you do here is directly related to the knowledge and skills required by the care sectors. Your teacher will make sure that the work you do is really relevant to your future career.

* **Generic learning** – during your course, you will also be working on maths, English and ICT functional skills that will be vital in getting the basics right for your career or further education. You'll also have the chance to develop your personal communication and thinking skills (known as personal, learning and thinking skills).

* **Additional learning** – in this part of your course you can choose to broaden your experience by choosing qualifications from areas outside the care sectors, or specialise even further in the care sectors.

It also includes a **project qualification** (see pages 232–247) and **work experience** (see pages x–xi). Your teacher will also support you in achieving these aspects of your diploma.

| Principal learning |
| --- |
| Principles, values and personal development |
| Working together and communicating |
| Safeguarding and protecting individuals |
| Growth, development and healthy living |
| Needs and preferences |
| Antisocial and offending behaviour |
| Supporting children and young people |
| Patient-centred health |
| The social model of disability |

*These are the units that you must do. Your teacher will set projects and assignments for each of them.*

## Practical work

The diploma will involve a lot of practical work. It is an active course in which you need to be an active learner. Your teacher will set up fantastic projects for you to work on, which may involve developing health promotional material, performing role-plays or creating an exhibition, and you will have to take on a range of roles and responsibilities.

### Activity

1 Think about the practical and creative work that you have been involved with in the past. Have you performed in a school play, carried out volunteer work, contributed to a student magazine or produced some posters? What sort of skills did you need to complete these tasks? Were some of them specific to the practical work that you were doing at the time and were some more generalised?

2 Think carefully about which parts of the diploma you are interested in and discuss the options that are available to you with your teacher.

# Get the basics right

In the care sectors, basic skills in English, maths and ICT are just as important as specialist or technical knowledge. Each unit of this book will give you opportunities to use and develop each of these three functional skills. You will need to reach the required standard in all three to obtain the diploma.

## Strengths and weaknesses

Think about each of the three functional skills (English, maths and ICT). What do you think your skill level is in each of these subjects? Which one is your strongest? Which one is your weakest? Will you need any extra help and support in any of the three areas?

These are all important questions that you will need to ask yourself and talk over with your teacher.

### Case study: Ryan

Ryan is very interested in public health and has chosen the Society, Health and Development Diploma because he hopes to learn more about this area and attend work experience in care settings, where he will meet some service users and members of the community. Ryan feels very confident about meeting and talking to people; however, he also realises that he will be using his reading and writing skills throughout his course when he needs to:

* research areas that are new to him, such as legislation relating to the care sectors
* learn how to use new equipment
* write accurate reports.

### Activity

1 Think about English first. Identify situations in which you will need to use both written and spoken English during your diploma and in your chosen career. Do the same for maths and for ICT.

2 How confident are you in each of the three areas?

### Case study: Amy

Amy feels confident in her use of both written and spoken English and is also able to use a number of different software programmes on her PC. She is looking forward to using her existing English and ICT skills in the work she will be doing on the diploma and learning some new skills as she goes along.

However, she has always struggled with maths and is worried that she won't be able to cope with this part of the course. She is surprised and worried that maths is an important part of the diploma, and hadn't realised how often she would need to draw on her maths skills in a career in care.

Amy's teacher has explained that she will need to use her maths skills when she has to:

* put together and manage budgets in a care home, hospital or primary school
* work out someone's body mass index as part of a health assessment
* carry out patient satisfaction surveys and analyse the results.

Her teacher has arranged for Amy to attend an extra maths workshop to get some help with the sums and calculations that she will need to do. He has reassured Amy that the calculations she'll work on will all be set within the setting of the care sectors and will link in with her project work.

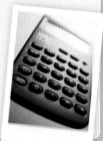

### Case study: Samuel

Samuel has basic ICT skills, but has always preferred to handwrite his work/use the library instead of the Internet for research, etc. However, he knows that the diploma might require him to use and develop his ICT skills further to:

* broaden his range of knowledge and research possibilities for his projects on the Internet
* manage his work and store his data electronically throughout the course
* format and create materials using applications such as Microsoft Publisher.

# Get ahead in the care sectors

To get ahead in the care sectors, you will need to develop skills to help you work effectively both alone and in a team. These skills are personal, learning and thinking skills, or PLTS. You will be able to use them in each stage of this qualification and take them with you when you progress on to the next level or get a job. They are the important skills in life, and important to pass this qualification and get the best out of your studies.

## Types of role

Each PLTS has been matched below to an example of one job in which it is important. However, it is important to remember that, for any role in the care sector, you will need strong skills in all six areas. Your teacher will be able to give you feedback on the progress you are making on your PLTS and highlight the areas that you need to develop further.

### Activity

1 Think back to a practical project you have worked on. Write down the words that best describe you and the way in which you like to work. Do you prefer to work alone or in a team? What motivates you? Are you a natural leader or do you prefer to let someone else take the lead?

2 Do you think that this description will change as you progress through the course?

### Team worker

**Teaching assistant**
Simon is a strong team worker who works in a collaborative way (i.e. with others) as a teaching assistant for a primary school. He feels confident working with other people and is able to take responsibility for his own role in a team. Simon is a good listener and is able to understand and relate to other people's views. These qualities allow him to form good working relationships with other people and to resolve issues so that the teaching team as a whole can meet their goals.

### Reflective learner

**Art therapist**
Floella has always been a strong reflective learner, as she is able to evaluate her own strengths and limitations and then set herself realistic targets for further improvement. She is happy to receive feedback from other people and is able to respond to this feedback in a positive way. Floella works very effectively on her own and is now self-employed as an art therapist.

### Independent enquirer

**NHS manager**
Anna works as an NHS manager. She is able to plan and undertake her own investigations and then process and evaluate the information. This allows her to take informed and well thought out decisions that also recognise that other people may well have different views and beliefs to her own.

### Effective participator

**Social worker**
At college, Yasmin could always be relied upon to engage with a range of different issues and play a full and leading role in getting things done. Yasmin is a good communicator and has used that skill in her role as social worker for a local authority.

### Self-manager

**Private residential care home manager**
Barbara was a very organised and committed student who displayed good levels of initiative, responsibility and perseverance at college. She now works as a care home manager and is responsible for the running of the home and ensuring it is up to government care home standards. Barbara responds positively to frequent changes to her schedule and organises her own time and resources effectively. She can prioritise and is able to balance many competing pressures and demands.

### Creative thinker

**Youth offending project officer**
Brian's role as a youth offending project officer means he works with a variety of young people from various backgrounds. His role involves him planning and organising activities to engage these young people within the community. He often comes up with imaginative ideas for activities and he is always keen to try out new and original ways of doing things.

# Get out to work!

Work experience is an important part of the Society, Health and Development Diploma and offers you the opportunity to apply and add to your knowledge, understanding, skills and experience of the world of work. Getting quality work experience may not be easy, as there is often a high demand for placements and the care sectors are often very busy and sensitive environments, but you will learn a lot through trying and even more when you succeed! So, go on, give it a go!

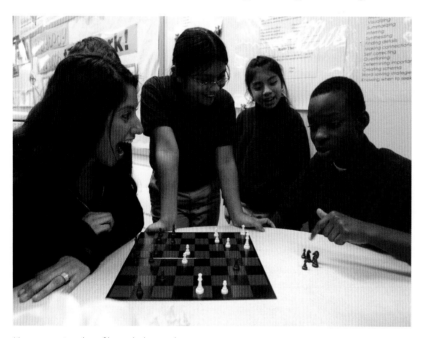

*You can gain a lot of knowledge and experience by finding a placement in a real-life working environment.*

## What's out there?

Although you don't *have* to do your work placement within a care environment, the sector is one of the largest, with approximately two million people working in health care alone in the UK. It is also the fastest growing, and there's a shortage of skills in some areas. So, by making sure you get the right experience and develop the right skills for the future, there's a huge range of jobs that you could do.

There's a whole range of jobs, roles and occupations the diploma could lead you to. It doesn't really matter what form your work experience takes; what's more important are the knowledge and skills that you get out of it and the insight that you gain into the world of work – there are a wide range of jobs that you could investigate, so start thinking creatively! These include:

* Adult care worker
* Art therapist
* Children's nurse
* Children's social worker
* Community safety warden
* Counsellor
* Dietician
* Educational psychologist
* Health care assistant
* Nurse
* Nursery nurse
* Occupational therapist
* Pharmacy technician
* Play worker
* Police community support officer
* Probation officer
* Prosthetics designer
* Speech therapist
* Teacher
* Victim support worker
* Youth offending team worker
* Youth worker

Work experience can come in lots of different shapes and sizes. Sometimes it is organised as a one-off two-week placement, but more often it can take the form of shorter, more regular activities that are linked in with the project work that you are undertaking in your school or college.

## Making contact

You will need to decide on the best way of making contact with the individual or organisation that you are trying to arrange a placement with. Sometimes the personal approach will be the best option – either talking to somebody who you already know face to face or by phoning them.

An email or a more formal letter might also be appropriate for some organisations, but you need to remember that some will receive lots of requests for work experience and you must be prepared to receive a letter or email back saying that they have no time available for you. They could be so busy that you might not even get a reply at all!

Don't let this put you off and don't take it personally. Working in the care sectors can be very busy and stressful, and people often have to work to very tight deadlines. This means that they have to prioritise their workloads, and sometimes answering letters, emails or phone calls from people wanting work experience is not at the top of their to-do list!

Your teacher should be able to advise you on the best course of action for your particular circumstances and it is best to talk it over with them first.

Some large care organisations will have staff dedicated to organising work experience and the best way to find this out is to ask for their human resources department. However, some care organisations are small and do not have a dedicated team to manage work experience. In this case enquire at the organisation whether they take students on work experience and if so who is the person that manages this.

### Remember

Remember that first impressions count. You need to communicate a positive image of yourself from the start. If you are writing to someone, check your spelling and grammar very carefully. If you are meeting somebody face to face, make sure you speak and dress in an appropriate way so you make the right impression.

* Work experience is your chance to make a great impression. Make the most of every opportunity!

* The care sector is made up of private, statutory and voluntary organisations.

### Activity

1 Discuss the work experience options that are open to you with the rest of your group and with your teacher. Write a list of the potential placements that are available.

2 Undertake some further research and decide on which ones you are going to contact. Good luck!

# How to use this book

This book has been divided into nine units to match the structure of the Society, Health and Development Diploma qualification Level 2. Each double-page spread covers an individual theme or topic.

## Features of the book

Throughout the book you will find the following features.

**Diploma Daily**
Newspaper-style features bring issues and topics to life, with built-in activities and questions.

**Personal, learning and thinking skills**
Elements of the generic learning (see page vii) are embedded in the principal learning. These features highlight opportunities to develop and demonstrate your personal, learning and thinking skills.

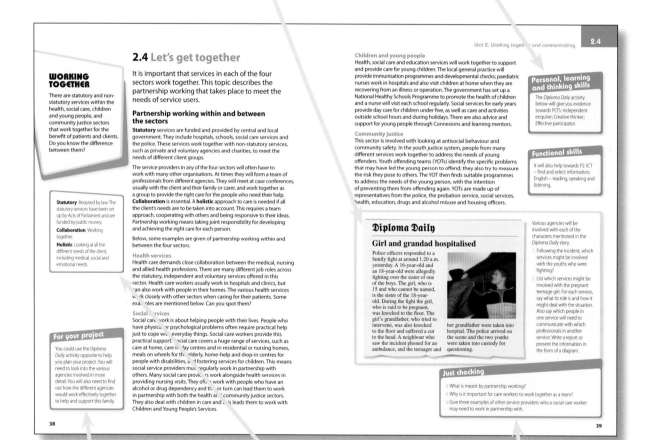

### 2.4 Let's get together

**WORKING TOGETHER**

There are statutory and non-statutory services within the health, social care, children and young people, and community justice sectors that work together for the benefit of patients and clients. Do you know the difference between them?

It is important that services in each of the four sectors work together. This topic describes the partnership working that takes place to meet the needs of service users.

**Partnership working within and between the sectors**
**Statutory** services are funded and provided by central and local government. They include hospitals, schools, social care services and the police. These services work together with non-statutory services, such as private and voluntary agencies and charities, to meet the needs of different client groups.

The service providers in any of the four sectors will often have to work with many other organisations. At times they will form a team of professionals from different agencies. They will meet at case conferences, usually with the client and their family or carer, and work together as a group to provide the right care for the people who need their help. **Collaboration** is essential. A **holistic** approach to care is needed if all the client's needs are to be taken into account. This requires a team approach, cooperating with others and being responsive to their ideas. Partnership working means taking joint responsibility for developing and achieving the right care for each person.

Below, some examples are given of partnership working within and between the four sectors.

**Health services**
Health care demands close collaboration between the medical, nursing and allied health professions. There are many different job roles across the statutory, independent and voluntary services offered in this sector. Health care workers usually work in hospitals and clinics, but can also work with people in their homes. The various health services work closely with other sectors when caring for their patients. Some examples are mentioned below. Can you spot them?

**Social services**
Social care work is about helping people with their lives. People who have physical or psychological problems often require practical help just to cope with everyday things. Social care workers provide this practical support. Social care covers a huge range of services, such as care at home, care in day centres and in residential or nursing homes, meals on wheels for the elderly, home-help and drop-in centres for people with disabilities, and fostering services for children. This means social service providers must regularly work in partnership with others. Many social care providers work alongside health services in providing nursing visits. They often work with people who have an alcohol or drug dependency and this in turn can lead them to work in partnership with both the health and community justice sectors. They also deal with children in care and this leads them to work with Children and Young People's Services.

**Statutory** Required by law. The statutory services have been set up by Acts of Parliament and are funded by public money.

**Collaboration** Working together.

**Holistic** Looking at all the different needs of the client, including medical, social and emotional needs.

**For your project**

You could use the *Diploma Daily* activity opposite to help you plan your project. You will need to look into the various agencies involved in more detail. You will also need to find out how the different agencies would work effectively together to help and support this family.

Unit 2: Working together and communicating   **2.4**

**Children and young people**
Health, social care and education services will work together to support and provide care for young children. The local general practice will provide immunisation programmes and developmental checks; paediatric nurses work in hospitals and also visit children at home when they are recovering from an illness or operation. The government has set up a National Healthy Schools Programme to promote the health of children and a nurse will visit each school regularly. Social services for early years provide day care for children under five, as well as care and activities outside school hours and during holidays. There are also advice and support for young people through Connexions and learning mentors.

**Community justice**
This sector is involved with looking at antisocial behaviour and community safety. In the youth justice system, people from many different services work together to address the needs of young offenders. Youth offending teams (YOTs) identify the specific problems that may have led the young person to offend; they also try to measure the risk they pose to others. The YOT then finds suitable programmes to address the needs of the young person, with the intention of preventing them from offending again. YOTs are made up of representatives from the police, the probation service, social services, health, education, drugs and alcohol misuse and housing officers.

**Personal, learning and thinking skills**

The *Diploma Daily* activity below will give you evidence towards PLTS: Independent enquirer; Creative thinker; Effective participator.

**Functional skills**

It will also help towards FS: ICT – find and select information; English – reading, speaking and listening.

**Diploma Daily**

### Girl and grandad hospitalised

Police officers responded to a family fight at around 1.20 a.m. yesterday. A 16-year-old and an 18-year-old were allegedly fighting over the sister of one of the boys. The girl, who is 15 and who cannot be named, is the sister of the 18-year-old. During the fight the girl, who is said to be pregnant, was knocked to the floor. The girl's grandfather, who tried to intervene, was also knocked to the floor and suffered a cut to the head. A neighbour who saw the incident phoned for an ambulance, and the teenager and her grandfather were taken into hospital. The police arrived on the scene and the two youths were taken into custody for questioning.

Various agencies will be involved with each of the characters mentioned in the *Diploma Daily* story.

1 Following the incident, which services might be involved with the youths who were fighting?

2 List which services might be involved with the pregnant teenage girl. For each service, say what its role is and how it might deal with the situation. Also say which people in one service will need to communicate with which professionals in another service. Write a report or present the information in the form of a diagram.

**Just checking**

» What is meant by partnership working?

» Why is it important for care workers to work together as a team?

» Give three examples of other service providers who a social care worker may need to work in partnership with.

38

39

**For your project**
These are useful things to consider when working on your project.

**Key terms**
Key concepts and new words are explained clearly and simply to make sure you don't miss anything important.

**Just checking**
Summary questions focus on important points covered in each double-page spread and check your understanding and knowledge.

# Want to achieve more?

Each unit ends with an assessment guide, which gives advice on getting the best from the assessment. It tells you how you will be assessed and how your work will be marked, and gives you useful reminders for key unit themes. Hints and tips give you guidance on how to aim for the higher mark band so you can use your new skills and knowledge to best effect.

## Starter stimulus
A discussion point or short activity that will introduce the key concepts of the double-page spread.

## Their story
Personalised case studies show the concepts covered in this book applied to the real world through scenarios. Questions and activities will encourage you to push your understanding further.

---

**THINKING POINT**

When you write notes in a lesson, can you understand them when you next look at them to type or write them up for your final piece of work? Or do you have to keep asking others if they know what you have written or should have written?

### 2.7 Get the record straight

It is important to be able to complete records accurately and legibly. This topic makes some recommendations on how to set out your writing.

*What a mess!*

**Activity**

Think about all the different types of writing you may do in a day at school and across different subjects.

1 Write a list. Which ones are notes or written in draft form?

2 Can you think of a piece of work you had to tailor to a particular audience or for a particular situation? What methods did you use to do this? Look at the language, the terminology. Was the writing formal or informal?

#### Writing that's right for the job
**The right language**
The aim of written communication is to give information; it is therefore important that the writing is clear and accurate. Service providers must be able to present information in different ways, depending on who they are communicating with and what they are writing about. You will need to be able to structure the material so that it is clear to the person you are communicating with. You must make yourself understood: if you are writing for a patient or client there is no point in using a lot of **jargon**, or terms that might cause confusion and worry. It is, however, important to use the correct **terminology**, especially when communicating with service providers in other sectors or if your records may be used in a court.

**Always check it**
People often make mistakes when they are writing; sometimes your brain seems to work faster than your pen and you miss words out, make spelling errors or use the wrong words. You should *always* read through what you have written before passing it on. Check that you have written in a clear and precise way, and check your spellings and punctuation. Make sure that what you have written makes sense and that your grammar is correct. If you don't do these things then, at best, what you have written might not make sense or, at worst, it could be very misleading to whoever is reading it, which could result in a serious mistake being made, such as the wrong medicine or the wrong advice being given.

**Research**
It may be that you will have to find out some information about a case, an illness or a piece of legislation. There are many ways of researching information. Depending on what you need to find out, you might use the Internet, books, letters or articles.

44

---

**Typing or handwriting?**
The information and communication technology (ICT) skills that you learn at school and college will be very helpful, as you will need to update client files and records, and prepare reports. A lot of this type of work is now done electronically, although there will still be times when you need to write things by hand. For example, a nurse will usually update medical records for patients on a ward by hand, with pen on paper. Similarly, a police officer will note about an incident. These will often have to be written up at a later date. Minutes at a meeting are often taken by hand.

**Presentation**
Because the records kept in the health, social care, children and young people and the community justice sectors are often so important, they must be accurate and legible. Make sure you:

• write clearly in pen or use a computer
• use the correct grammar, spelling and punctuation
• write for the audience, and use the correct and appropriate terminology
• use headings, subheadings and paragraphs
• make sure your reports and letters are dated and signed.

**Jargon** Specialist words and expressions when used inappropriately, with people who won't understand them.

**Terminology** Specialised words or expressions that are used by people in a particular work setting.

**Minutes** A record of what is said and decided at a meeting, made at the time.

**Functional skills**

The case study tasks will help you towards FS: English – writing.

#### Case study: Emma's story

Emma is 15 years old. She had become very interested in dieting when she was 14 and lost a lot of weight. Her mother became worried about her. She put some weight back on over the summer holidays but since starting school again in September she has lost weight again. Her periods have stopped. She complains about being too tired to do her homework and has lost interest in school and her friends there. Her mother can't understand why, as she could do well at school if she put her mind to it. Her mother insists she goes to see their GP.

The doctor measures Emma's weight and height and calculates her body mass index (BMI) (see topic 8.4) as 17, which is very much underweight. He thinks she may be suffering from anorexia.

People with anorexia have extreme weight loss as a result of strict dieting. In spite of this, they believe they are fat and are worried about what is in reality a normal weight or

shape. People with low self-esteem are more vulnerable, as are girls in mid-adolescence. A diagnosis of anorexia nervosa is based on the person's BMI, the individual having a distorted body image and abnormal attitudes to food and weight, amenorrhoea (which is the absence of menstruation) and other signs of starvation, such as tiredness, slow pulse rate and gaunt face.

1 Imagine you are Emma's GP. You want a hospital colleague to confirm the diagnosis and to take on the case if necessary. Write a brief referral letter to this colleague, giving your findings and requesting help. Use the appropriate language and terminology for a formal letter to a professional colleague.

2 Write a short letter to Emma's mother explaining your findings and the referral. Think carefully how you will word this letter.

#### Just checking

• List four types of sources of information you could use in researching a case you were working on.
• Why and when might you need to write notes or fill in forms by hand?
• What kind of work might you do electronically in a hospital, at a school or in a community justice agency?

45

---

## Activity
These activities test your understanding and give you opportunities to apply your knowledge and skills.

## Functional skills
Functional skills (see page vii) have been built into many of the activities in this book. These features highlight opportunities to develop and practise your functional skills in English, ICT or maths. Remember, you will need a pass in all three functional skills to achieve the full diploma.

## Introduction

This unit is about the importance of following good practice in caring for others. The workers in the four main sectors covered in this qualification will often be referred to as 'service providers' and the people who use the services as 'service users'.

### THINKING POINT

Service providers base the way they work on their values and beliefs about caring for others. What do *you* believe in? If you go on to have a career in one of the four main care sectors, how do you think your beliefs will help you care for other people?

### Diploma Daily

#### Parents' joy as Toby is brought back to life

Mr and Mrs Ashley appeared on television last night to thank the police and all others involved in helping save their youngest son, Toby, from drowning. Mrs Ashley had been changing her baby daughter's nappy at a fund-raising picnic when Toby wandered off and fell in the river. A search was launched and he was pulled out of the water by a community police officer on duty at the event. Toby wasn't breathing and had to be resuscitated by paramedics. A tearful Mrs Ashley said: 'I cannot thank everyone enough. If the

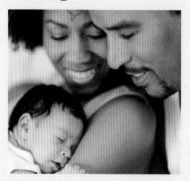

police officer hadn't spotted Toby when he did, and if everyone else had not acted so promptly and efficiently, things could have ended very differently.'

1 Write down as many different groups of people, such as the police, who will have helped the family during the time between Toby falling in the river and being collected from the hospital by his parents.

2 When they were working to find, revive and return Toby to his family, what do you think all these people believed was important for:
(a) Toby
(b) his family
(c) society in general?

**Sector** The care industry is divided into sectors that are responsible for different aspects of the care of people, such as the social care sector and the health sector.

### The main sectors

The main four **sectors** covered in this qualification are health, social care, children and young people, and community justice.

### The health sector

The role of a health worker is to help people stay healthy and to treat them if they become ill, physically or mentally. Health workers include doctors, nurses, dentists, opticians and pharmacists. The Department of Health is responsible for the National Health Service, which provides most health care in the United Kingdom.

### The social care sector

The role of a social worker is to enable people to live more successfully within their local communities. Social workers not only work with individuals but also build relationships with their families and friends.

They also work closely with organisations such as the police, the health service, schools and the local housing department. Ensuring that all workers in the sector follow high professional standards is the responsibility of a public body called the General Social Care Council (GSCC).

### Children and Young People sector

People who work in this sector help children and young people reach their full potential. This sector covers education services, adoption and foster care and children's homes. The sectors overlap considerably and social workers also work in this one, where they help to keep families together and support young people who are in trouble with the law or who have problems at school, for example.

### Community justice sector

The community justice sector helps to reduce re-offending. Another word for community justice is restorative justice. The crimes can range from **antisocial behaviour** to domestic violence, or from serious motoring offences to substance misuse. Not all of the offenders will have served a prison sentence. Agencies involved in community justice include local authorities, the police, the probation service and the Youth Justice Board.

## What underpins good practice in the care sectors?

Workers in the care sectors share a set of **values**, which form the value base. To provide a high standard of care, service providers follow a set of **principles**.

To ensure that workers stick to a set of values and principles, they are provided with **legislation**, **codes of practice**, **policies** and **procedures** to follow. These are looked at in topic 1.9.

## How you will be assessed

For this unit you will be assessed by one assignment, consisting of three tasks. The tasks will cover: the principles and values that are at the heart of the work of the four sectors; key legislation, codes of professional practice, policies and procedures that relate to principles and values of the four sectors; and a reflective account – you need to reflect on your own values, knowledge and skills and then relate these to the work of the sectors.

## What you will learn in this unit

You will:

* Understand the meaning of the terms diversity, equality, culture and belief systems, individuality, rights, choice, privacy, independence, dignity, respect and partnership
* Know how equality and diversity are promoted within and across the sectors
* Understand what is meant by inappropriate behaviour, how to recognise it and how it can be constructively challenged
* Know how key legislation, codes of professional practice, policies and procedures support an individual's rights, and provide a framework to maintain and improve quality of practice
* Be able to assess your own values, knowledge and skills
* Understand what is meant by 'reflective practice' and how practitioners develop their knowledge and skills to continually develop and improve practice and quality of service provision
* Be able to identify sources of information for professional development

---

**Antisocial behaviour** A wide range of selfish and unacceptable activity that spoils the quality of community life.

**Values** Beliefs about what is important and worthwhile in life and what is morally right.

**Principle** A basic guide to the right way to behave, for example that you should try to treat everyone fairly.

---

**Legislation** A law or group of laws as passed by Parliament.

**Codes of practice** Sets of standards of conduct for workers and employers across the four care sectors.

**Policy** A document that tells service providers how to deal with particular situations in the workplace.

**Procedure** A list of steps to follow to complete a particular task in the correct way.

# 1.1 Principles and values

In this topic you will learn what 'diversity', 'equality' and 'individuality' mean. You will also find out how a person's culture is taken account of when they use services and why it is important to value diversity.

**SHOP TILL YOU DROP**

Do you think it is fair to treat everyone equally? Write down an example of how everyone is treated equally when visiting a shopping centre. Can you think of any examples where certain shoppers should be treated differently? Explain why you think this.

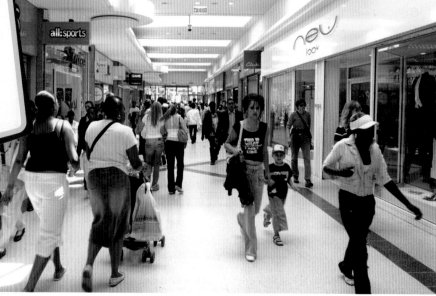

*Is everyone treated equally when they visit a shopping centre?*

**Ethnicity** The fact that someone belongs to a particular ethnic group. An ethnic group means people who share the same way of life and culture.

**Culture** A set of beliefs, language, styles of dress, ways of cooking, religion, ways of behaving and so on shared by a particular group of people.

**Discriminate** Treat a person or group unfairly or differently from other persons or groups of people (e.g. on the basis of prejudice).

**Prejudice** An unreasonable feeling against a person or group of people, especially not liking a particular group of people.

## What is diversity?

People are different in many ways, such as age, gender, sexuality, **ethnicity**, **culture** and beliefs. Diversity means a variety. To value diversity means to respect the cultures and beliefs of other people. If we dismiss or ignore other people's beliefs and cultures, we will not be able to learn about and understand them.

Good service providers get to know the people they work with. They will be open to other people's life experiences and differences, and they will value their diversity. They will form good relationships with both colleagues and service users. A team of service providers who have different interests and skills is more likely to be able to tackle the range of tasks required to help a service user.

## What is equality?

Equality means everyone having the same chance as everyone else to obtain or achieve something, for example access to a service they need. Different people see the world in different ways. Our way of thinking might seem as strange to other people as theirs does to us. We should value and learn from these differences rather than treat people unfairly because of them.

4

When people **discriminate** unfairly against someone else we say they are **prejudiced**. Service providers have to adopt an anti-discriminatory approach to service users, by recognising and responding to their individual needs.

## Diploma Daily

**Dear Dorothy**
I have just been in the Citizens Advice Bureau. A traveller told me he was asking for help to get benefits, medical care and education for his children.

How can this be right when he doesn't live in the area and hasn't contributed any money towards our services?

*Name withheld*

1 Write an answer to the letter from the problem page of the *Diploma Daily*. Include the words *diversity* and *equality* in your answer.

2 Now think about people who immigrate to this country. Discuss with a friend how you feel about people moving in and having use of various services. Then write a letter and an answer for the problem page, explaining why they should have full access to all services.

## Treating people as individuals

Everyone should receive a service of equal quality that meets their personal needs. This is not the same as everyone receiving the same service. For example, everyone should be able to register with a doctor but a sick person will require more of the doctor's time. Similarly, everyone has the right to a fair hearing in court if they have been accused of a crime, but someone with, say, a speech impediment may need an extra service, such as an advocate (someone who speaks on their behalf), in order to have a fair trial.

Treating people as individuals by taking into account their different beliefs, abilities and so on is crucial when caring for others. Service providers need to acknowledge an individual's personal beliefs even if they do not share those beliefs. For example, if Manny is Jewish and only eats kosher food at home, it is only right that he is given kosher meat if he is in prison or in hospital. This will make him feel that his identity has been valued and may also help his rehabilitation or recovery.

**Activity**

Choose a culture that is different from your own.

1 Find out what people from that culture eat, how they dress and what their beliefs are (for example that it is right to pray at particular times of day, or that it is wrong to have a blood transfusion). Find this information from your library or on the Internet.

2 How should these beliefs be acknowledged when a person of your age uses the residential services provided by one of the four main sectors (that is, a care home, a hospital, a young offender institution or a boarding school)? Write down your ideas.

3 To help people from that culture, produce a leaflet which explains their needs.

**Functional skills**

The activity will help with FS: ICT – find and select information; English – reading and writing.

**Just checking**

✳ Why is it important to value diversity?

✳ What is the difference between culture and ethnicity?

✳ Why is it correct to treat people in an anti-discriminatory way?

# 1.2 Belief systems

This topic covers what belief systems are, and the difference between belief and knowledge. It also tells you more about values, which are important to both service users and service providers.

## COURT IN THE ACT?

Look at the picture of a young person in court on trial for a minor crime. She has been advised by her lawyer that she should remove her piercings, but she feels they reflect her identity. What effect might her appearance have on the jury? Do you think she is more likely to be found guilty? Why is this? Is this fair? What advice would you give her if she were to appear in court again?

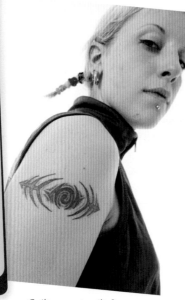

*Guilty or not guilty?*

## Belief systems

Belief systems are strongly held opinions that determine how you see life. Many people don't reflect much on what they believe, but their beliefs still influence their everyday thoughts, words, feelings and actions. People's beliefs usually stem from their upbringing, the events that happen in their lives, and the influence of family and friends.

A belief system may be based on religion, family values or personal experiences. It can affect everything that a person does, and even a person's health. A person who worries all the time and is constantly under stress will have increased blood pressure and will be more likely to have headaches and stomach problems.

A person's belief system will affect how they access services. For instance, if someone believes they are not very bright they are less likely to try hard at school, believing they can't do the work, and so lose out on the education they deserve.

## What is the difference between belief and knowledge?

A belief is something that a person accepts as true without proof. For example, they may believe that God exists even though no one has ever seen God. A belief may be true or false.

Knowledge is always true and can be a proven belief. For example, a detective might believe that a person is guilty of a crime; that belief would become knowledge if evidence from the forensic laboratory proved it to be right.

### When is knowledge important in the care sectors?

While it is important to respect service users' beliefs, to make sure they feel valued, it is also important to know certain things when dealing with people. For example, a doctor would need to know whether a person is allergic to, say, penicillin. It is also crucial to know the home contact details for a person in hospital, in a care home, a school or in prison, in case of an emergency.

# The value base

Some values common in the care sector have already been mentioned in this unit – valuing diversity and treating people equally. Other values that are of the utmost importance are respect and having regard for people's privacy, independence and dignity.

## Respect

Respect for a person means showing them consideration and courtesy. Even if a person has been convicted of a serious crime, they should not be treated with a lack of respect, because this makes the service provider look unprofessional.

## Privacy

Privacy means being free from intrusion in your personal life. For example, the residents of a care home for elderly people will feel very upset if carers walk into their room whenever they want without knocking first. A lack of privacy will undermine their **self-esteem** and make them feel they have lost their identity as **independent** people in control of their own lives. It is also important that carers keep any information they have about service users **confidential**, as this shows that they respect and value them, and can be trusted with confidences.

## Independence

It is important that people have control of their own lives. Workers in all care sectors aim to help people develop or maintain their independence. This will be discussed in topic 1.8.

## Dignity

Service providers should help people maintain their dignity. For example, a child at primary school who accidentally wets herself will be embarrassed if it is pointed out to everyone else. A good nursery teacher will simply take the child somewhere private, reassure her and get her clothes sorted out. This allows the child to maintain her dignity rather than feeling ashamed.

## Activity

Think of something you have learned recently in another subject and decide whether it is a belief or knowledge.

---

**Self-esteem** How highly you think of your abilities and yourself.

**Independent** Not having to rely on someone else to do things for you.

**Confidential** Private and secret.

---

## Case study: Aesha's story

Aesha is 84 years old and still lives in her own home. However, she can be lonely and so goes to a day care centre twice a week. There she helps other older people with small things and she leads games such as bingo. Because she was physically fit, the care assistants used to let her take the tea trolley round, but recently she broke her ankle. She now needs help going to the toilet and is helped to have a bath while she is at the centre, although she is expected to make a good recovery.

1 State which of the values mentioned in this topic are being applied in the care Aesha receives at the centre.

2 Explain how each of these will make her feel about herself.

3 Construct a spider diagram with Aesha in the centre and put the ways in which she is being helped at the day care centre on it. Add suggestions for how her family and friends can apply the same values as the service providers to help Aesha.

---

## Personal, learning and thinking skills

The case study tasks will provide evidence of PLTS: Creative thinker.

## Just checking

✳ What is a belief system?

✳ Give an example to show why it is important to have knowledge of facts about a person, as well as a respect for their beliefs, when caring for them.

✳ What could be the effects on a person if they were not treated with respect?

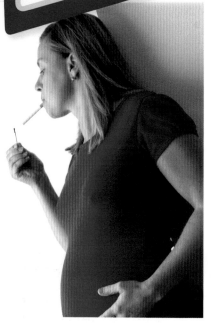

*Does everyone have the right to smoke?*

# 1.3 Rights and choice

In this topic you will find out about the difference between rights and responsibilities, and the importance of being able to have choice in life. The topic also explains some of the individual rights that are important to both service users and service providers.

## Rights and responsibilities

A right is something that a person can claim is due to them. A responsibility is a burden of obligation. People have the right to have their own beliefs and lifestyles, but no one has the right to damage the quality of other people's lives. This means that rights often come with responsibilities towards other people.

The easiest way to understand this is to consider a specific example. In this country, adults have the right to drink alcohol, even though there is a danger of it damaging their health and shortening their life. However, drinkers have a responsibility not to drive while under the influence of alcohol, so that they do not put other lives at risk. Other examples of rights and responsibilities are shown in the table.

*Examples of the rights and responsibilities of people using services in the care sectors*

| Rights | Responsibilities |
| --- | --- |
| Not to be discriminated against | Not to discriminate against others |
| To have control and independence in your own life | To help others to be independent and not to try to control others |
| To make choices and take some risks | Not to interfere with others or put others at risk |
| To maintain your own beliefs and lifestyle | To respect the different beliefs and lifestyles of others |
| To be valued and respected | To value and respect others |
| To live in a safe environment | Not to endanger others |
| To have personal matters kept confidential | To respect the confidentiality of others |

## Choice

It is important that people have choice in their lives so they can maintain as much independence as possible. For example, people who have a disability should be able to choose whether to live in a residential home or to live in their own home with a service provider going to help them each day. A person with a life-threatening illness may face a very difficult choice:

* undergo treatment that will give them a few more months of life but which will make them feel very ill during that time

* not receive the treatment but have a better quality of life for the short time they have left.

Should anyone else be allowed to make that choice for them?

Giving a person as much choice and control over their lives as possible increases their self-esteem. People should be allowed access to information about themselves, so that they can make informed choices. Good communication therefore often underpins choice.

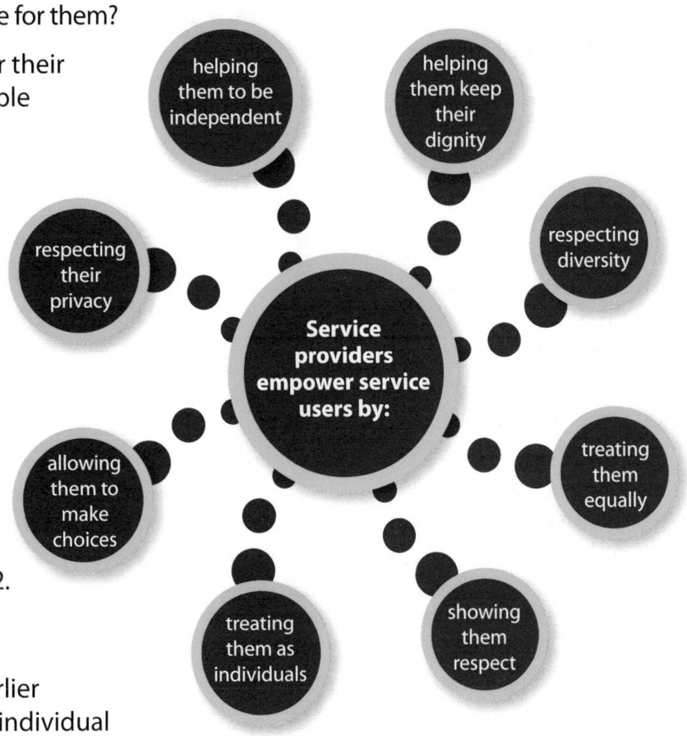

## Communication

It is vital that service providers communicate effectively with service users. This will allow good relationships to be formed. It will also empower the users, as they will feel that their opinions about their care are valued, that they are respected and that they can take part in decisions that affect their own care. The need for service providers to promote effective communication is covered in more detail in Unit 2.

# Individual rights

When we pull together all the ideas from the earlier topics, we see that some of the most important individual rights are those to be:

* respected
* treated equally and not discriminated against
* treated as an individual
* treated in a dignified way
* allowed privacy
* protected from danger and harm
* allowed access to information about yourself
* able to communicate using your preferred methods of communication and language
* cared for in a way that meets your needs, and that takes account of your choices and protects them.

## Health and safety

Health and safety issues affect both service providers and service users in the care sectors. Both have the right to be in a safe environment away from harm and there is considerable legislation around this issue. It is now part of a worker's daily routine to assess the safety of all situations.

All service providers try to base their work on a set of key values, which include those in the diagram above. This is called the value base in the social care sector. These key values are reflected in Clinical Governance and Essence of Care guidelines in the health sector, and in similar guidelines in the community justice and Children and Young People's sectors.

**Service providers empower service users by:**
- helping them to be independent
- helping them keep their dignity
- respecting diversity
- respecting their privacy
- treating them equally
- allowing them to make choices
- treating them as individuals
- showing them respect

## For your project

You could consider the different aspects of the key values and why they are important in providing consistently high-quality care.

## Just checking

* What is the difference between rights and responsibilities?
* Why is it necessary to allow people to have choice in their lives?
* Why is it vital to have effective communication between service providers and users?

# 1.4 Putting the value base into practice

This topic recaps the principles and values discussed so far in this unit. It looks at how these can be put into good practice in the social care sector. Good practice in the community justice sector is covered in Unit 6, the children and young people sector in Unit 7 and the health sector in Unit 8.

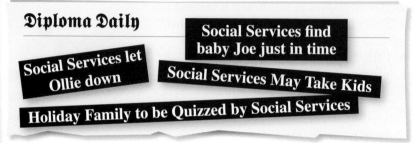

*Why might stories about the social services be of interest to the press?*

## The aims of social care

Social care covers a wide range of services that help people to carry on with their daily lives. The aims of all social services are:

* to support independence and respect dignity
* to meet the service user's specific needs
* to organise and finance social care in a fair, consistent manner
* to ensure that children in care get the same opportunities as other children
* to ensure that every user is safeguarded against abuse
* to provide a skilled, trained workforce
* to provide care to the highest standards.

The Department of Health states on its website (www.dh.gov.uk) that 'at any one time up to 1.5 million of the most vulnerable people in society are relying on social care workers and support staff for help.... There are now 25,000 employers with over one million staff providing social care.'

### Activity

1 Copy the mind map from the page opposite.

2 The branch for elderly people has branches coming off it showing some of the services provided, but most of the other branches have been left incomplete. Do some research (on the Internet or at the library) on the social services provided in your local area and add them to your mind map as smaller branches off the correct main branch.

3 One such service is the drug and alcohol team. Do research on how this service operates in your area. Make an information leaflet to tell people about this service.

## Case study: Amir's story

Amir is 16 and a young carer. His mother is single; her marriage failed after her drinking problem brought shame on her husband's family. Amir often comes home from school to find her slumped on the bed, having passed out from drinking too much. Despite being a very bright young person, he only just got the grades in his GCSEs to stay at school to study for his A-levels. He has to do the housework, shop and cook, as well as look after his mother. He does not have many friends, does not join in activities after school and will not go out at night, fearing for his mother's safety if he leaves her on her own. She loves Amir and when she is sober apologises and promises to try to stop drinking, but it never lasts. When she is drunk she sometimes lashes out at him in temper and says hurtful things to him, but Amir loves her and does not hit back, because he knows she is only behaving like this because of her drink problem.

His teachers do not know why his grades have suffered or why he seems quiet and withdrawn. His mother makes the effort to stay sober enough to go into school on review days, when she is presentable and charming. The sixth-form tutor asks to see Amir after school one day, but Amir is so worried about getting home later than usual that he gets agitated and upset. The tutor therefore lets him go, but she makes an appointment to see him in a free lesson instead. He finally breaks down and tells her the whole story. She alerts social services, who visit Amir and his mother at home. Because he is 16 they do not remove Amir from home but put services in place to support him and his mother.

1 Write down all the services you think Amir and his mother need help from, including the drug and alcohol team you have researched for the activity on page 10.

2 How do you think each of these service providers will support Amir's independence and dignity, and those of his mother?

3 Write down: (a) Amir's needs; and (b) his mother's needs. How can social services and other services such as education support their specific needs?

4 In what ways is Amir's mother abusing him? How can social services stop this?

5 Look at the value base diagram on page 9. Which other values besides those already looked at in this case study can the social services put into practice and how?

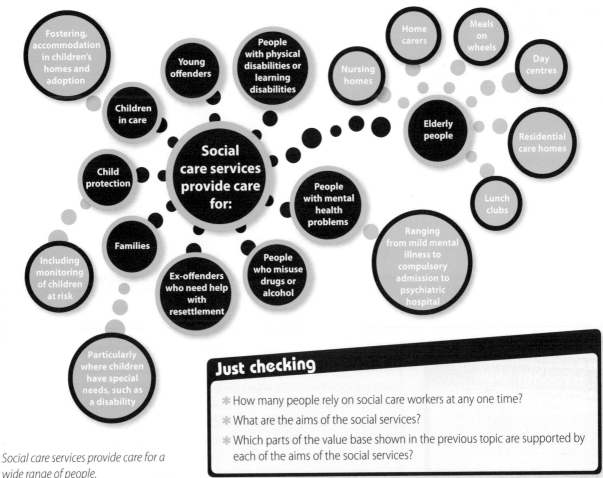

Social care services provide care for a wide range of people.

## Just checking

* How many people rely on social care workers at any one time?
* What are the aims of the social services?
* Which parts of the value base shown in the previous topic are supported by each of the aims of the social services?

# 1.5 Partnerships

This topic looks at how services work together in partnership to promote equality and diversity across the sectors. These partnerships may be between different service providers or between service users and providers. Topic 2.10 looks further at partnership working.

## Case study: Sam's story

Sam is 14 years old. He has a severe hearing impairment and uses a hearing aid and sign language. Before he started at high school, someone from the peripatetic hearing service visited to show the teachers and other staff how to help Sam as much as possible.

Recently Sam was crossing the road at pedestrian lights opposite the school when a car that was travelling too fast knocked him down and failed to stop. One of his teachers was at the crossing and immediately called the emergency services. Another teacher made a note of the names of those who had witnessed the accident. An ambulance took Sam to hospital while one of the teachers rang his parents. Sam was X-rayed and it was found that both his legs were broken. He was seen by an orthopaedic surgeon, who decided to operate. Sam is a Jehovah's Witness, so his parents would not allow him to have a blood transfusion; however, the medical team had a blood substitute on hand.

Sam's legs were set in plaster and he was given medication to ease the pain. He was allowed home the following week. His parents asked the school to provide some work so that Sam would not fall too far behind. His head of year regularly collected work from each of Sam's subject areas and called at Sam's home to drop it off and see how he was.

Sam had follow-up appointments at the hospital, including for physiotherapy. A lady from occupational health got him a wheelchair and helped his parents arrange the house to allow Sam to move about as much as possible. He continued to visit the hospital as an outpatient until he was discharged. After that he visited his own GP if he needed any pain relief.

On the same day as the accident, the police interviewed the teachers and students who witnessed the hit-and-run. They later interviewed Sam in hospital, with the help of a nurse who knew some sign language. They found that the driver was a local youth called Wayne, who lives in a care home. He had only recently passed his driving test and had not stopped because he panicked. The police arrested him but could tell that he was ashamed of what he had done and treated him sympathetically, helping him with a duty solicitor and calling his social worker. When Wayne appeared in court he pleaded guilty. He received a suspended sentence and community service, and his driving licence was cancelled. He was also given an appointment to appear in front of the local youth offenders panel, with his social worker and probation officer to support him. Sam and his parents were also invited. Sam was able to explain how the accident had affected him and Wayne apologised and vowed not to behave so irresponsibly again. He made amends to his victim, did his community service and went on to be a responsible citizen. The police asked him to go into local schools to talk to students about his experiences.

1 Working with a partner, make separate lists of all the different people, such as teachers and the police, who helped: (a) Sam; (b) Wayne. Do this down the left-hand side of a large sheet of paper. This list will include many, such as receptionists, who are not mentioned above. You need to imagine each stage of what happened to them both. Draw on your own experience of visits to the hospital and so on. Think about programmes you have seen on the television, such as *Casualty*.

2 When you have completed your lists, write by each person what service they provide and which of the four main sectors they work in.

3 Look at the list of individual rights presented in topic 1.3 and identify how each of these rights were met for: (a) Sam; (b) Wayne.

## Functional Skills

The case study tasks will provide evidence of FS: English – thinking and listening, writing.

## Partnerships

Service providers build effective relationships both within and across sectors. A good example is the care of someone with a physical disability. Instead of different people repeatedly assessing their needs, one professional will do so and pass on the relevant information to all the other organisations. The service user may need help in getting up and washed each morning, moving around the house and doing things like cooking a meal. One professional, maybe an occupational therapist, will go to the house, look at its layout, and talk to the individual and family to assess their needs. That one professional will then pass on the information and recommendations to all the relevant agencies.

One challenge facing workers in these sectors is to achieve the correct balance between action and inaction, between getting involved in people's lives and not. It may be that if a service does not take a certain action, both individuals and other members of society or the family could be at risk. Take as an example a teacher who spots a bruise on a child who is changing for PE and has seen other bruises previously on the same child. They may decide to report their concerns to social services. The child may be considered to be at risk and taken away from the family for some time. The bruises might have been caused by a family member or friend abusing the child, in which case the child has been removed from harm and put into a safe environment. On the other hand, the bruises might be the result of the child being particularly clumsy when playing out. By the time this has been proved, the child and family concerned will have suffered and relationships within the family may be irretrievably damaged.

## Promotion of equality and diversity

Within and across the sectors, service providers work in partnership to promote equality and diversity. They do this by:

* embracing (valuing) diversity and recognising equality
* respecting individuality
* respecting and promoting rights
* offering choice
* communicating effectively
* acknowledging personal beliefs and identity
* adopting non-judgemental attitudes
* ensuring anti-discriminatory practice.

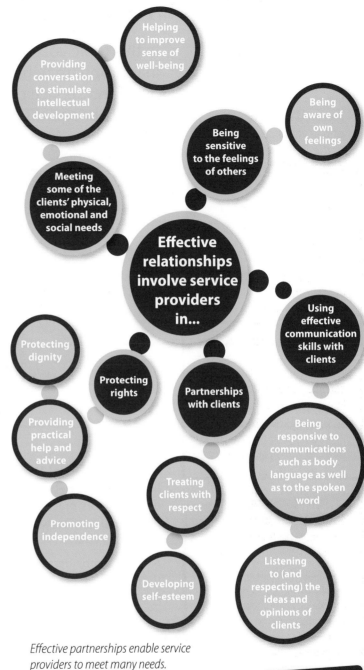

Effective partnerships enable service providers to meet many needs.

## Just checking

* What are the dangers of someone in the police force not taking action or taking action when they suspect someone of taking and dealing drugs?
* Why is it important for the different care sectors to work closely together? Give at least three reasons.
* What are the four general reasons why individuals need services within the care sectors? Give examples of when you, members of your family or friends have used services within two or more of the four main sectors (i.e. social care, health, children and young people, and community justice) to support your answer.

## HOW WOULD YOU FEEL?

How would you feel if a member of your family was spoken to like the older person pictured right? Which of the values covered in the first five topics of this unit are not being shown by this care worker? What do you think a witness to this behaviour should do about it?

**Inappropriate behaviour** Behaviour that is not suitable or proper.

**Judgemental** Making decisions or forming opinions on the basis of something such as appearance, without proper evidence, and being too critical.

## Activity

1 Think of any occasions when you feel you have been judged unfairly and treated unfairly because of it. This might be by a family member, a friend or a teacher. Discuss this with a friend.

2 Tell your friend how you dealt with each of these situations. Discuss whether this was the correct way to respond, now you are looking back at the situation.

## Personal, learning and thinking skills

The activity will provide evidence of PLTS: Reflective learner.

# 1.6 We need to talk about that

In this topic you will start to learn what we mean by inappropriate behaviour, on the part of both service users and service providers. It includes judgemental behaviour and discriminatory practice.

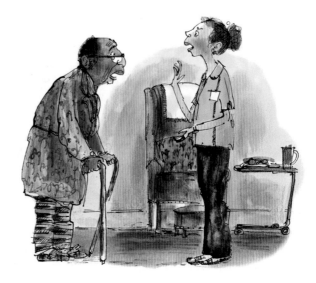

*This isn't good enough.*

## Inappropriate behaviour

**Inappropriate behaviour** includes **judgemental** behaviour, discriminatory practice, breaching confidentiality, abusing others and putting up barriers to services, such that people find it hard to access those they need.

All service providers have a *responsibility* to behave appropriately, but they also have the *right* to be treated properly themselves. It is for this reason that 'zero tolerance' posters now appear in places such as school offices, accident and emergency departments and on buses.

## Judgemental behaviour

This is when we make unfair judgements about someone else and react accordingly. Imagine a group of young people walking down the street, looking a bit scruffy, having a laugh, and one of them bumps into a woman, causing her to drop her phone. An onlooker thinks that this was done to steal the phone. When one of the group bends over to pick it up and return it to the woman, the onlooker accuses him of being a thief. This is an example of judgemental behaviour.

## Discriminatory practice
### Discrimination and prejudice

There are several kinds of discrimination. Someone may have a *prejudice* (a bias) against a person or a group of people for reasons such as age, gender, ethnicity, class, religion, sexual orientation, disability or appearance. They may then *discriminate* against that person or group.

There are four different kinds of discrimination:

* *Unfair discrimination* is when a person is treated unfairly in comparison with somebody else. One example of such behaviour is if someone is not being considered seriously for a job because they are older than another candidate, even though they have better qualifications and experience.

* *Direct discrimination* is when a person is rude, hostile or offensive to someone because they see them as different. An example is an overweight child being called names such as 'Fatty' and 'Blobby'. This form of discrimination is easy to prove because it is heard by other people.

* *Indirect discrimination* is harder to prove. It is where everyone is treated in the same way but particular groups are still disadvantaged. Asking that job applicants have a minimum height, for example, can mean that women and people from some ethnic groups will be less likely to be able to apply.

* *Positive discrimination* is when a decision is made in a person's favour for the exact reason that there is something different about them. Sometimes this is done quite openly. For example, someone may ring a casting agent and say they want a very short person to play the part of a dwarf in *Snow White*. At other times it is done less openly. It may be that a particular service has very few managers from one ethnic minority, so they appoint someone from that minority.

If medical professionals argue that people who are obese should not receive certain types of hospital treatment, they are discriminating against them. A member of a jury assuming that because the defendant is a traveller she is guilty is using discriminatory practice. Service providers need to be anti-discriminatory by recognising and responding to the needs of service users. Discriminating against people can affect their health and well-being, and cause them stress, anxiety and a loss of confidence.

While service providers need to have the correct attitude, it is also right that service users treat the providers in an anti-discriminatory way. It may be that providers have to challenge the attitudes of some of their service users.

There is much legislation to protect people from discrimination and to help those who feel they have been discriminated against. These include the Sex Discrimination Act 1975 and the Race Relations (Amendment) Act 2000. Legislation is discussed further in topic 1.9.

### Stereotyping and labelling

People can also discriminate against others unknowingly, by **stereotyping** and **labelling** them. If someone meets a mother pushing her teenage son in a wheelchair and speaks to the mother about him as though he weren't there, that person has subconsciously labelled the son as someone who is disabled and therefore cannot speak for himself. In fact, the son is likely to have problems only with walking. Another example is when people talk to older people slowly, loudly and patronisingly because they assume they are deaf and intellectually less able. This is stereotyping older people.

**Labelling** Identifying or describing someone with a label rather than as an individual. Labelling is linked to stereotyping, as people are expected to conform to the behaviour associated with the stereotype with which they have been labelled.

**Stereotyping** Thinking a group of people will all have the same attributes, for example, that all older people will be deaf and have memory problems.

### Just checking

* What is meant by the term 'judgemental behaviour'?
* What are the four main types of discrimination?
* How can discrimination affect people? Give at least five ways.

# 1.7 Privacy, dignity and abuse

This topic continues to look at inappropriate behaviour. This includes not allowing someone privacy and dignity. It also covers the related topics of confidentiality and abuse.

## WHO'S BEHAVING INAPPROPRIATELY?

In pairs, discuss how the patient in the picture could very easily be given privacy and so retain some dignity. Discuss occasions when you have personally been embarrassed and how that embarrassment was overcome. Then discuss ways in which you have embarrassed other people and why it was wrong.

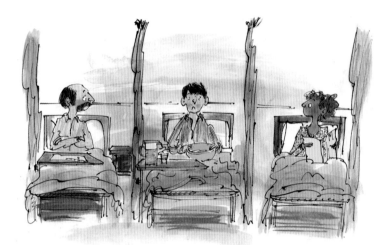

*Not so private or dignified.*

## Confidentiality

Confidentiality is one aspect of privacy. It means respecting the privacy of your personal information. Think about the information your doctor has about you. This includes not only facts, such as your address, date of birth and details of any illnesses and treatments you have had. It also includes things you may have shared with your doctor in conversation, such as worries about your weight, or an embarrassing problem, or advice about contraception. Some of the information held about you will depend on which service provider you are using, but in each case there is likely to be a lot of it. Now imagine the huge amount of data that might be held, for example, on an elderly resident in a care home.

Carelessly or unnecessarily breaking **confidentiality** is inappropriate behaviour and can have many consequences, some of which are shown in the table below.

**Confidentiality** Keeping sensitive information secret.

*Consequences of breaking confidentiality*

| Consequence | Service users may be: |
|---|---|
| Loss of trust | Less likely to say how they really feel or to share a problem |
| Lower self-esteem | Likely to feel unvalued and as though they don't matter |
| Being put at risk | Feeling their property and personal safety are threatened |
| Loss of professional reputation | Feeling the provider is unprofessional |
| Law breaking | Likely to sue the provider |
| Discrimination | Treated differently by others |

### Necessary breaches of confidentiality

Maintaining the confidentiality of information communicated by a service user is very important. There are times, however, when it is appropriate to breach confidentiality. Examples include when service users might harm themselves or others in some way, or if they have broken, or are about to break, the law. It is therefore inappropriate for service providers to promise to keep everything confidential; they should explain that there may be times when it becomes necessary to pass the information on to an appropriate colleague or authority.

## Abuse

**Abuse** can happen for a variety of reasons, such as frustration with a person, loss of temper, a desire to exert power over someone else, prejudice or discrimination.

There are several different forms of abuse:

* *physical abuse* is when someone is physically assaulted in some way, such as being hit
* *sexual abuse* is when someone interferes with a person's body in a sexual and unwanted way
* *verbal abuse* is when someone assaults a person verbally, such as insulting them and calling them names
* *neglect* is when a person is ignored or not given the help they need
* *exclusion* is when someone is stopped from getting help or maybe the company that they need
* *avoidance* is when someone deliberately avoids contact with another person
* *devaluing* is when someone ignores a person's ideas and opinions or denies them something others are allowed, so making them feel less valued.

It is inappropriate behaviour for a service provider to fail to protect a service user from abuse, just as it is inappropriate for the service user to abuse the provider. There are, however, circumstances where service users won't understand what they are doing, as may be the case with some people who have a mental illness. In such instances, steps may need to be taken to protect the provider, for example by having two workers in a room instead of one.

A service provider needs to look out for signs of abuse in service users, such as bruises, mood swings, becoming withdrawn and feeling worthless. Many support organisations and telephone helplines offer help, protection and advice about abuse, in addition to the police and social services. A service provider should report signs of abuse to the appropriate agency.

---

### Activity

Explain the possible consequences of the following breaches of confidentiality:

1 A worker tells someone about a person who lives near them who has been mentally ill but now has the illness totally under control.

2 A worker chats too loudly about the holiday plans of the family of someone held in a young offender institution.

3 A worker tells someone about a person who has committed a crime involving children and who is about to be released from prison.

---

### Personal, learning and thinking skills

The activity may help you to produce evidence of PLTS:

Independent enquirer;
Reflective learner.

---

### Functional skills

It will also help with FS:
ICT – find and select information, English – reading and writing.

---

**Abuse** To treat wrongly, harmfully or inappropriately.

---

### Just checking

* What is meant by breaching (breaking) confidentiality?
* Why is it inappropriate behaviour to not allow someone privacy and dignity?
* What are some of the reasons for abuse happening? Give at least five.

# 1.8 Promoting independence, challenging inappropriate behaviour

In this topic you will find out more about the importance of developing and maintaining service users' independence. You will then go on to look at how to challenge inappropriate behaviour.

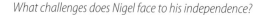

*What challenges does Nigel face to his independence?*

## Why is independence so important?

In order to have **independence**, a person needs to be able not only to do very basic things, such as to move, feed themselves, reproduce and excrete, but also things such as washing and shopping. If we lose the ability to do any of these we have to have help from others.

Loss such as Nigel's in the situation above often leads to despair, loss of confidence and a feeling of being a burden.

Nigel may now rely on others to wash him, dress him and cut up his food. He may have had to give up his job. He won't be able to play football with his children or drive them around anymore. He may have lost some of his acquaintances, although his real friends will continue to support him. He is now more likely to be discriminated against and become a victim of abuse. It is therefore crucial that service providers work in partnership to do everything they can to help Nigel regain control over his life.

**Independence** Freedom from the control and influence of others and from the need for their support; the ability to make your own decisions.

## Barriers to access to services

It is important that Nigel gets access to all the services he needs. Service providers should remove any barriers to those services.

* *Physical barriers*. Nigel will need a wheelchair, ramps and lifts to get into buildings that house the services, as well as doors that are wide enough, handles that are low enough and facilities such as adapted toilets.

* *Psychological barriers*. Nigel may become so used to hospital that he is reluctant to leave it, and then become reluctant to leave the house to access services. He may hide some of his problems because he is too proud to ask for more help. He may also be afraid of pain, or change.

* *Financial barriers*. Nigel may need help applying for benefits so that he can afford transport to services, some of which may be quite a distance from where he lives.

* *Geographical barriers.* Nigel may live in the countryside, with no easy means of transport to access services such as physiotherapists and doctors.

* *Cultural barriers.* Although Nigel does not face cultural or language barriers, this could be the case for others. For example, a child whose first language is not English will find schooling difficult.

* *Resource barriers.* Nigel may need access to specialist equipment, staff or information that are not available in his area or there may be too much demand for a particular service, so he will have to go on a waiting list.

* *Communication barriers.* Nigel may find it hard to understand what some service providers are saying to him, perhaps because the language is too technical. The attitude of some service users may not be wholly sympathetic, which will not encourage Nigel to communicate.

## Challenging inappropriate behaviour

A series of steps can be taken to challenge inappropriate behaviour.

### Step 1. Challenge the person yourself

To do this you need to be assertive. This means being firm, without losing your temper or becoming aggressive. Ask to have a word with the person. Ask someone else to be present as a witness. Explain what the problem is, without starting by saying you are sorry (which would make it sound as though it is you who has done something wrong). State your case firmly but quietly. If the person is answering back and not accepting your point, keep repeating the same point in the same calm way until they apologise, in which case you need take the matter no further.

This is the best way of challenging inappropriate behaviour because it is constructive. The person concerned does not get into trouble with anyone else, so doesn't lose face, and will hopefully change their behaviour. If they will not accept that they have behaved inappropriately, move to step 2.

### Step 2. Follow the complaints procedure

Every organisation or agency in any of the sectors is required by law to have a complaints procedure. Following it may mean filling in a form or getting someone to speak or write on your behalf (an advocate) if you are unable to do so. Someone more senior than the service provider you are complaining about may interview you. If you are still not satisfied by the outcome, move to step 3.

### Step 3. Take your appeal to the law

Look at the relevant legislation and, if need be, get a lawyer. You could even end up taking your case to the European Court of Human Rights! More detail about the relevant legislation is given in topic 1.9.

More detail about the relevant legislation is given in topic 1.9.

### Activity

1  Elaine is in prison in the countryside, many miles from her family. Write about how each type of barrier affects her and how this will make her feel.

2  Elaine's family believe her to be innocent and are campaigning to have her released. What barriers might stop the family accessing all the services they need to attempt to appeal against her conviction?

### For your project

You could explore the importance of independence. Make a list of barriers to independence and ways to overcome these barriers.

### Just checking

* What are five possible effects of loss of independence on a person?
* What is meant by the phrase 'barriers to access to services'?
* How can a lack of resources be a barrier to access to services?

# 1.9 We all need guidance

This topic looks at key legislation, codes of practice, policies and procedures. These all support people's rights and help them to challenge inappropriate behaviour if the need arises. They also provide a framework to maintain and improve the quality of practice.

**Professional bodies**
Organisations that set standards for and look after the interests of their members, who all do one type of job. An example in the health sector is the Royal College of Nursing.

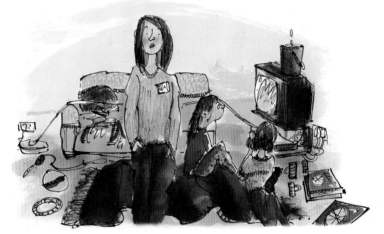

*Who cares?*

## Guidelines

All care settings have guidelines. These come in four main forms, namely legislation, codes of professional practice, policies and procedures.

### Legislation

This is a law or a set of laws, as passed by Parliament. If legislation is not adhered to, the person or group of people responsible can be either sued in court or charged with a crime. Some of the key pieces of legislation for the four care sectors are set out in the table.

*What the law says*

| Legislation | Brief details |
| --- | --- |
| Sex Discrimination Act 1975 | Prohibits sex discrimination against individuals in areas including employment, education and provision of services |
| Convention on the Rights of the Child 1989 | A set of human rights (basic standards) that protects children below the age of 18 against all forms of discrimination |
| Race Relations (Amendment) Act 2000 | Promotes race equality as central to the way all public services work |
| Human Rights Act 1998 | Incorporates the European Convention on Human Rights into UK law |
| Data Protection Act 1998 | Gives rights to individuals in respect of personal data held about them |
| Care Standards Act 2000 | Passes responsibility for overseeing care services from local authorities to the National Care Standards Commission (now the Commission for Social Care Inspection) |
| Criminal Justice Act 2003 | Reforms the criminal justice system, from crime prevention through to the punishment and rehabilitation of offenders |

| Legislation | Brief details |
|---|---|
| Children Act 2004 | Creates clear accountability for children's services, enables better joint working and secures a better focus on safeguarding children |
| Disability Discrimination Act 2005 | Gives disabled people more rights, for example in relation to public transport, employment and education. It also requires public bodies to promote equality of opportunity for disabled people |
| Mental Capacity Act 2005 | Provides a framework to empower and protect vulnerable people who are not able to make their own decisions |
| Employment Equality (Age) Regulations 2006 | Prohibit unjustified direct and indirect discrimination and all harassment and victimisation on grounds of age, of people of any age, young or old |

## Codes of professional practice

All **professional bodies** and services should have a code of practice, sometimes called a code of conduct, that gives guidelines for workers to follow. A code helps to make sure that workers are adhering to the values of that profession. An example is shown to the right. It is an extract from the Nursing and Midwifery Council's Code of Professional Conduct.

A code of practice will advise service providers how to behave, not only to promote the rights of the service users but also to protect themselves. It will also set out the standards of practice and conduct workers should meet.

## Policies

A policy is different from a code of practice in that it relates to a particular service (rather than a profession as a whole, in general terms). A policy tells service providers how to deal with a particular situation in their own workplace. Every service has its own policies, covering areas such as work practices, staff training, quality and confidentiality.

## Procedures

A procedure is a list of steps for a service provider to follow to complete a particular task in a certain way. Procedures are closely tied to the value base. For example, a prison officer will follow a particular procedure when doing a full body search on a prisoner. This will be written so that, when followed correctly, the prisoner is searched with as little embarrassment as possible. Almost every policy that a service provider has is supported by one or more procedures.

### Code of professional conduct

As a registered nurse, midwife or health visitor, you are personally accountable for your practice. In caring for patients and clients, you must:

- respect the patient or client as an individual
- protect confidential information
- co-operate with others in the team
- maintain your professional knowledge and competence
- be trustworthy
- act to identify and minimise risk to patients and clients.

These are the shared values of all the United Kingdom health care regulatory bodies.

*Extract from the Nursing and Midwifery Council's Code of Professional Conduct.*

## Activity

1 Draw up a table to match the one above but in the right-hand column write how you think each piece of legislation applies to your school or college and how it affects you.

2 Pick one of the key pieces of legislation listed and do some further research into how it affects service providers in one of the four main care sectors.

## Functional skills

The activity will help with FS: English – writing.

## Just checking

* Why do we have legislation, codes of practice, policies and procedures?
* Why is the Children Act important for both children and those providing services for children?
* What is the difference between a policy, code of practice and procedure?

**Interests** Those things that draw your attention, that you want to get involved with and spend time on.

# 1.10 Who am I?

In this topic you will start to learn about self-exploration. You will be encouraged to look at your own interests, values and knowledge.

## Self-exploration

Deciding on a career is a very important process and takes time. Career planning involves learning about yourself, your **interests**, values and abilities, and relating that information to a choice of occupation. For this you will also need to learn about the job.

### Interests

Ask yourself what kind job you would enjoy doing, one in which you would want to work hard and do well. This could be cooking, childcare, working outdoors, in an office, making or fixing things, working with facts, people or animals, performing, selling, travelling… the list of possibilities is endless. Go to your careers library or use an online careers service to find out what sort of jobs match your interests. If you want to work with people and to help them, a job in the care sectors may appeal to you.

### Your values

Your values will have a large impact on whether you feel a particular career is right for you. Knowing your values will help you to decide whether it is important to you to have a job helping other people, or whether you would prefer to work alone, maybe for yourself, or with numbers, or machines, or books. You may like to have lots of variety in your job or you may prefer stability. Another choice may be whether you want to have a job which involves taking responsibility for others. Is this simply because you want to be in charge, so you have power over people and earn lots of money, or because you feel you will be able to help others? Some people prefer a job where they are told what to do.

### Knowledge

The knowledge that you gain through studying subjects like maths, science and English at school is needed for most jobs. In addition, though, you will also need to know about the actual career: what qualifications, qualities and skills you will need; what the prospects, salary and working conditions are; where the job will be based; and how the particular service provider fits into the overall structure of the sector. This you can find out from websites, from your Connexions advisers or from the service provider.

*Some of the service providers within each of the four main sectors (there are many more)*

| Social care | Health | Children and young people | Community justice |
|---|---|---|---|
| Residential home | Hospital | School | Police |
| Day care centre | Medical centre/GP surgery | Nursery | Court |
| Domestic help agency | District nurse | Child protection agency | Youth offenders panel |
| Social services | Community health care | Early years centre | Probation service |
| Home care | Dental practice | Play service | Prison service |
| Physical disabilities team | Optician | Family placement | Young offender institution |
| Learning disabilities team | Occupational health | Residential care | Drug and alcohol service |
| Palliative care | Physiotherapist | Day care | Liaison officer |
| Support group | Psychologist | Support group/helpline | Education |
| Citizens Advice Bureau | Hospice | Foster care | Behaviour support |
| Helpline | Chiropodist | Youth worker | Physiologist |
| Housing | Nursing home | Playgroup | Community safety agency |
| Refuge | Pharmacist | Crèche | Youth Justice Board |
| Counselling support | Mental health team | Child guidance | Community outreach |

## Snapshot

Most general practices have at least one practice nurse; some have nurse practitioners and health care assistants as well. Receptionists will advise patients when a nurse rather than a doctor can help.

Practice nurses can do things like taking blood and urine samples, and checking blood pressure. They are often responsible for wound care, immunisations and taking cervical smears. They provide information on things like contraception and travel health. Practice nurses can also refer people to other health professionals.

Many practice nurses are qualified to monitor chronic disease, such as asthma and heart disease, working to agreed procedures. Some are qualified to prescribe drugs, suggest changes to treatment plans, or to provide phone consultations. Nurses are also involved in monitoring standards, training and developing services. Good nurse practitioners offer a real choice for patients, and reduce pressure on doctors.

Adapted from *Woman's Weekly*, 22 May 2007, written by Dr Melanie Wynne-Jones.

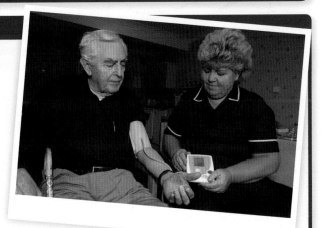

*The practice nurse.*

## Just checking

* What are the main things you need to know about yourself when looking into whether you would be suitable for a particular career?
* What are the main pieces of information you need to know about a job before deciding if it is one you could apply for?
* How do a person's values affect their choice of career? Give some examples.

# 1.11 Wanted, people like you

This topic continues to look at self-exploration, focusing on qualifications, qualities and skills. It gives you a further opportunity to reflect on yourself and a possible choice of career.

## NURSERY NURSE WANTED

Have you got the skills and qualities asked for in the job advertisement from the *Diploma Daily*? How do you know? Try to find similar advertisements for a variety of jobs in the care sector.

---

## Diploma Daily

### Little People's Nursery

We are looking for a dedicated nursery nurse to join our team in delivering the highest possible quality childcare to our little people. The successful candidate will have a childcare qualification at level 2 or 3 and a thorough knowledge of 'Birth to 3' issues and the Foundation Stage. We are looking for someone who:

- is a warm, committed individual with initiative
- has a desire to enhance the lives of children
- can be flexible, works well as part of a team and is highly motivated
- is positive and sensitive
- is literate and numerate
- has a current first-aid qualification.

If you would like to apply please send a CV and a covering letter to Miss Little, Little People's Nursery, Littledon, London, SW111 6TJ

Rates of pay will depend on experience and qualifications. Closing date is 20th August 2008.

---

**Reflection** Looking at yourself or back on something you have done, deciding whether you like what you see or have done well (or not) and using that to improve yourself.

**Interpersonal skills** Skills that allow us to interact successfully with others.

---

### For your project

You could consider the qualities, qualifications and skills needed for a particular career in the care sectors.

---

## Self-exploration continued

### Qualification

A qualification is something you gain through schooling or training and may be a GCSE, A-level, NVQ, degree, diploma or certificate. You may already have some. When you have decided on a particular career, you will have to find out what specific qualifications are needed and you may have to go on a course to gain them.

### Quality

These are part of your nature or personality, such as being sensitive to the feelings of others or being a caring person. These are to do with *how* you do things rather than *what* you do. You may be logical, rational and a clear thinker; you may be kind, caring and trustworthy; or you may be self-confident and assertive. Some of the qualities you need to work in the care sectors are shown in the table on page 25.

### Skills

Skills refer to what you do. Some skills need natural talent, while others have to be learned. Usually they require a combination of the two. You may not think you have many skills but in fact everyone does. There are two types of skill: transferable and job-related.

*Transferable skills* are those that you have been developing throughout your life and that you can use in a wide variety of situations. These include literacy, numeracy, use of ICT, **reflection** and **interpersonal skills**.

*Job-related skills* are those that are used in a particular job. Examples include using or repairing particular tools, vehicles or machines, raising plants or animals, keeping records or analysing data.

You may have some of the skills you need for the career you have in mind. You may have got these skills from jobs you have already had, courses you have taken, or hobbies and family experience. You will be taught others on training courses. A nurse, for example, will need to be able to take temperatures and measure blood pressure, draw up charts, dress wounds and bandage limbs.

## Activity

1  *Self-assessment.* Draw up a table on a large sheet of paper using the headings shown below and complete it to show your own qualifications, qualities and skills.

| Qualifications studying for or already got | Qualities | Transferable skills | Job-related skills |
|---|---|---|---|
|  |  |  |  |

Leave a line between each row. In that space write down the evidence you have to prove that you have got that qualification, quality or skill, such as a certificate, example of a piece of work, photo or a reference.

2  *Peer assessment.* Now ask a partner (a) to say whether they agree with how you see yourself and (b) to add any quality or skill that they think you have but that you have missed out.

3  Continue to work with a partner. Look at those qualities for which you have no evidence. Each partner can then write the other a witness statement saying that they have the quality and giving several examples of where they have seen them use it. Write this neatly and it can be added to other evidence you may already have in something like a progress file or record of achievement.

## Qualities and interpersonal skills needed in all jobs in the care sectors

| Qualities | Patient, able to get on with people, cooperative, tactful, sensitive, energetic, trustworthy, kind, reliable, adaptable, committed, calm, caring, respectful, observant, cope under stress, outgoing, assertive, flexible, dependable, sincere, motivated, friendly, good sense of humour, optimistic, cheerful, open minded, punctual, understanding |
|---|---|
| Interpersonal skills | Communication (listening, speaking, other methods), negotiating, teamwork, leadership, ability to work on your own, time management, ability to meet deadlines, ability to prioritise, problem solving, taking responsibility, advocacy, organising, planning |

### Beliefs and attitudes to the work of the four care sectors

Your interest in a career within one of the four care sectors will have been influenced by your own experiences of them, as well as those of friends and family. You will also have been influenced by images in the media. Think carefully about these experiences and images, and do not let one negative one affect your judgement. Negative events are often reported in the media, while so much excellent day-to-day care goes uncommented on.

You will spend a large proportion of your life at work, so it is vital that you think carefully before making a decision. When choosing your career, you should reflect fully on your own values, beliefs, principles, knowledge, qualifications, qualities and skills. Take a look with an unbiased eye at each service provider before making an informed decision.

## Just checking

✳ Why does someone need good interpersonal skills to work in the care sectors?

✳ What is the difference between a skill and a quality?

✳ How might a person's choice of job in one of the care sectors be influenced by their own and their family's experiences of contact with these sectors?

# 1.12 Pause for reflection

## LOOK IN THE MIRROR

Pause for a few minutes to reflect on yourself as a student at your school or college. How do you think you are doing? What do you think of yourself? How do you think others, both teachers and students, see you? Write down what you think your attitude is towards your studies and describe your behaviour on a normal day. What do you think will be the consequences for you of the way you have tackled your education so far? Is there anything you would do differently if you could repeat the whole experience?

This last topic in Unit 1 looks at what is meant by reflective practice and how service providers develop their knowledge and skills throughout their working lives. It also looks at sources of information for professional development.

## Reflective practice

Reflective practice is about learning from experience. This involves service providers thinking about and critically analysing their own actions. One method of reflective practice (called Rolfe's framework) uses three simple questions to reflect on a situation: 'What, so what and now what?' For example, teachers would first ask themselves, '*What* teaching model have I been using?' They would then ask, '*So what* has it achieved?' (That is, how well is it working and has it helped the students to learn more effectively?) Very importantly they next ask, '*Now what* do I do to move on and do things even better?'

The reflective process is a continuous one. Experience is the basis of learning and learning cannot take place without reflection. Reflection makes sense of an experience. More experience and learning then follow, and more reflection.

An example of a 'reflective practice tool' is shown in the table below. A nurse has been told to complete the table for encounters he has with patients and issues that arise at work.

*Reflective practice tool*

| Date | Patient or problem | Issue/what happened? | Ideas for learning/ what have you learned? | Action plan/what are you going to do about it? |
|------|--------------------|----------------------|---------------------------------------------|------------------------------------------------|
| 01/01/2001 | Mrs S | Unable to use inhaler device despite showing her once already<br><br>Patient does not remember what was shown to her | Need to find ways of reinforcing how to use her inhaler<br><br>Learned that I can't just rely on showing a patient once and expect them to remember forever; continual reinforcement and education are necessary | Make sure that their inhaler technique is checked on every clinic visit, whether with myself or with another member of the practice. Have a prompt put up on the computer screen |

Source: www.wipp.nhs.uk/tools_gpn/toolu4_eg_reflective.php (Crown copyright September 2006)

## Professional development

Service providers should always try to improve the quality of their care. Continuing professional development (CPD) is how professionals ensure that they keep up to date with new theories, treatments, procedures and so on. There are various types of CPD, and the main ones are looked at opposite.

### Induction

When someone starts a new job or moves to a new department, they take part in an induction session or course. This introduces them formally to the workplace and teaches them all the policies, procedures and codes of practice they need to follow.

### Mentoring

A person new to a job may be assigned a mentor. This is a trusted person who can show them what to do and help them with any problems.

### Work-based learning

This is when someone learns knowledge and skills in the workplace, rather than in a school or college. An apprentice will be being taught the job as they go along, by others in the workplace, as well as by a trainer or teacher, perhaps, coming into the workplace. A surgeon will learn new operating techniques and procedures by watching another surgeon and helping them.

### Courses and qualifications

Most job advertisements ask for specific qualifications. For example, an advert for an alcohol project worker might state that applicants need a degree or a diploma in social work, nursing or addiction studies.

Practitioners are expected to continue to learn and improve their practice after they have started the job. They will therefore be sent on courses. These may be run in-house (i.e. within their own workplace) or by other professional bodies and organisations. Many one-day courses give the participants a certificate of attendance. Longer courses often lead to the participants being assessed in some way; if they do well enough, they will gain a qualification.

## Sources of information on professional development

Sources of information on professional development include:

* Colleagues in the same or similar service.
* Professional bodies. These organisations, which are usually non-profit, maintain and enforce standards of training and ethics in their professions, to protect both the public interest and the interests of the professionals. The General Teaching Council (GTC), for example, is a professional body for teachers. It seeks to improve standards of teaching and the quality of learning.
* Sector skills councils (SSCs). These are independent organisations that work together to improve services. They are employer-led but also involve trade unions and professional bodies.
* Professional journals. These magazines will have articles on all aspects of that profession, as well as adverts for jobs and resources. Examples are *Nursery World* for nursery nurses and the *GTC* magazine for teachers.

> **Activity**
>
> 1 Think about a lesson or an educational visit you have enjoyed recently. Draw up a table with columns headed: Lesson or visit; What worked well; What did not work; What will I do differently next time?
>
> 2 Complete the table, thinking about the learning you took part in.
>
> 3 Devise your own reflective practice tool for a receptionist at your doctor's surgery to use. Imagine some encounters they have with a variety of service users, in different moods, asking for prescriptions, appointments and help with a variety of problems, and how the receptionist might respond. Enter some of them on your reflective practice tool.

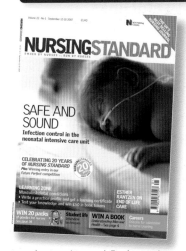

*A professional journal. Find some in your local library in the areas that interest you most.*

> **Just checking**
>
> * What is meant by 'reflective practice'?
> * How is reflective practice a continuous process? Include a flow or circle diagram in your answer.
> * List five possible sources of information on professional development.

# Unit 1 Assessment guide

This unit is assessed by an assignment which is marked by your teacher. You will need to show that you understand how organisations from the health, social care, community justice and children and young people sectors treat the individuals they work with in a fair and equal manner, while still appreciating that everyone is different, with different needs. You will need to show in your assignment that you know how employees' guidelines in the form of laws, policies and codes of practice are used in different situations. You will also have the opportunity to learn about yourself, what you value and what your views are about people who are different from yourself. You will need to show that you can reflect in this way upon your own values, knowledge and skills and how these can help you when you work in a sector that offers care and support.

## Time management

* Ensure that you keep any class work safely. You may be given copies of legislation (laws), organisational policies and professional codes of practice, and asked to give examples of how they are used in different organisations. File these away in a folder where you can find them easily if you need to use them. This will save time and show that you are well organised. Being well organised shows that you are able to manage your own learning and will help you to fully meet the requirements of the diploma. You could highlight important points with a highlighter pen on these documents – your teacher will see that you have read and understood them and it will be easier for you to find the information you need when you are writing your report.

* Be prepared with a list of questions that you could ask if your teacher arranges for a speaker to come and talk to your class. For example, if a nurse comes to talk to you from an organisation that provides care for older people, you could ask how they make sure that people are given choice in their everyday lives. Make notes of the answers they give, as this will provide you with some examples of how principles and values are promoted, which will help with your assignment. If you visit an organisation that provides care and support for children, ask the same question and compare the answers.

## Useful links

* You may do some work experience in organisations that care for people who cannot communicate how they want their needs to be met. Ask the people who work there how they make sure those individuals are treated fairly and how their organisation's policies helps them.

* You may want to arrange to talk to other workers that you meet from the four sectors, such as the practice nurse at your GP's surgery or your police community support officer, about how they ensure that people are treated fairly. You could also ask how they develop their knowledge about diversity, and whether or not they had an induction when they started their job or if they have received any training about equality and diversity.

* A useful website is www.nmc-uk.org, which contains information about the way nurses promote the rights and choices of their patients.

## Things you might need

* ICT equipment to produce your report, as it is important that your assignment is well presented and this may help to produce the evidence required for the ICT functional skills element of the diploma. You could also research current legislation and codes of professional practice on the Internet.

* You may hear or see information which is private to individuals when you are visiting an organisation that cares for or supports people. You may hear information from your peers in the classroom about how they have been treated unfairly. This information must be treated sensitively and must remain confidential.

* A dictionary and a health and social care glossary, for looking up important terms.

# How you will be assessed

| You must show that you *know*: | Guidance | To gain higher marks you must *explain*: |
|---|---|---|
| What the principles and values are that are used by the sectors that look after health, social care, community justice and children and young people. | Find out what the terms diversity, equality, culture and belief systems, individuality, rights, choice, privacy, independence, dignity, respect and partnership mean. You could use a dictionary and a glossary in the back of a health and social care textbook and compare the definitions – are they the same? You might find examples of these in case studies given to you by your teacher, from your or friends' personal experience, or from workers in organisations that provide care and support.<br><br>To find out how equality and diversity are promoted, you could talk to a worker from one of the sectors, who could give you some examples.<br><br>You also need to investigate what is inappropriate behaviour and how it should be dealt with. An example of this might be a vegetarian given the same meal as others but with the meat removed. You should describe why an example like this does not promote people's rights nor respect their beliefs and values. You could present this work in the form of a report or written account. | What the terms diversity, equality, culture and belief systems, individuality, rights, choice, privacy, independence, dignity, respect and partnership mean and give examples.<br><br>How equality and diversity are promoted, with some examples from each sector.<br><br>What inappropriate behaviour is, e.g. discrimination, stereotyping, labelling and prejudice, and how it is dealt with. You may see examples of this when you are on work experience. Try to talk to at least two workers from different sectors about this. |
| How legislation, codes of practice, policies and procedures are used to support individual rights. | You do not need to have a detailed knowledge of the legislation (laws) that help to prevent discrimination and promote equality and diversity. You should investigate one piece of legislation, one code of professional practice, and one policy or procedure that relate to the promotion of individual's rights in each sector. You might look at the Children Act 2004, which looks at all aspects of improving children's lives. How has your school or college implemented this? Do they have their own policy? Nurses and social workers have their own codes of practice which tell them how to recognise discrimination and what they should do about it. You could present this work as a table and give a written explanation. | How legislation, codes of practice and resulting policies and procedures are used in each of the four sectors to support rights and improve practice, making links between the sectors.<br><br>How your chosen examples of a piece of legislation/a code of professional practice/a policy or procedure support an individual's rights in each sector. |
| How to assess and reflect upon your own values, knowledge and skills and relate these to the work of the four sectors. You also need to investigate the different ways of professional development of the workforce in the sectors. | You need to identify your own values, knowledge and skills. What are your own values and beliefs – do they come from your family, culture, community, the media or a combination of these things? Do you think your own values and beliefs are more important than anyone else's? Would they be appropriate to allow you to work with people who may not be able to voice their own beliefs in an organisation that provides care and support?<br><br>To 'reflect' means to think about what we have done and how we could have improved. Why is reflective practice a useful way of learning? How do practitioners develop their own skills? Present your evidence as a reflective account, where you think about your own views and values and how others may be affected by these. You should also reflect upon the skills and qualities you have – are they the right ones for working with people who need care and support? | Examples of your own values, knowledge and skills and compare these to those needed to work in the four sectors.<br><br>What reflective practice means.<br><br>How practitioners use induction, training and qualifications, mentoring, updates from professional bodies and work-based learning to help them develop their own practice, considering at least three of the sectors. |

## Introduction

In this unit you will discover that there are many ways of communicating with others, both verbal and non-verbal. You will also learn about the different methods that are used to communicate with clients and other care workers in various agencies. The unit also covers partnership working and team working.

### WHAT ARE YOU SAYING?

Your body language is a very important part of what you are saying to a client, patient or colleague. How would you respond to someone who doesn't speak your language?

### The importance of good communication

Communication is fundamental to our lives. How long could you cope without communicating with anyone, that is, without talking to, smiling at, or even looking at or listening to anyone? It would be difficult if not absolutely impossible! Communicating, in whatever way – a word, a smile, a small gesture such as touching someone's hand, is vital to our relationships with others. So it makes sense that you need good communication skills to develop positive relationships with other people.

We use different methods of communication for different situations and purposes. You may have thought that communication is just speaking, but there are many other ways of communicating our views, needs and feelings. You will learn that professionals in the care sectors need to be able to communicate with a wide variety of people, including service users, relatives, colleagues and professionals in other organisations. There may be many reasons why it is difficult to communicate with these different individuals and organisations. You will gain an understanding of the types of barriers that prevent us communicating effectively and the skills involved both in working with others and in good communication.

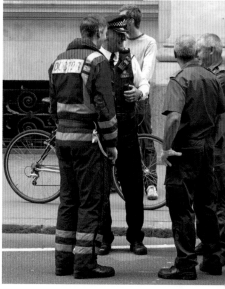

*It is important that people working in different ser and agencies communicate well with each other. facilitates partnership working.*

### Working together

As a service provider you will be dealing with **clients** of a wide age range, from babies to older adults, as well as people with disabilities, people from different cultural and ethnic groups and people from different professions. In this unit you will begin to develop the skills you will need to provide the right support for each individual you come across.

If you work in any of the sectors you will need to communicate with **colleagues** and workers from other **agencies**. The sharing of information between teams is very important, as it helps to ensure that services work efficiently. You will develop an understanding of how partnerships work together to improve the support they give, the impact of legislation and how workers overcome barriers that may prevent users, colleagues and organisations working together successfully.

**Agencies** Organisations that provide a government or local authority service.

**Clients** People who use the services or professional advice of the health, social care, community justice and children and young people sectors.

**Colleagues** The fellow professionals you work with.

This unit links with others to give you knowledge and understanding of good working practice. You will begin to develop skills that you can apply in your work placements. It will give an insight into how colleagues work collaboratively in the different sectors.

Most service providers, whatever their jobs or responsibilities, will need to work with a wide team of people. Problems that arise with clients or other members of staff will be discussed in meetings. This makes the service provision a shared responsibility between all participants, including the service user, to ensure an effective service for all.

## How you will be assessed

For this unit you will be assessed by one assignment, consisting of four tasks. The first task will involve the production of a report on the use of different methods of communication. The second task again involves the production of a report; this one will be on record keeping and information sharing in the sectors. The third task involves the production of leaflets or case studies about at least three examples of partnership working in your local area. The fourth task is to work in a team and organise an event, then produce an account.

## What you will learn in this unit

You will:

* Understand the use of different methods of communication and how to overcome or minimise barriers to communication
* Be able to use different methods to communicate effectively for different purposes and situations
* Understand the purpose of recording and reporting arrangements for a range of settings and know the ways in which information is shared within teams and between organisations, including inherent difficulties and risks
* Understand why confidentiality, accuracy and security of records are important
* Be able to complete records accurately and legibly
* Understand what is meant by successful partnership working, including statutory and non-statutory partnerships, and the importance of working in partnership to provide effective services
* Be able to work effectively as a member of a team

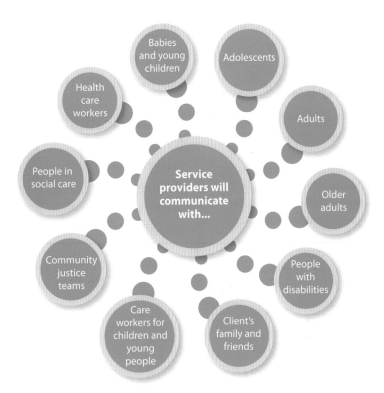

*Who do service providers need to communicate with?*

## Activity

1. Make a list of the different methods people use to communicate with each other.

2. Describe how you could make someone feel more comfortable by your style of communication alone.

3. What might you do that could be seen in a negative way?

# 2.1 Communication

## BODY LANGUAGE

When you meet someone for the first time, what impressions do you think you are giving by the way you are dressed or how you hold yourself and the expressions on your face? Do you communicate what you mean by what you say or how you look?

This topic looks at both verbal and non-verbal communication, especially body language. Different methods will be required for communication to be effective when used for different purposes and in different situations.

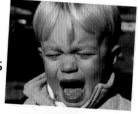
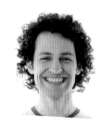
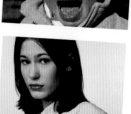
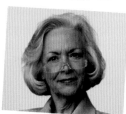

*What feelings and attitudes do you think are being expressed by the people in this picture?*

**Communication** The giving or exchange of thoughts, opinions or information by speech, writing or signs.

**Effective** When something produces the intended or expected result.

**Non-verbal cues** Methods of communicating other than talking, mainly body language and facial expressions.

## What do you mean?

We communicate with other people all the time, at home with our family, at school, when socialising, when shopping and on holiday. Sometimes we communicate without even realising it. Think about how you judge people by what they are wearing, for example, without even speaking to them. Our ideas are sometimes based on what we see rather than taking the time to understand the person.

We use different methods for different situations and purposes: verbal, body, touch, facial expression, dress, listening, silence, use of pictures/symbols, use of technology.

It is very important for service providers to communicate well with their clients, otherwise their relationship could be damaged. Clients will not feel supported and the service providers will not be as **effective** as they could be. As a professional, you will need to develop many ways of communicating with other people – your clients and their families, as well as colleagues and workers in different sectors.

There are three main types of **communication**:

* ⁕ the spoken word
* ⁕ **non-verbal cues**
* ⁕ the written word.

Let's look at the first two of these.

### Verbal communication

Verbal (or oral) communication is the ability to explain and present your ideas in clear English, to a range of audiences. This includes using styles and approaches appropriate to the particular audience you are speaking to. Verbal communication also requires you to use the skills of listening and being aware of the person you are talking to, especially their body language.

## Non-verbal communication

Non-verbal communication is the ability to express ideas and concepts without talking, through the use of body language, gestures, facial expression and tone of voice, and also with the use of pictures, icons and symbols.

In each of the sectors you will come across people from different countries where certain gestures may mean something different to what you have learned. For example, in European countries eye contact is seen to be polite, and to look away is thought to show that you are bored or not interested, whereas in some other countries it is respectful to look down when talking to someone and eye contact is seen to be rude and defiant.

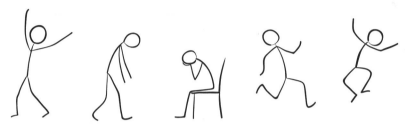

*What would you say each of the expressions suggested by the stick people is showing?*

'Body language' is an important part of how we communicate. When we respond to other people we take into account the following factors:

* 55 per cent is judged from body language
* 38 per cent is drawn from tone of voice
* 7 per cent is based solely on the words.

This shows that it's not *what* we say, but *how* we say it that really counts.

We will all greet our friends with a smile and a wave. When you do this, your face and body work together to show your friends that you're happy to see them. But what happens if your face and body send mixed messages? Would someone be more likely to believe the look on your face or the way you hold your body? These issues are very important when you are dealing with clients who may be in pain, anxious or worried.

Your body language is also important if you are dealing with someone who is deaf. For people with hearing impairments in the UK, the primary method of communication is **British Sign Language** (BSL). This is a language of signs, gestures and expression. Each country has its own sign language, just the same as with spoken languages.

### Activity

1 Create a collage using pictures of people based around a feeling (e.g. happy, angry, worried).

2 In a presentation to others, describe how each image in your collage gives the impression of the feeling/ attitudes being expressed. What other factors would you take into account (e.g. dress, hairstyle, gestures)? Do others agree?

**British Sign Language** This is the language many deaf people prefer. The language makes use of space and involves movement of the hands, body, face and head.

### Just checking

* What are the three different ways in which we communicate with each other?
* Think of five different ways in which we communicate without speaking.
* What methods could you use to explain something to someone who is hearing impaired?

**Empower** Allow someone to make decisions for themselves.

**Empathise** To understand another person's feelings.

# 2.2 Individual needs in communication

This topic looks further at the nature of communication and at why good communication is so important. It highlights the importance of tailoring the means of communication to the needs of the service user.

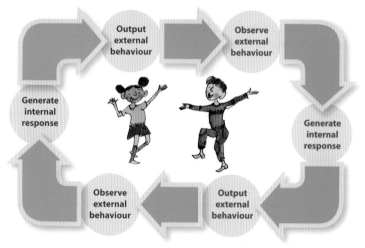

*Communicating is like dancing – whatever you are doing will affect the person you are communicating with.*

## Communication as a dance

When we communicate with someone else we are aware what the other person is saying and doing (their external behaviour). We hear what they say, think about it and have an internal response before we show our own external behaviour. The other person watches our behaviour and this generates an internal response in them and they reply back. This forms a communication cycle, as shown in the figure. It's a bit like a dance.

The idea of communication being a bit like dance between two people is important because it will help you understand the role you play when communicating with another person.

Good communication is very important to service providers because they must develop good relationships with others, to gain their trust and respect. They need to make clients feel supported and to provide information. Good communication helps them to understand and meet the needs of others. It will also **empower** clients. It enables service providers to respect clients' preferences and beliefs, to promote confidentiality and privacy.

Good communication skills will also support your own personal development.

Understand the communication dance

Be aware of the needs of others

Understand non-verbal messages – eyes, touch, face, gesture, tone of voice, body posture and movement

**Communication skills**

Use listening skills to help you understand the other person

Use non-verbal messages to communicate

Know how to ask questions effectively

Understand cultural differences

*Think about your communication skills.*

# Who needs what?

As we saw in the previous topic, there are many ways of communicating. As people have different needs, the service provider will have to choose the best methods in each case. For example, health and social care workers will often touch patients and clients. This helps to reassure them and make them feel that these workers are interested in them, and will support them and understand the way they are feeling. However, you do need to be aware that there are acceptable and unacceptable ways of touching. Arms and hands are usually seen to be appropriate areas of the body to touch. There are cultural differences that you must also be aware of. For instance, many Asian women would not want to be touched by a man. You need to be aware of the appropriate use of touch.

### Communicating with people with disabilities

Clients and patients who are physically disabled will often require different ways of communicating. People with a visual disability may need written information provided in Braille so they can read it for themselves. To take into account the difficulties often faced by people with visual impairments, care workers might use large clear text, bright images, easy-to-use controls, and voice accompaniment; they will also take care to face the client so their face can be seen clearly. These are all ways to make communication easier.

People who are hard of hearing or deaf may need you to speak clearly or they may need a sign language interpreter. British Sign Language (BSL) uses space and involves movement of the hands, body, face and head. Many thousands of people who are not deaf also use BSL – for example, hearing relatives of deaf people. Makaton is another method hearing-impaired people may use. This method also uses signs made by the hands. It is often used as a means of communication with children who have learning disabilities. Be aware that someone who uses a hearing aid will not want to be shouted at or talked to as if they are unintelligent.

You may also come across older people who suffer from dementia and you will need to show kindness and patience when dealing with them. Speaking clearly and gently, you may have to repeat what you have said several times and your body language needs to show care and support, not frustration.

### Empathy and sensitivity

If someone is agitated or aggressive you will only make the situation worse if you become impatient. It is important to speak slowly and clearly, and remain in control of the situation. Always aim to calm the client by the way you are behaving.

Think about how you feel when you are unhappy or stressed. What do you think would upset or annoy you most at these times? Look at the key word **empathise**. As a service provider you may need to try to understand how your client feels in order to communicate with them effectively and help.

## Personal, learning and thinking skills

The activity will give you evidence towards PLTS: Independent enquirer; Creative thinker.

## For your project

You could use the material produced in the activity below and develop it more fully for your project.

## Activity

1 Choose one group of people with specific needs or a particular age group and draw up a list of all the aspects of communication with which they may have difficulty.

2 Prepare a presentation that gives advice on how you should and should not communicate with a person from that group.

## Just checking

* Why is it important that there is good communication between service providers and their clients?
* Describe three different ways in which you can communicate without words.
* What types of communication would you use to put at ease someone who is in pain and doesn't speak your language?

# 2.3 How to overcome barriers

Service providers need to understand that there may be barriers to communication with clients and other colleagues. This topic is about these barriers and how they can be overcome or minimised.

## Barriers to communication with service users

If we are going to care for clients and patients, we need to understand what it must be like to try to communicate with someone who doesn't understand what we are trying to say or for some reason is getting the wrong message. Service users will not be able to contribute to a discussion about their care or planning their future if they do not understand what is being said.

There are many ways a service user may not be able to access the care they need. Some of the reasons may affect them for many years or all their life, or barriers may arise out of specific situations. The following may all impair communication between a service provider and a service user:

* sensory impairment, particularly of hearing or vision
* a different preferred spoken language
* jargon used by the service provider or slang spoken by the service user
* cultural differences (e.g. eye contact in Western culture is seen as showing respect but in some cultures is seen as being rude and defiant)
* misinterpretation of messages resulting from confused readings or use of body language
* differing ideas regarding the use of humour
* emotional issues, especially worries or distress (these often cause people to behave in ways that they would not normally)
* the use of inappropriate behaviour, especially aggression
* learning disabilities (both because people with a learning disability will by definition have problems with understanding, but also because they often do not respond in an 'acceptable' manner)
* environmental factors such as stairs and high work surfaces.

## Overcoming barriers to communication

Barriers to communication with service users can be overcome or at least minimised by:

* adapting the environment to the needs of the clients – for example, installing lifts or ramps
* understanding language needs and appreciating preferences and differences in dialect and use of slang
* using the person's preferred language (most leaflets that are produced by the government or organisations within the four care sectors will be available in various languages so that people who do not speak English very well can still access the information)
* using interpreters for people who do not speak English (there are also BSL interpreters for people who are deaf)

* using **active listening** with the client on a one-to-one basis
* using and being aware of body language, eye contact and sitting close without invading the individual's space
* talking quietly but firmly to someone who is agitated or aggressive, to try to calm the situation
* allowing sufficient time to get to know and understand the person's needs (take time to listen, give time for the client to respond)
* repeating the message yourself, and getting the other person to repeat the message you have given
* confirming information
* using technological aids
* using alternative forms of communication, such as sign language, lip reading, signs and symbols, pictures and writing.

> **Active listening** A structured form of listening and responding in which the listener attends fully to the speaker, and then repeats, in their own words, what they think the speaker has said, to check on understanding.

Individuals who have social or health problems may come to depend on other people to meet their needs. By talking to service users and understanding their needs a solution can be found that empowers the client.

## Barriers to partnership working

Many agencies will work together to provide care for an individual. This is called partnership working, which is looked at in more detail in topics 2.4, 2.10 and 2.11. Good communication is key to partnership working, but there are many types of barrier to it. In particular, problems can occur when:

* one partner dominates
* the various agencies or teams involved have different ways of working or different priorities
* there is a lack of communication
* there are 'hidden' or different agendas
* there is an unequal balance of power
* the partners are separated geographically (although such barriers are these days overcome more easily through the use of technology such as email and fax)
* budgetary constraints impose problems.

If service providers do not try to overcome these barriers, the outcome will mean a poorer service for the client.

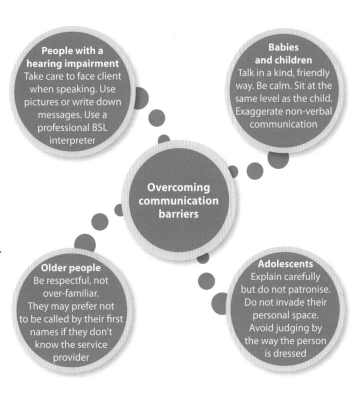

**People with a hearing impairment** Take care to face client when speaking. Use pictures or write down messages. Use a professional BSL interpreter

**Babies and children** Talk in a kind, friendly way. Be calm. Sit at the same level as the child. Exaggerate non-verbal communication

**Overcoming communication barriers**

**Older people** Be respectful, not over-familiar. They may prefer not to be called by their first names if they don't know the service provider

**Adolescents** Explain carefully but do not patronise. Do not invade their personal space. Avoid judging by the way the person is dressed

*Some examples of ways of overcoming barriers to communication.*

> **Just checking**
>
> * What methods could you use to communicate with someone who doesn't speak English?
> * How would you comfort a three-year-old who is afraid of the hospital?
> * Why might emotional issues impair communication between a service provider and a service user?

There are statutory and non-statutory services within the health, social care, children and young people, and community justice sectors that work together for the benefit of patients and clients. Do you know the difference between them?

**Statutory** Required by law. The statutory services have been set up by Acts of Parliament and are funded by public money.

**Collaboration** Working together.

**Holistic** Looking at all the different needs of the client, including medical, social and emotional needs.

**For your project**

You could use the *Diploma Daily* activity opposite to help you plan your project. You will need to look into the various agencies involved in more detail. You will also need to find out how the different agencies would work effectively together to help and support this family.

# 2.4 Let's get together

It is important that services in each of the four sectors work together. This topic describes the partnership working that takes place to meet the needs of service users.

## Partnership working within and between the sectors

**Statutory** services are funded and provided by central and local government. They include hospitals, schools, social care services and the police. These services work together with non-statutory services, such as private and voluntary agencies and charities, to meet the needs of different client groups.

The service providers in any of the four sectors will often have to work with many other organisations. At times they will form a team of professionals from different agencies. They will meet at case conferences, usually with the client and their family or carer, and work together as a group to provide the right care for the people who need their help. **Collaboration** is essential. A **holistic** approach to care is needed if all the client's needs are to be taken into account. This requires a team approach, cooperating with others and being responsive to their ideas. Partnership working means taking joint responsibility for developing and achieving the right care for each person.

Below, some examples are given of partnership working within and between the four sectors.

### Health services

Health care demands close collaboration between the medical, nursing and allied health professions. There are many different job roles across the statutory, independent and voluntary services offered in this sector. Health care workers usually work in hospitals and clinics, but can also work with people in their homes. The various health services work closely with other sectors when caring for their patients. Some examples are mentioned below. Can you spot them?

### Social services

Social care work is about helping people with their lives. People who have physical or psychological problems often require practical help just to cope with everyday things. Social care workers provide this practical support. Social care covers a huge range of services, such as care at home, care in day centres and in residential or nursing homes, meals on wheels for the elderly, home-help and drop-in centres for people with disabilities, and fostering services for children. This means social service providers must regularly work in partnership with others. Many social care providers work alongside health services in providing nursing visits. They often work with people who have an alcohol or drug dependency and this in turn can lead them to work in partnership with both the health and community justice sectors. They also deal with children in care and this leads them to work with Children and Young People's Services.

### Children and young people

Health, social care and education services will work together to support and provide care for young children. The local general practice will provide immunisation programmes and developmental checks; paediatric nurses work in hospitals and also visit children at home when they are recovering from an illness or operation. The government has set up a National Healthy Schools Programme to promote the health of children and a nurse will visit each school regularly. Social services for early years provide day care for children under five, as well as care and activities outside school hours and during holidays. There are also advice and support for young people through Connexions and learning mentors.

### Community justice

This sector is involved with looking at antisocial behaviour and community safety. In the youth justice system, people from many different services work together to address the needs of young offenders. Youth offending teams (YOTs) identify the specific problems that may have led the young person to offend; they also try to measure the risk they pose to others. The YOT then finds suitable programmes to address the needs of the young person, with the intention of preventing them from offending again. YOTs are made up of representatives from the police, the probation service, social services, health, education, drugs and alcohol misuse and housing officers.

### Personal, learning and thinking skills

The *Diploma Daily* activity below will give you evidence towards PLTS: Independent enquirer; Creative thinker; Effective participator.

### Functional skills

It will also help towards FS: ICT – find and select information; English – reading, speaking and listening.

# Diploma Daily

## Girl and grandad hospitalised

Police officers responded to a family fight at around 1.20 a.m. yesterday. A 16-year-old and an 18-year-old were allegedly fighting over the sister of one of the boys. The girl, who is 15 and who cannot be named, is the sister of the 18-year-old. During the fight the girl, who is said to be pregnant, was knocked to the floor. The girl's grandfather, who tried to intervene, was also knocked to the floor and suffered a cut to the head. A neighbour who saw the incident phoned for an ambulance, and the teenager and

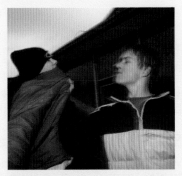

her grandfather were taken into hospital. The police arrived on the scene and the two youths were taken into custody for questioning.

Various agencies will be involved with each of the characters mentioned in the *Diploma Daily* story.

1 Following the incident, which services might be involved with the youths who were fighting?

2 List which services might be involved with the pregnant teenage girl. For each service, say what its role is and how it might deal with the situation. Also say which people in one service will need to communicate with which professionals in another service. Write a report or present the information in the form of a diagram.

### Just checking

❋ What is meant by partnership working?

❋ Why is it important for care workers to work together as a team?

❋ Give three examples of other service providers who a social care worker may need to work in partnership with.

**Partnership** People or organisations working together towards a common goal.

**Respect** A feeling or attitude of admiration and regard for somebody or something.

**Skills** Abilities you have when you become expert at something.

## For your project

If you decide to use the case study opposite as the basis for your project, then submit your video as part of your work.

# 2.5 Working with other people

This topic explains what skills you will need to work as part of a team, and how, as a service provider, you must involve clients in deciding on their own care.

## Involving the client

Because many service users have a wide range of needs, the service providers in the four sectors will have to overlap in the care they provide. It is therefore important for each service provider to work successfully with others and to ensure they are meeting their clients' needs. To do this they must talk to each other and work in **partnership**.

Many organisations may have to work together on any one case. Each will have the client's best interests at heart but it may be that all do not have the same approach; however, they will agree that the needs of the clients should always be paramount, and this is often the basis of partnership working.

It is important for the client that each service provider communicates and cooperates with other providers, as well as with the client, to find solutions to problems. All service providers must **respect** the beliefs and preferences of their clients, be they families/carers, children and young people, victims, offenders or patients. It is their job to give their clients the confidence to have a say in their own care. Service providers use different techniques to involve individuals in making decisions and participating in their care:

* providing choices for the client
* giving accurate information on treatment, available resources and procedures
* sharing ideas
* empowering individuals.

They can do this by being aware of the individual's needs and preferences, by observing, questioning and looking at past records.

## Skills needed to work as part of a team

Working in partnership with other agencies will mean you have to develop **skills** so that you are working together to solve problems or promote care. These skills will include: communication and listening; diplomacy; respect; consideration and fairness; and being able to adapt to different situations and roles.

If the team of service providers does not work together effectively, clients may become confused about who is looking after their needs. This could lead to distress or anger and the client will distrust the very services that are trying to help.

The agencies providing services will vary in a number of ways, and the workers will operate in different styles, depending on the following influences:

* the legislative frameworks that define their powers and responsibilities
* lines and degrees of political accountability

* funding regimes and financial accountability
* agency norms, language and career structures
* geographical areas of jurisdiction
* how data and information are collected and how they indicate progress made.

By working together and using the expertise and resources within the statutory, voluntary and community sectors these agencies can increase clients' well-being.

## Case study: Mr Butler's story

Mr Butler, the grandfather of the pregnant girl and one of the boys in the *Diploma Daily* article from the previous topic, suffered a blow to the head when he tried to break up the fight between the two boys. An ambulance was called by a neighbour and the 64-year-old man was taken to hospital. The hospital was concerned that he may have suffered a stroke as well as the cut to his head.

The nurse discovers, through talking to him, that Mr Butler is the sole carer of the pregnant girl and the 18-year-old boy, and he is now afraid that if he is ill he will not be able to look after the girl and her baby.

1 How might you involve Mr Butler in the decision making about his care?

2 Role-play a meeting with all agencies involved to show what skills would be used to promote Mr Butler's health care and to address the concerns he has for his family. How would you empower Mr Butler? Video the role-play, play it back and evaluate your performance.

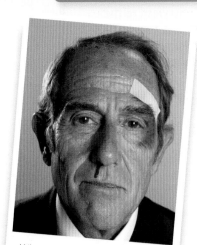

*What immediate and longer-term needs will Mr Butler have?*

## Our Health, Our Care, Our Say

The government has placed increasing emphasis on partnership working between individuals and agencies. In its 2006 White Paper *Our Health, Our Care, Our Say*, the government set out how it would provide people with high-quality social care and health services in the communities where they live. NHS services are putting into practice a plan to become more responsive to patient needs and prevent ill-health by the promotion of healthy lifestyles. Social care services are also changing to give service users more independence, choice and control.

The government wants to introduce more personalised care, so that service users become customers. For example, elderly people will be able to choose whether to be cared for in a residential home or to have the support they need from a range of services to continue living at home.

## Just checking

* List five skills a care worker needs to work effectively as part of a team.
* Give three examples of how service providers involve clients in making decisions about their care.
* What should always be paramount in making decisions about a service user's care?

## 2.6 Purpose of recording and reporting information

Written communication is a central aspect of the work of any service provider. This topic covers the different forms and purposes of records and reports.

### Why write it down?

Service providers have to write down information about the jobs they do each day and about the clients in their care. They need to be able to write effectively in a range of contexts and for a variety of different audiences and purposes, and so to tailor their writing to a given audience. This means using appropriate styles and approaches, depending on who they are writing to and what type of writing they are doing. Written communication also encompasses electronic communication, such as SMS, email, discussion boards, chat rooms and instant messaging.

It is important, therefore, that you have a good command of the English language. Here are some of the tasks you may have to do in a care setting that would require you to write something either by hand or at a computer:

* producing a diet chart for your patient to take home
* producing a care plan for your client
* writing up case notes and medical notes
* writing out prescriptions
* recording data
* taking statements from offenders and witnesses
* taking minutes at a meeting
* reporting on health and safety checks within the workplace.

Different types of communication will demand different styles of writing. If it is a formal piece of writing, to another professional or to be used in court for example, it will need the correct terminology, whereas an informal note may not. Notes may not require full sentences to be used, whereas a longer, more formal piece of writing, perhaps a **record** of a meeting or a **report** on a problem at work, should use full sentences, although the writing should still be **concise**.

It is also important to present information clearly in your records. You may know what kind of night a patient has had but the worker on the next shift can only know this if your hand-over notes make the facts plain. You have to make sure you are not writing an essay but, equally, that what you have said is not too vague and lacking in information.

*How tidy is your writing, and how clear are your notes? Would somebody else be able to understand them if they had to use them?*

## Justice sector

If a 15-year-old boy were brought in for speeding down the high street in a car, a police officer at the station would need to take a statement from him and record the incident, possibly with the inclusion of witness statements. The police officer would also need to share the information with other agencies. The parents or carers would need to be told what had happened; social services might need to be involved because the individual is under age. The types of paper evidence that may be admitted in court include:

* written statements
* documents
* maps, plans and photographs (which need a written statement saying when and where the photograph was taken or that the plan has been drawn correctly)
* business records
* print-outs of digital images.

All statements must be signed and dated by the defendant or witnesses. It is obviously important that facts are stated clearly and the notes can be read and understood. Most of the information given to others will be in written form. There are many other occasions when you might be required to complete notes or fill in forms, as mentioned above.

## Using written communications with service users

There may be times when service providers want to communicate information to clients, family or visitors. Ways in which this could be done might include making a poster (e.g. to promote a fund-raising event) or creating a leaflet.

If you are trying to get a message across or inform people of a particular healthy eating campaign, or to give advice on how to stop smoking, you have to think about your target audience and what will attract their attention. Producing a diagram to help clients, particularly children, keep a record of their progress would be more appropriate than a written record. This will help the care worker to check progress in a particular area while being fun and encouraging for the child.

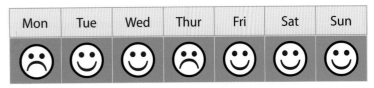

*A picture chart could be used for a young child to show how they are feeling on that day.*

> **Record** A written account of what has happened or been achieved, for example in a meeting or by a student.
>
> **Report** A structured account of a particular subject matter, or of something that has happened.
>
> **Concise** Brief and to the point.

**Activity**

1 Find out how records are kept at school.

2 Then find out which agencies might need to know some of the information held on those records. What happens to that information?

**For your project**

Describe the different ways information is passed between colleagues and agencies.

**Just checking**

* What two different written tasks might you have to undertake for a patient in a hospital ward?
* What written evidence might you have to produce in a court of law if you were a police officer?
* Name two types of written communication you could use to get clients interested in a healthy-eating campaign.

# 2.7 Get the record straight

It is important to be able to complete records accurately and legibly. This topic makes some recommendations on how to set out your writing.

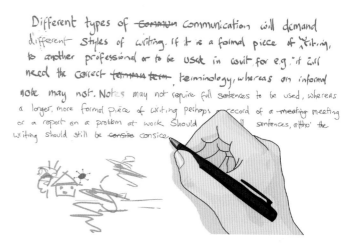

*What a mess!*

## Writing that's right for the job

### The right language

The aim of written communication is to give information; it is therefore important that the writing is clear and accurate. Service providers must be able to present information in different ways, depending on who they are communicating with and what they are writing about. You will need to be able to structure the material so that it is clear to the person you are communicating with. You must make yourself understood: if you are writing for a patient or client there is no point in using a lot of **jargon**, or terms that might cause confusion and worry. It is, however, important to use the correct **terminology**, especially when communicating with service providers in other sectors or if your records may be used in a court.

### Always check it

People often make mistakes when they are writing; sometimes your brain seems to work faster than your pen and you miss words out, make spelling errors or use the wrong words. You should *always* read through what you have written before passing it on. Check that you have written in a clear and precise way, and check your spellings and punctuation. Make sure that what you have written makes sense and that your grammar is correct. If you don't do these things then, at best, what you have written might not make sense or, at worst, it could be very misleading to whoever is reading it, which could result in a serious mistake being made, such as the wrong medicine or the wrong advice being given.

### Research

It may be that you will have to find out some information about a case, an illness or a piece of legislation. There are many ways of researching information. Depending on what you need to find out, you might use the Internet, books, letters or articles.

## Typing or handwriting?

The information and communication technology (ICT) skills that you learn at school and college will be very helpful, as you will need to update client files and records, and prepare reports. A lot of this type of work is now done electronically, although there will still be times when you need to write things by hand. For example, a nurse will usually update medical records for patients on a ward by hand, with pen on paper. Similarly, a police officer will take notes about an incident. These will often have to be written up at a later date. **Minutes** at a meeting are often taken by hand.

## Presentation

Because the records kept in the health, social care, children and young people and the community justice sectors are often so important, they must be accurate and legible. Make sure you:

* write clearly in pen or use a computer
* use the correct grammar, spelling and punctuation
* write for the audience, and use the correct and appropriate terminology
* use headings, subheadings and paragraphs
* make sure your reports and letters are dated and signed.

**Jargon** Specialist words and expressions when used inappropriately, with people who won't understand them.

**Terminology** Specialised words or expressions that are used by people in a particular work setting.

**Minutes** A record of what is said and decided at a meeting, made at the time.

### Functional skills

The case study tasks will help towards FS: English – writing.

## Case study: Emma's story

Emma is 15 years old. She had become very interested in dieting when she was 14 and lost a lot of weight. Her mother became worried about her. She put some weight back on over the summer holidays but since starting school again in September she has lost weight again. Her periods have stopped. She complains about being too tired to do her homework and has lost interest in school and her friends there. Her mother can't understand why, as she could do well at school if she put her mind to it. Her mother insists she goes to see their GP.

The doctor measures Emma's weight and height and calculates her body mass index (BMI) (see topic 8.4) to be 17, which is very much underweight. He thinks she may be suffering from anorexia.

People with anorexia have extreme weight loss as a result of strict dieting. In spite of this, they believe they are fat and are worried about what is in reality a normal weight or shape. People with low self-esteem are more vulnerable, as are girls in mid-adolescence. A diagnosis of anorexia nervosa is based on: the person's BMI; the individual having a distorted body image and abnormal attitudes to food and weight; amenorrhoea (which is the absence of menstruation); and other signs of starvation, such as tiredness, slow pulse rate and gaunt face.

1 Imagine you are Emma's GP. You want a hospital colleague to confirm the diagnosis and to take on the case if necessary. Write a brief referral letter to this colleague, giving your findings and requesting help. Use the appropriate language and terminology for a formal letter to a professional colleague.

2 Write a short letter to Emma's mother explaining your findings and the referral. Think carefully how you will word this letter.

## Just checking

* List four types of sources of information you could use in researching a case you were working on.
* Why and when might you need to write notes or fill in forms by hand?
* What kind of work might you do electronically in a hospital, at a school or in a community justice agency?

**'Need to know' basis** Giving only that information which is needed, and only to those who need to know.

# 2.8 Safe and secure

The records kept by service providers, as well as being accurate and legible, must always be confidential, accurate and securely held. This topic looks at these issues.

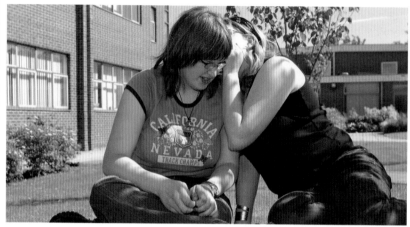

*Can you keep a secret?*

People have physical needs, such as food, warmth and medical care if they are ill. Service providers can at times concentrate on these but forget that everyone also has emotional needs. Care workers should respond to these needs, taking into account the client's age, culture, disability and the situation.

## Promises of secrecy should never be given!

Information may need to be shared across services working in partnership; however, the client must give consent first. To break this trust between the carer and the client would be disrespectful and upsetting. Sometimes information is shared with another person on a **'need to know' basis**. An example might be at a nursery where the break-up of a relationship might affect the way a child behaves: the nursery nurse responsible for the child will need to know so that they can keep an eye on the child and monitor any changes in behaviour.

In most circumstances confidentiality should be maintained. These are times when things are said or incidents happen that are right for you to deal with yourself and not speak to anyone else about. For instance, if an older woman has had 'an accident' in bed, you would do your best to stop her feeling embarrassed, change the bedding and make sure she is clean and comfortable. You would not moan about it or tell other people and make the woman feel even more uncomfortable than she does already.

There are times, however, when confidentiality must be broken. These are situations in which you have been told something in confidence but do need to report it, usually to a more senior colleague. For example, if a 15-year-old who has been taken into custody tells you they have had several bottles of lager, you would need to report that information to someone more senior, as the child is drinking under age. It would be right to tell the 15-year-old that you had to do so.

If a client is in danger, has committed a crime, is unconscious or any type of abuse has taken place, you will usually need to report it to a senior colleague. You should never promise to keep something secret before you know what you are about to be told.

## Confidential files

Medical and other written records must be kept confidential. They must be locked away in filing cabinets. The 1998 Data Protection Act gave patients the right to be able to see their medical and social service records. You have to give notice that you want to see them and doctors will charge a fee. There are exceptional circumstances when clients may not be able to see their records; this is usually to protect clients, for example some with mental health problems.

Information is also kept on computer. The 1998 Data Protection Act means that all organisations which keep records in this way must be registered and there are **data protection** guidelines that must be followed, such as:

* people have to give their consent to their data being used
* the information must be obtained legally
* it can be used only for the purpose for which it was collected
* it must not be given to anyone else
* there must be a proper security system that has a password for access.

The National Health Service is developing a lifelong electronic medical record for each patient. This can then be accessed by GPs and hospital doctors, who will be able to see the patient's information at the press of a button. Certain information will not be available for service providers to see without the client's permission (e.g. patients who are HIV positive, or someone who has been treated for sexually transmitted diseases). However, there are some who are concerned about confidentiality and whether this system could be abused.

> **Data protection** Legal safeguards to prevent misuse of information about an individual that is stored on a computer.

> **Personal, learning and thinking skills**
>
> The activity should help towards PLTS: Independent enquirer; Creative thinker; Reflective learner.

### Case study: Grace's story

Grace, a young woman, is brought into casualty. You are her nurse. She is very drowsy but she tells you she has just arrived in this country from Africa. Before boarding the plane she swallowed a quantity of drugs and is expected to pass them on to another person at an address in the city. She is afraid of anyone finding out and has asked you not to tell anyone. Can you keep this a secret?

1 Discuss with a partner what you would do if you were the nurse. What do you think are the dangers for Grace? How would you explain to her what your decision would be? Are there other people or agencies that you would inform?

2 Think of two other situations. Use examples from your work experience if possible; otherwise, use the examples of a child in a nursery and a conversation with an older person in a residential home. In each situation, say whether you would be able to maintain client confidentiality. Explain why.

### Just checking

* What is meant by giving information on a 'need to know' basis?
* What legislation governs how organisations keep clients' records on computer?
* Give two advantages and two disadvantages of the electronic medical patient record.

# 2.9 Sharing information

This unit covers why and how information is shared between service providers and the risks involved.

## Who shares information and how

Local authorities, police authorities, health and social care services, services for children and young people and others need to be able to share personal data in order to comply with their statutory duties to work together in support of their clients. Staff in all agencies will have to write up case notes, produce care plans, record and present data, and so on. For clients who are using two (or more) separate services, and there are many such clients, it is important that information is shared, so that the services know what each other are doing and that they are not duplicating some aspects of care. Good communication between service providers is crucial to the delivery of high-quality, effective care.

The sharing of this information is likely to be both written and verbal. Sharing information verbally is an effective and adequate way of communicating with a colleague in some circumstances. When changing shifts, for example, you might tell your colleague that Mr Perry had a really good night. In other circumstances and for many other purposes, information *must* be in written form. Details of Mr Perry's medication and the results of monitoring would have to be noted on the patient record sheet. In multi-agency meetings, service providers will discuss at length the best way forward for their client but notes will be taken and written up in detail later, usually electronically, and then circulated to all the members of the team. This will often be done by email. If the information is confidential, practitioners should always password-protect electronic files. Meetings and case conferences with other colleagues and with the client must be minuted, as the information may need to be shared and may be called upon at a later date, for example if a case goes to court.

Sharing information between professionals and agencies helps to ensure that people with health, educational and social care needs receive appropriate care, protection and support. This can be seen among practitioners working with children and their families, as it is only when information from a range of sources is put together that a child can be seen to be in need or at risk of harm.

The aims of sharing information are:

* to promote the welfare of service users
* to ensure that the needs of the clients are assessed effectively, so the correct services and care are provided

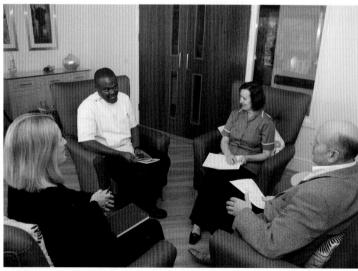

*Gathering and sharing information with clients and other service providers.*

* to ensure **integrated** care planning
* to avoid **duplicating** the information gathered.

This clearly requires agencies to work effectively and efficiently together to provide the best services for the particular circumstances of each individual. Sharing personal data in both manual and electronic format with colleagues, family and partner agencies is vital to them providing coordinated care.

## Risks in sharing

There are always risks to sharing information. Remember the time you told a friend something personal and all of a sudden the whole world knew about it? There can also be risks involved with sharing information between care services, whether it is verbal or written. These risks fall into three categories:

* risks to service users, for example if unauthorised people gain access to a client's personal, medical or financial data
* risks to the agency, which could include a financial risk if information about costs are shared
* risks to practitioners, for example misunderstandings, misinterpretation and breaches of confidentiality.

Most risks are overcome and people work very hard to ensure that the risks are kept to a minimum. Records can be shared between agencies if the information in the records is necessary to protect the health and safety of any individual. However, there are important rules and safeguards that have to be taken into consideration. Service providers work to a suitable framework so that sharing relevant information between agencies can be done effectively, with confidence and trust, while also making sure they maintain the confidentiality of their clients.

Each organisation within the four sectors will have its own codes of conduct, charters and policies that govern what service providers can and cannot do in relation to the sharing of information. In addition, the Data Protection Act will help to ensure confidentiality and respect (see topic 2.8).

The key pieces of legislation that relate to the sharing of information are:

* Data Protection Act 1998
* Access to Health Records Act 1990
* Crime and Disorder Act 1998
* Criminal Procedures and Investigations Act 1996
* Human Rights Act 1998
* Freedom of Information Act 2000
* Children Act 2004.

**Integrated** When all the different elements are combined as one.

**Duplicating** Doing something more than once.

### Activity

1 While you are on a work experience assignment, or in your school or college, follow a piece of information (this could be a note, record or file) from receipt and then from one department to another. Record what happens.

2 Make a list of all the workers who have had access to that information. What risks have been involved?

### For your project

As a team, organise a school event for young children or older people. Collect all letters, emails, logs, planning notes, invoices, records of sharing information with the team, feedback from people attending the event.

### Just checking

* Give one reason why meetings should be minuted.
* What are the aims of sharing information among your colleagues at work or between agencies?
* By what means can the confidentiality of electronic files be enhanced?

Have you had to work as a team on a project at school? How well did you all work together? Were there differences of opinion? If so, how did you resolve them – did everyone contribute or was it left to a few to do most of the work? Imagine that sort of situation in any of the care services. How would it affect a patient who has suffered a stroke, is left in the corridor and no one takes responsibility for making sure they are getting the right treatment and going to the correct department for care? If health and social services do not work together to provide support and care at home, how would this affect the patient and their family?

# 2.10 The importance of partnerships

This topic covers shared care and partnership working.

## Working together

Have you ever watched *Casualty* or *Holby City*? You will have seen how successful and positive it can be for different service providers to work collaboratively. Each person has different skills and contributes ideas based on their various experiences and expertise.

You will also have seen that sometimes people and groups do not always work together effectively. A lot depends on the organisation and size of departments, the management, and how individuals and groups interact on a personal and professional level.

It is essential for service providers to work together as a team and to share the risks and responsibilities for the care of their clients. Partnership working aims to promote a more 'joined up' way of working. It should help reduce bureaucracy and give clients as well as the public, private, voluntary and community sectors more power to participate and share in the care of the individual and society.

Some examples of partnerships include:

* crime and disorder reduction partnerships, which are a combination of police, local authorities and other organisations and businesses who together develop and implement strategies for tackling crime and disorder at local level
* youth offending teams, which are present in every local authority in England and Wales, and are made up of representatives from the police, probation service, social services, health, education, drugs and alcohol misuse and housing officers
* Connexions (see snapshot)
* voluntary and community sector organisations (see below).

### Snapshot

Have you seen Connexions at your school? Maybe you have already had an interview. Connexions is an agency that works together with schools and gives advice on a wide range of issues, from learning and careers to healthy lifestyles and relationships. It works with 13–19-year-olds but also provides support up to the age of 25 for young people who have learning difficulties or disabilities (or both).

## Shared care

**Shared care** is a **partnership** between professionals and others where they work towards a common goal. For example, the services will work together to find the best way of helping a client who wants to take a large degree of responsibility for their own care, or where the life of a disadvantaged person is improved by the joint efforts of a social service and another provider. The partnership between the service user and each of the services involved is equal. Consider the case of a young

**Partnership** Care workers, professionals, the service user and families working together.

**Shared care** Professionals and others sharing in the care of an individual.

offender who needs to return to education. A case conference may be called that would probably include professionals from social services, the education service as well as the offender and their family or carers. The clients who benefit from this type of care are of all age groups, and may have all types of disabilities or social problems.

Other examples of shared care may include charities or voluntary services and faith groups that provide short breaks for disadvantaged children or those that help enlist families for short-term fostering. In each case there is significant input from the non-professional, in the latter case the foster carer, who is supervised by the professional.

## Voluntary and community sector

Partnership working between local government and the voluntary and community sector (VCS) has benefits for everyone. All organisations in an area can come together to improve the lives of people and communities. Bringing the statutory and non-statutory organisations in an area together to set priorities and discuss the issues that are particular to them in their neighbourhoods can strengthen society.

It is important for statutory agencies working within an area to work with their local communities. The VCS can play three main roles locally:

* It can provide information and advice to individuals and communities, which empowers local people and brings them together.
* It enables people's voices to be heard by those who make decisions and other members of the community.
* It can provide activities or services, funded either publicly or independently.
* Non-statutory partners can bring different perspectives, expertise and knowledge.

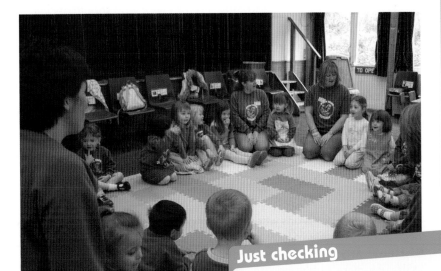

*People from a variety of backgrounds may be involved in running a children's playgroup, and they will network with a wide range of services.*

### Activity

1 Take the case of an older person who has had a stroke. List all the agencies that might be involved in their care.

2 Which agencies and individuals might be involved if there was repeated antisocial behaviour in your local area?

3 Role-play a case conference that had brought together representatives of all the different agencies for one of the above cases.

### Personal, learning and thinking skills

The activity should help towards PLTS: Creative thinker; Reflective learner; Effective participator.

### For your project

Look at the different agencies that might work together on a case. Use the tasks in the activity to help with your work. Perhaps take one case in particular that you have had some experience of in your work placement and show how care workers and agencies have worked together on it.

### Just checking

* Give an example of a situation where different agencies work together with a service user and name the agencies.
* What are the three main roles that the voluntary and community sector can play in your community?
* Give three examples of partnership organisations.

# 2.11 Work as a team and be effective

This topic looks further at partnership working.

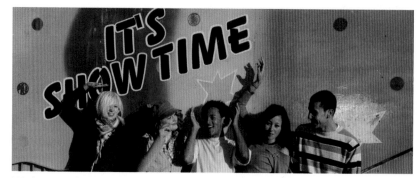

*Working together can be enormously rewarding as well as effective.*

## Partnership working with clients

A good example of partnership working is the suppport given to vulnerable older people who want to continue living in their own home. Charities and voluntary services often work together with health and social care services, as well as with older people themselves, to decide on the type of care needed and to provide practical as well as emotional support.

For example, the health and social services offered to an older client who had become frail might include: an occupational therapist, to assess any adjustments in the home; a physiotherapist, to help with mobility concerns; a community nurse; placement at a day centre for maybe one day a week, to allow the person to socialise with others; meals on wheels; and home-help. Importantly, it is the client who should decide what precisely is wanted from the range of services that can be offered.

## Partnership working with other agencies

Each agency may have a different **perspective** that it will bring to the team. For example, the criminal justice sector may be concerned that an offender has the care and supervision needed to stop the person from re-offending, while a social care worker may think the person needs to be independent and have the freedom to become more responsible for their own actions. Whatever their views, each member of the team must support the others to work towards the common goal, which is the health and well-being of the client, as well as society.

There are many occasions when teams of people from different agencies need to get together to look at particular issues relating to individuals and the local community. Partnerships are formed between organisations in the voluntary, public, private, statutory and non-statutory sectors. Here we will look at one example, from the justice sector.

The Crime and Disorder Act 1998 established crime and disorder reduction partnerships, mentioned in topic 2.10. The aim is for everyone to work together to reduce crime, disorder and the fear of crime locally, in order to improve the quality of life and to create a safer living and working environment.

By working as a team, partnerships establish what the particular crime and disorder problems are in their area. The different services work with local communities to make sure that the partnership's **perception** matches that of local people, especially minority groups, such as gay men and lesbians, or members of ethnic minorities, to ensure their crime and disorder concerns are considered and incorporated in any crime reduction work.

Partnerships then devise a **strategy** to tackle the problems that are seen to be a priority. This includes setting targets for each of the priority areas and providing feedback to all concerned.

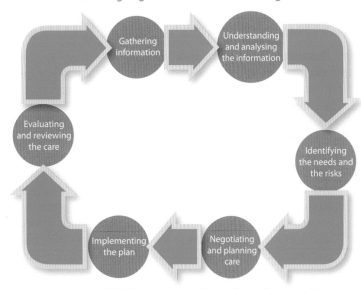

*Working together to plan and provide appropriate care.*

Crime and the fear of crime are very real issues for many people, especially the elderly and vulnerable groups. Even in an area of low crime, disorder, drugs and antisocial behaviour can have a huge effect on residents' quality of life. All agencies need to work together to ensure that their policies and actions take full account of crime. For example, local authority planning departments will now consider the crime impact that a new development may have on its surroundings. By working with the crime and disorder reduction partnerships they can recommend alterations, such as additional lighting, to ensure that the new developments do not increase crime levels.

> **Perception** Understanding of the issues.
>
> **Strategy** A plan or a method of getting results.

## 𝕯𝖎𝖕𝖑𝖔𝖒𝖆 𝕯𝖆𝖎𝖑𝖞

### Gamesville against litter

In response to the city-wide litter problem, Gamesville City Council and other key agencies affected have established a partnership called 'Gamesville Against Litter' to tackle the messy issue. The aims of this partnership are to encourage community pride and participation, and to reduce litter dropping in the city.

The Mayor, Mr Mumble, said: 'By including residents and local businesses this partnership approach encourages each and every one of us to contribute and ensures a better use of resources and time. Here's to a cleaner city!'

1 Name four groups of people that might get together to tackle a litter problem.

2 Discuss as a team the groups you've named. Why should they be involved in this partnership and how can they make a difference?

## For your project

Expand on the work from topic 2.10. Show how and why different service providers collaborate and support each other. Give examples and show the role of the client and the advantages of clients being involved in their own care.

## Just checking

✳ What is the aim of the Local Government and Public Involvement in Health Act 2007?

✳ Name a voluntary sector organisation that campaigns for elderly people.

✳ Which Act established crime and disorder reduction partnerships?

# Unit 2 Assessment guide

This unit is assessed by an assignment which will be marked by your teacher. You will need to show that you have good communication skills and can communicate effectively with different types of people in many different situations. You will need to show that you have interacted with one other person and a group of people, preferably of different ages. Some people have barriers that make communication more difficult, such as visual or hearing impairments or a speech problem. You will need to investigate some of these barriers and suggest ways of improving communication. You will need to show that you understand why record keeping is important and why confidentiality is important but why information needs to be shared between professionals and organisations at times. When different organisations work together to provide care and support for people, this is called partnership working. You will need to think about some of the problems that may occur in partnership working and how they can be overcome. You will also gain personal experience in working and communicating with a team, when you and your peers organise an event for a group of people. You will need to show the role you played within the team and how you communicated to ensure the success of the activity.

## Time management

* It is important that you participate in class activities that demonstrate how communication skills are used, as this will allow you to practise your own skills in preparation for the two interactions.

* Be well organised. This will involve storing useful information that you need in a file or folder so that you can easily find it. This may include notes that you have made about how you planned, participated in and evaluated your one-to-one interaction and group interaction.

* By being well organised you can show that you are a team worker and a self-manager, which will contribute towards achievement of your personal, learning and thinking skills.

* You will also need to keep documents that show you are able to complete them correctly and legibly and understand their purpose. You may be given these by your teacher or by an organisation.

* It is important that you keep a record of all the meetings you have attended when planning your activity. These are called 'minutes' and should contain basic information about the date and time of the meeting, its purpose, who attended and the points discussed.

* Be prepared with a list of questions that you could ask if your teacher arranges for a speaker to come and talk to your class or if you go to visit an organisation. Make a note of the answers like a reporter would.

## Useful links

* There are lots of useful websites that will help with your investigation into partnership working. An example of this is www.respect.gov.uk, which shows the people involved in working together to reduce antisocial behaviour.

* Work experience will also be useful, as you may get the opportunity to communicate with people who have communication difficulties; for example, you may interact with toddlers and small children at a nursery or older people at a day centre. Remember that anything you see or hear in an organisation is confidential.

## Things you might need

* Forms or documentation used by organisations to communicate information which you need to fill in to show that you can complete them correctly and in clear handwriting.

* Craft materials or use of ICT to produce your leaflet on partnership working, showing that you understand the different organisations that work together. One example may be the different organisations that look after an older person at home. These may include the GP and community nurses from the statutory health care sector, social care workers from either the statutory or the private social care sector and the Age Concern day centre from the voluntary sector.

* Minutes from planning meetings, notes about your role and any evaluation material used when organising your event. If you take photos of your event, remember you should not take pictures of anyone who is not part of your team, to ensure confidentiality is met.

# How you will be assessed

| You must show that you *know*: | Guidance | To gain higher marks you must *explain*: |
| --- | --- | --- |
| The methods of communication. These will include verbal and non-verbal methods, e.g. speech, listening, gestures, facial expression, posture, touch, silence and proximity.<br><br>The barriers to communication. These will include physical or learning impairments, age, cultural, environmental and language barriers.<br><br>What verbal and non-verbal communication skills you need to use in a one-to-one and a small-group interaction and how you can overcome any communication barriers. | ✳ You need to conduct your investigation in two settings that provide services for health, social care, community justice or children and young people. You also need to take part in two interactions (a one to one and a small group) that demonstrate your communication skills. This may include a nursery for children or a day centre for adults or within your school or college. | ✳ The methods of communication that are used.<br><br>✳ At least four potential barriers to communication and how they can be overcome in each setting to ensure effective communication.<br><br>✳ How you will participate in 2 different interactions; explaining the different communcation methods you will need to use and assessing your communication strengths and the areas for improvement.<br><br>✳ Your effective participation in a one to one and a group interaction. |
| Why record keeping is important and how information is stored safely. Why is it important that records are accurate and confidentiality is maintained?<br><br>Why is it important that information is shared only with the people who need to know? | ✳ You need to carry out your investigation in at least three different settings. You might do this by asking questions at your work experience placement.<br><br>✳ You also need to complete three different documents or forms that give information in different situations, describing what the form and the information are used for. You must complete these in handwriting that is neat and tidy and can be read by someone else. You should not use any records that identify people. | ✳ The purpose of reporting and recording arrangements, giving at least three examples of how information is shared within teams and between organisations. You might consider examples such as when teams hand over to the next shift within a hospital, or when schools work with Connexions. Why are confidentiality, accuracy and security of records important in these examples? What is the purpose of recording the information accurately and legibly? |
| Partnership working means when different organisations or professions work together to provide a service. How do they work together to provide an effective service? | ✳ Produce a leaflet that shows three examples of partnership working in your local area, using at least one organisation from the statutory sector and one from the private or voluntary sector.<br><br>✳ The statutory sector is paid for by the government. The private sector is formed by businesses, which aim to make a profit and may include private hospitals, dentists and complementary therapists. The voluntary sector is formed by charitable organisations, which generally do not receive government funding. | ✳ What the factors are that enable partnership working to be successful. You might consider the communication skills needed within a meeting or a case conference where each member of a different organisation has a different point of view.<br><br>✳ Who is involved in the partnerships.<br><br>✳ What the potential barriers are that need to be overcome to provide a good service for an individual. |
| How to organise an event as part of a small team and then write an account of it. | ✳ You could organise an event for children or older people. It does not need to be a fund-raising event but could be a simple activity.<br><br>✳ You need to show that you can work well in a team and you should collect evidence of this, e.g. minutes from meetings or planning notes. | ✳ How you planned, participated in and evaluated the event, reflecting on your role and the roles of others in the team. You must play a full and active role within the event, as this will also help you to gain higher marks. |

# 3 SAFEGUARDING AND PROTECTING INDIVIDUALS

This unit is about the importance of safeguarding and protecting individuals from harm and abuse. Within your workplace, you will be required to keep yourself, colleagues and those you are caring for safe and secure. The unit aims to help you develop an understanding of how to assess various situations and decide what to do if you feel a person or a group of people is at risk.

## Gathering information

In order to understand how to protect yourself and others you need to be able to gather information relevant to a particular situation. There are two different types of sources of information: **primary** and **secondary**.

To collect primary information, you could use research techniques such as questionnaires and interviews. Secondary sources of information include the Internet, books, journals and leaflets. You will have a chance to use such tools in some of the activities in this and other units.

## What helps to keep people safe in the care sectors?

You have already come across some examples of legislation, policies, procedures and codes of practice in Unit 1 and will do so in other units. If you have forgotten the meaning of any of these terms, look back at page 3, and read the key word definitions.

This unit looks at laws such as the Health and Safety at Work Act 1974 (HASAW). It says that every employer has to protect the health, safety and security of staff, service users and other visitors. It requires employers not only to draw up safety policies and procedures but also to put them into practice and to **review** them regularly. This may seem to be an old law but it still applies to every workplace in all sectors and helps an organisation maintain a safe working environment.

## How can you ensure your own safety and that of others?

Your own roles and responsibilities as a service provider will include following organisational policies and procedures for safety and security, and identifying hazards and carrying out risk assessments. It is important that you know how to record, report and share information. You should always operate within the limits of your own role and responsibilities.

> ### THINKING POINT
> On your way to school or college today did you take any risks? Think about that journey. Did you have to cross the road? How did you reduce the risk to yourself and other road users? This is an example of a simple risk assessment.

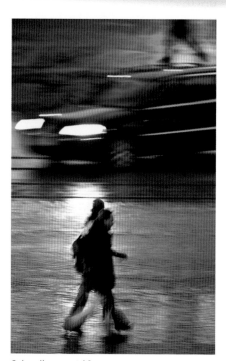

*Schoolboy at risk?*

> **Primary information**
> Information obtained by asking a person directly.
>
> **Secondary information**
> Information gained at second-hand, such as from books.
>
> **Review** To look at something again with a view to improving it.

## Emergencies and how to respond to them

The possible range of emergencies includes injury, fire, flooding and security breach. There must be procedures in place in all workplaces to make sure service providers respond to emergencies swiftly and in a way that minimises any risk to themselves and others.

## Infection prevention and control

Infection can be caused by bacteria, viruses or fungi. You will learn what these are and how infections can be spread in topics 3.7 and 3.8. There are standard precautions to take, such as hand hygiene, personal protective equipment and general cleanliness.

## Trust and abuse

It is vitally important to establish and maintain a trusting relationship with individuals if you are not only to care for them in some way but also to safeguard and protect them. To do this, you need to set up boundaries for the relationship, promote independence, support individuals by communicating effectively with them, be consistent, reliable, helpful and enabling, promote rights, be non-judgemental and maintain privacy and confidentiality. You will recognise many of these things as part of the key values discussed in Unit 1.

You also need to be able to recognise the signs that an individual is at risk of harm or abuse. Abuse can be physical, emotional, sexual or financial. Individuals can suffer from self-abuse as well as abuse by others. Some of the signs of abuse are failure to thrive, some things that you can easily see, such as bruises, and complaints, either in writing or verbal.

## How you will be assessed

For this unit you will be assessed by one assignment, involving the production of a training pack for new workers. You will need to plan and carry out investigations into health, safety and security issues at two settings and produce a training pack based on your findings. You should choose settings in two of the four sectors. The overall investigation may be a group activity, but your training pack should be your own work. The investigation will enable you to develop personal, learning and thinking skills such as those of an independent enquirer, a creative thinker, and a self-manager.

## What you will learn in this unit

You will:

* Be able to research and gather information
* Know the key legislation that supports safe practices and maintains standards of health and safety
* Understand the role of legislation, regulations and codes of practice in governing health, safety and security so as to protect individuals
* Understand how following policies and procedures in an organisation helps to maintain a safe environment and working conditions
* Know how to ensure your own safety and the safety of others
* Know a range of emergencies and the appropriate responses that should be taken
* Understand the main causes of infection and the importance of standard precautions in infection prevention and control
* Understand the role of risk assessment within and across the sectors
* Be able to carry out an assessment of risk in a specified situation
* Understand the importance of establishing and maintaining a trusting relationship with individuals
* Know how to recognise the signs that an individual is at risk of harm or abuse

In this topic you will learn and develop research skills, to help you, for example, carry out an investigation in the workplace.

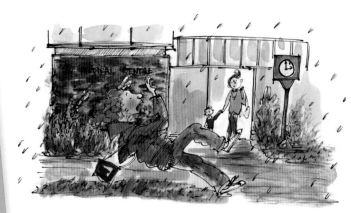

*Whoops!*

## Primary research – straight from the horse's mouth

### Questionnaires

A questionnaire is simply a set of questions designed to collect the same kind of information from a large group of people in the same way, so that the answers can be analysed systematically.

There are several steps to take when designing a questionnaire:

1 Decide what your research aims are. That is, what are you aiming to find out by asking people to complete a questionnaire?

2 Pick your population and sample. Who are you going to ask, and how many people will you ask, to complete your questionnaire?

3 Decide how to collect the replies. Are you going to ask people to write their own answers down or are you going to ask the questions and write their answers down? Some questionnaires are sent by post or email, with an accompanying letter or introduction explaining the purpose of the survey and the importance of returning it.

4 Write the questions:

  ✳ make them relevant, concise and clear

  ✳ use short, simple sentences

  ✳ ask for only one piece of information at a time

  ✳ ask closed questions (e.g. 'Do you like chocolate?') if you want a 'yes', 'don't know' or 'no' type of answer, and use open questions (e.g. 'What do you think about the suggestion that chocolate is bad for you and should be banned?') if you want to explore a range of possible ideas arising from an issue

  ✳ start with easy questions, going from closed to open questions

  ✳ ask them in a logical order

  ✳ avoid negatives if possible – express questions in a positive way

  ✳ don't write too many questions, because long questionnaires often give a poor **response rate** and so do not provide enough reliable information.

---

### THINKING POINT

A patient complains to her doctor that the surface of the health centre car park is unsafe when it is wet. She has slipped several times on her way in. What would you have to know in order to determine whether the surface is unsafe? How would you find out the information you would need to determine this?

---

**Response rate** The proportion (percentage) of questionnaires that are returned to you completed.

5  Lay the questions out clearly. If the questionnaire is to be used with a large number of people, have a trial run with a few people first to make sure the questions are good enough to collect the information you are looking for.

After you have carried out the questionnaire survey, you will have to analyse the data – that is, look at the answers, decide what they show and draw some conclusions.

### Interviews

Interviewing involves asking someone questions to collect information. To do this effectively you need to do the following:

* Prepare your questions beforehand but be prepared to ask supplementary questions if the person being interviewed does not quite answer the question (e.g. 'Could you just explain what you meant by that in a little more detail please?').

* Ask the person if they wouldn't mind being interviewed and explain what you want to interview them about.

* Be polite – say please when you ask them to be interviewed and thank you when appropriate, especially at the end.

* If possible, conduct the interview somewhere where there will be no distractions.

* Start with closed questions and build up to open ones.

* Do not ask personal questions that will make the interviewee uncomfortable or annoyed.

See also the important safety tip on page 241 regarding interviews.

### Observation

This technique to gather information can be used when you are able to look at something for yourself, such as whether a building has a wheelchair ramp or not.

## Secondary research

Secondary research involves gathering 'second-hand' information, for example from the Internet, books, magazines, newspapers, journals and leaflets. Effective use of secondary information can save a lot of time. Remember:

* When using the Internet use a search engine such as Google, and select the option 'pages from the UK' if this will make the search results more relevant to you.

* Use the index at the back of the book to find the section you need rather than spending ages flicking through. Journals have a contents page and leaflets are usually short enough to just flick through.

* Reject any information that is written at a level that is too high for you – if you don't understand it, you will be unable to use it properly.

* If you are going to include certain pieces of information in a report, put it into your own words rather than copying chunks of text – it is always obvious that the information is written in a different style or to a different standard from the rest of the report.

### Activity

1  As a group, conduct a survey of the safety of your school or college. You will need to use primary research skills for this task – a questionnaire, interviews and observation.

2  Write a report of your findings, having first decided as a group how you are going to do this.

3  Make some recommendations based on your findings. Use secondary sources such as the Internet to help you find facts and costings to support these recommendations.

4  Have a group discussion to decide how effective each of the techniques used has been in gathering useful information. What could you improve upon next time you carry out such an investigation?

### Personal, learning and thinking skills

The activity should help towards PLTS: Independent enquirer; Creative thinker; Reflective learner; Team worker; Effective participator.

### Functional Skills

It should also help towards FS: English – writing.

### Just checking

* What is the purpose of using a questionnaire?
* What is the difference between an open question and a closed question?
* Why should you never copy blocks of text from secondary sources of information?

Have you seen adverts like this in newspapers or on television? What do you think of companies that persuade people to sue their employers or the local council? What do you think the short- and long-term effects are on our society as a whole?

# 3.2 Safe in the arms of the law

This topic looks at some of the key legislation that supports safe practices and maintains standards of health and safety.

## Key health and safety legislation and regulations

There are numerous pieces of **legislation** and **regulations** concerning health and safety. Some of these are shown in the table opposite.

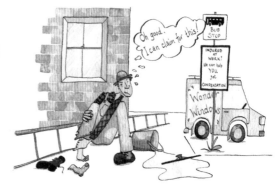

*Is it good that he can claim for this?*

### HASAW Act 1974

This important piece of legislation helps safeguard and protect individuals. It requires employers to provide:

* a safe working environment
* health and safety policy and procedures
* information on health and safety
* a risk assessment of potential hazards.

Risk assessments are covered in more detail in topics 3.9 and 3.10.

The HASAW Act also requires that you, as an employee:

* take reasonable care of your own health and safety, as well as that of others, such as visitors and other employees
* cooperate with your employer on health and safety issues
* make sure that any health and safety equipment is not intentionally damaged.

The Act is important because it is like an umbrella covering all the other legislation applying to the workplace, in that all of these help enforce and reinforce the requirements above.

## Personal, learning and thinking skills

The activity should help towards PLTS: Independent enquirers.

## Functional skills

The activity will also help towards FS: ICT – find and select information.

## Activity

1 Read the table opposite. Use a dictionary to look up any words you don't understand.

2 Draw up a table with three columns. In the first, copy the left-hand column from the table opposite, and head the other two columns 'Students' and 'Staff'. In these columns say how you think the legislation or regulations affect students or staff or both in your school. Remember that staff includes not only teachers but also support, administrative and kitchen staff, as well as caretakers and cleaners.

3 Pick any one of the key pieces of legislation (except the HASAW Act) or regulations and do some further research into how it affects service providers and users in one of the four main sectors covered by this qualification.

## Key health and safety legislation and regulations

| Legislation/regulation | Brief details |
|---|---|
| Health and Safety at Work (HASAW) Act 1974 | Lays down wide-ranging duties for employers to protect the health, safety and **welfare** of all their employees as far as is reasonably practicable |
| Food Safety Act 1990 | Lays down rules which apply to everyone involved in the production, storage, distribution or sale of food |
| Food Safety (General Food Hygiene) Regulations 1995 | Cover general requirements for the design, construction and operation of food premises |
| Manual Handling Operations Regulations 1992 | Seek to reduce the incidence of injury and ill-health arising from the manual handling of loads at work |
| Reporting of Injuries, Diseases and Dangerous Occurrences Regulations (RIDDOR) 1995 | States that employers, the self-employed and those in control of premises must report specified workplace incidents |
| Data Protection Act 1998 | Seeks to protect individuals with regard to the processing of personal **data** |
| Management of Health and Safety at Work Regulations 1999 | Cover the way the duties laid down in legislation such as the HASAW Act are managed in the workplace |
| Care Standards Act 2000 | Transfers regulation of all social care and independent health care services to the National Care Standards Commission (now the Commission for Social Care Inspection) |
| Criminal Justice Act 2003 | Modernised many areas of the UK's criminal justice system, including police power, bail, sentencing and release on licence |
| Control of Substances Hazardous to Health (COSHH) Regulations 2002 | Seek to make safe the handling of chemicals in the workplace |
| Children Act 2004 | Updated the law with regard to children, including those being cared for by local authorities |

**Legislation** A law or group of laws as passed by Parliament.

**Regulations** Government orders (rules) which have the force of law, made to control conduct.

**Welfare** Health, happiness, well-being.

**Data** A collection of facts about a person or organisation.

### For your project

When you are on work placement, do a study of how your workplace manages each of the requirements of the HASAW Act. Remember to ask your supervisor for permission first. The study should look at this from the perspective of both your employer and you, as an employee. In relation to the former, try to get copies of your employer's policies and procedures, as well as some risk assessments in the area you are working. For the latter, think about how you took care of yourself and others, and how you cooperated with your employer on health and safety issues. Ask one of your work colleagues to take photos of you doing this (e.g. wearing the correct protective clothing or lifting things correctly).

### Just checking

* Name three key pieces of legislation or regulations that would apply to a prison.
* What aspect of an employer's business do the COSHH Regulations cover?
* What does the HASAW Act 1974 expect employees to do?

# 3.3 Protection of individuals

In this topic we will look at some policies regarding health, safety and security, and how they help maintain a safe environment and safe working conditions. This will help you understand the role of legislation, regulations and codes of practice in protecting individuals.

<br />

## THINKING POINT

Imagine the government said that people no longer have to drive on the left side of the road. Imagine what would happen if people could drive on whichever side of the road they wanted to! What would happen at points such as roundabouts and pedestrian crossings?

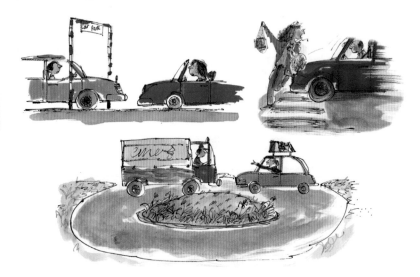

*Chaos on the road.*

## Why do we have health and safety laws and rules?

Imagine if there was no referee and no rules in a football match. Fights and arguments would quickly break out and people would get injured. The same applies in the area of health and safety. If there were no rules and procedures to follow, many more people would be injured or killed and life would be much more dangerous.

We are going to look at some examples of policies and procedures in different settings to illustrate how following these in an organisation helps to maintain a safe working environment.

### Health

Childcare settings, such as nurseries and playgroups, are reinforcing the basic skill of hand washing from an early age. Washing hands helps to prevent **infections**. Childcare settings have guidelines on how to do this, such as having signs up that encourage children to wash their hands after they have been to the toilet. The Welsh Assembly has produced a policy document called 'Mind the Germs! Infection Control for Nurseries, Playgroups and Other Childcare Settings', which can be found on the website of the Hospital Infection Society (www.his.org.uk).

In hospitals, anyone entering a ward is encouraged to wash their hands and again when they leave. Staff always 'scrub up' before entering an operating theatre. This is to control the spread of infections such as MRSA (methicillin-resistant *Staphylococcus aureus*).

**Infections** Illnesses that are spread by the passing of microorganisms between people.

## Safety

Every organisation has a policy and rules to follow in the case of the fire alarm going off. Similarly, every organisation has to have procedures in place to control hazardous substances such as chemicals. The COSHH Regulations require employers:

* to ensure the safe storage and disposal of substances that are harmful to health
* to check that hazards from all substances are assessed
* to ensure that appropriate control measures are implemented
* to ensure that staff receive training on safe procedures and the use of protective clothing
* to check that procedures for spillages are in place
* to check that new staff are trained before they use hazardous substances.

All teachers, technicians, cleaners or cooks in a school who handle chemicals follow these regulations, as do people in all workplaces in all sectors.

## Diploma Daily

### Caught in the act

Two men were found guilty of dumping more than 5 litres of toxic chemical waste outside a recycling centre in Betherton at court today. The council said it cost more than £1,000 to sort the situation out when the container leaked and the chemicals let off toxic fumes. The fly-tippers were caught after CCTV footage was studied and David Molyneux, 26, and Philip Trafford, also 26, will be sentenced later this month. A spokesman for the council said 'If the label showing what the chemical was hadn't been left on the container the situation would have been much worse.'

1 Why would it have been much worse if the label had not been left on the container in the *Diploma Daily* story?

2 Do some research into the various symbols put on bottles and other containers of chemicals, such as tankers. Produce a leaflet showing the various symbols, and what they mean, to provide information for the general public.

## Security

All service providers have rules concerning security. In any nursery, for example, doors are kept locked once all the children have arrived, so they cannot wander off and no one can come in, unless they ring a bell and identify themselves. Also, when it is time to go home, the staff will only allow a person known to them as being in charge of a particular child to take that child away. In schools, the only way in and out is usually via a reception office, so that visitors can be screened and not allowed to wander around unaccompanied. All computer rooms have bars at the windows to stop theft and only school staff are allowed keys to the school building.

### Activity

1 Look at your school's or college's fire procedures. A copy should be on the wall in the room you are in. Draw up a table with two columns. In the first column write the different steps to be taken when the fire alarm goes off. In the right-hand column write down why that step is necessary to keep you and the staff safe.

2 Imagine a fire alarm going off in a hospital. With a partner, write a step-by-step set of rules for what to do when a fire alarm goes off. Use the school rules to give you some ideas, but remember to include rules for people who are really ill in bed, maybe fighting for their lives in the accident and emergency department, or who are in the middle of being operated on, and so on.

3 Now repeat this exercise for evacuating a prison when the fire alarm goes off, remembering that the prisoners and staff must be kept safe from the fire but also that no prisoners should be given the chance to escape, so security must be maintained.

### Personal, learning and thinking skills

The activity should help towards PLTS: Creative thinker; Reflective learner; Team worker; Self-manager; Effective participator.

### Just checking

* Why does every organisation need health and safety rules?
* Give an example of what all organisations have to have a policy on regarding health and safety.
* Why should everyone be encouraged to wash their hands?

Have you ever thought
'They just don't want me
to have any fun!' when
you were told to be home
by a certain time, or not
to go to certain places?
Have you ever fallen out
with your parents when
they have given you
instructions like this?
Imagine you had children
and they wanted to do
the things you want to
do. Would you react any
differently?

### Activity

1 With a partner, write down a list of things you do during a typical weekend. Next to each one, write down: (a) what you do to keep yourself safe; (b) what you do to keep others safe, such as friends; and (c) what your family do to keep you safe.

2 Produce a safety poster that could be put up in local clubs and other places where people of your age go, showing teenagers how to stay safe. Think about issues such as alcohol and drugs, walking home in the dark, mobile phones and so on.

**Implement** To carry out something, follow it through.

**Risk** The chance of suffering harm, loss, injury, danger or some other bad consequence.

**Hazard** Anything that has the potential to harm someone in some way.

# 3.4 How to stay safe

This topic is all about how you can ensure your own safety and the safety of others. It also investigates your own roles and responsibilities for this.

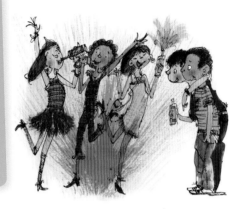
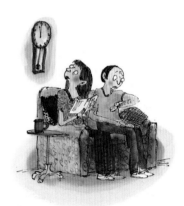

*Girls just want to have fun.*

## Roles and responsibilities

We need to keep ourselves and others safe not only at home and when we are out socially, but also in the workplace. Health and safety is a shared responsibility between employers and employees; that is, both employers and employees have their own roles in ensuring their own safety and that of others.

### Organisational policies and procedures

In topic 3.3 we looked at some examples of these and why we have them. It is the responsibility of the employer not only to provide a health and safety policy but also to make sure that employees **implement** it. The policy must include:

* a statement of intent to provide a safe working environment

* the 'named person' in the workplace who is responsible for implementing the policy

* the names of individuals responsible for any particular health and safety hazards which have been identified

* a list of potential health and safety hazards and the procedures which must be followed when working with these

* the procedure for recording accidents and illnesses at work.

It is the role and responsibility of the employee to follow the policy and procedures. Failure to do so can result not only in someone being hurt but also dismissal.

### Identifying, assessing and minimising health, safety and security risks

It is the responsibility of the employer to identify **risks**, assess them and act to minimise them, either by removing the **hazard** or by putting procedures in place to cope with the hazard so that people remain safe.

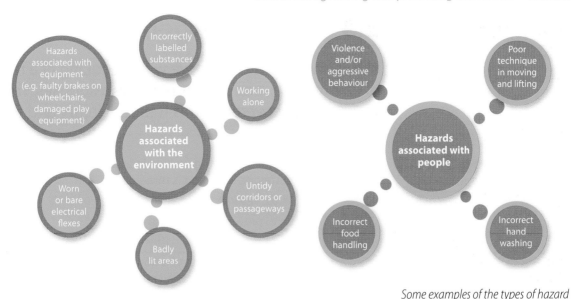

*Some examples of the types of hazard in the workplace. Can you think of any more in each category?*

Hazards in the workplace fall into two groups: those associated with the environment and those associated with people.

Risk assessment will be covered in more detail in topics 3.9 and 3.10.

### Recording, reporting and information sharing

As a worker in a care sector, it will be your responsibility to react to any potential hazard. This could be by dealing with it by yourself, if it is something like wiping up a spilt drink, moving a trailing flex out of the way or tidying up anything you have been using that could be a risk, such as a paper cutter or some cleaning fluid.

On other occasions you will have to record, report and share information on a risk. One example is if you find that a piece of equipment is faulty. This would have to be reported to your manager so it could be repaired; often there will be a special form on which to note the fault, which is then handed to the appropriate person. Other colleagues will need to be told the equipment is faulty so that they don't use it and hurt themselves or others. It is your employer's responsibility to put a warning sign up once you have reported the fault, but it is your responsibility to warn an individual if you see them about to use it before it has been fixed. Another example is if you see someone on the premises who should not be there.

### Operating within the limits of your own role and responsibilities

It is important that employees don't do anything that falls outside their own role and responsibility. To take a simple example, if you find a piece of electrical equipment is faulty and either ignore the fact or attempt to mend it yourself, someone could be electrocuted. There can also be more difficult instances. Imagine a young girl asks you to keep something a secret and then tells you she is being abused; you keep the secret and something unthinkable happens, such as the girl committing suicide. Teachers cannot say to children that they will keep a secret, as they might have to pass the information on to the school's child protection officer.

### For your project

When you are on work placement, identify your own role and responsibilities as regards health and safety. Look at the various health, safety and security procedures at your workplace and write down the possible consequences for yourself, other employees and your employer if you do not follow them.

### Just checking

* What are the five things a health and safety policy must include?
* Name the two different types of hazard and give three examples of each.
* Why is it important to act within the limits of your own role and responsibilities in the workplace?

# 3.5 It's an emergency

In this and the next topic we will be looking at a range of emergencies and the appropriate responses. The emergencies covered in this topic are injury and fire.

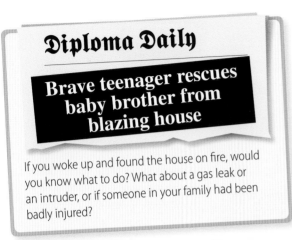

## Diploma Daily

### Brave teenager rescues baby brother from blazing house

If you woke up and found the house on fire, would you know what to do? What about a gas leak or an intruder, or if someone in your family had been badly injured?

**Emergency** A sudden unforeseen crisis (usually involving danger) that requires immediate action.

## Injuries

The aim of giving first aid in an **emergency** when someone is injured is threefold:

* to preserve a casualty's life
* to prevent further harm
* to promote or help their recovery.

It is important that you don't rush to help without doing certain things first – you might make the person's injuries worse or get injured yourself. You need to prioritise, and the correct order of actions to take is often referred to as 'DR ABC', where the letters stand for: danger, response, airway, breathing, circulation.

### Danger

The first thing to do is to assess the situation, so you don't put yourself or others in danger. If possible, make the area safe. If more than one person is injured, attend to any unconscious ones first. Send or ring for help immediately.

### Response

When treating someone, you need first to check for a response, by gently shaking the casualty's shoulders and speaking to them loudly. If there is no response you proceed with the ABC of first aid.

### ABC

* *A: Airway.* Open the airway. To do this, place your hand on the forehead and gently tilt the head back while lifting the chin with your fingertips.
* *B: Breathing.* Check for normal breathing by looking for chest movement, listening for breath sounds and feeling for air by putting your cheek by their mouth. If the person is breathing, place them in the recovery position. While waiting for help keep checking to make sure they continue breathing.
* *C: Circulation.* Check for a pulse or heart beat. If the person has none and is not breathing, start CPR (cardiopulmonary resuscitation) by leaning over them with your arms straight and your hands on top of each other and pressing down on the breast bone, releasing again, pressing down again, and so on, at a rate of about 100 times a minute. After 30 compressions, pinch the person's nose so the mouth opens and seal your mouth around their mouth, blowing steadily into the mouth and watching their chest rise. Then remove your mouth, watch the chest fall and repeat once. Then do another 30 compressions followed by two breaths until either they start breathing normally again or help arrives and someone takes over.

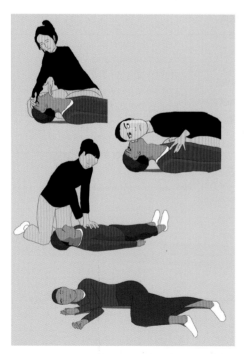

*A (airway), B (breathing), C (circulation) of first aid, and the recovery position.*

**First aid at work**

All workplaces must have at least one first-aid kit, as well as notices showing its whereabouts and a list of qualified first-aiders. If you have to deal with an injury in the absence of a qualified first-aider, the following points are important:

* If someone is bleeding badly, you should apply direct pressure to the wound. Raise and support the injured part unless it is broken, and firmly apply a dressing and bandage if you have one.

* If you suspect the casualty has a broken bone or a spinal injury, don't move them unless they are in immediate danger.

* If they have anything embedded in their eye, do not remove it but wash out any loose material or chemicals with clean water.

* If someone has been burnt by fire, cool the affected parts with cold water for at least 10 minutes.

* If the casualty has been burnt by chemicals, flood the area with water for at least 20 minutes, being careful to avoid getting any chemical on your own skin or clothes.

The Reporting of Injuries, Diseases and Dangerous Occurrences Regulations (RIDDOR) 1995 require that the details of any accident or injury that occurs at work must be recorded in the workplace's accident book.

# Fire

Workplace arrangements for fire safety must comply with the Fire Precautions (Workplace) Regulations of 1997. You should get to know your work setting's procedures for fire safety and go to fire training at least once a year.

Fire is responsible for many deaths each year. It can be prevented by:

* the use of smoke alarms

* unplugging unused electrical equipment at night (e.g. televisions)

* keeping fire doors closed

* making sure that all electrical and gas appliances have been properly checked for safety.

If a fire starts you should:

* raise the alarm – use the fire alarm and/or dial 999 for the fire brigade

* close all windows and doors, to help prevent the fire spreading

* use designated fire exits and escape routes, closing the doors behind you as you go, without running if possible

* not use any lifts, unless you are told to do so by the fire brigade

* check that everyone is accounted for and report this to the fire brigade

* not return to the building unless the fire brigade says it is safe to do so.

**Activity**

1 In pairs, decide what you would do in each of the following situations: (a) a colleague faints at work; (b) after two colleagues collide and bang heads, both fall to the ground, one groaning and the other unconscious; (c) someone slips on a wet floor and crashes through a glass door panel.

2 Do a role-play for each of the situations above and be prepared to show one of them to the rest of the group.

**Personal, learning and thinking skills**

The activity should help towards PLTS: Creative thinker; Team worker; Self-manager; Effective participator.

**Just checking**

* Why should you not rush in and start helping a casualty as soon as you see an accident?

* What does DR ABC stand for?

* Why should you not use any lifts when you hear a fire alarm?

# 3.6 More emergencies

In this topic we will continue to look at a range of emergencies and the appropriate responses to them. The emergencies covered in this topic are flooding and a security breach.

## Flooding

Floods can be caused either by severe weather or by a water leakage. In the case of rising floodwaters (at work or at home) you will need to take the following steps to keep yourself and others safe:

* Keep an eye on what is happening with the weather and what other people are doing.

* Move any vehicles to higher ground, to stop them being washed away.

* Check on those with you or in your care. Help them if they need help to move upstairs or to some other place of safety.

* Do as much as you can in daylight. Doing anything in the dark will be a lot harder and more dangerous, especially if the electricity fails.

* Block doors and airbricks with sandbags. If you cannot get hold of sandbags through your local council, use carrier bags or pillow cases filled with earth or sand.

* Turn off power supplies at the first sign of floodwaters reaching the property.

* Try to keep warm and dry. A flood can last longer than you think; take some warm clothes and blankets upstairs to a safe place, as well as a thermos and food supplies too.

* Pile up furniture if you can and put valuable items like photographs or electrical equipment and any information such as records as high as possible. Tie up the curtains and roll up the carpets if you can.

* If you or people in your care are taking regular medication, make sure you have it with you.

* Don't forget to secure and seal all your rubbish and any chemicals if you have time.

If the flooding is due to a water leak from a burst pipe, say, or an overflowing bath or washing machine, you need to stay calm. Turn off the **stopcock** – if you don't know where it is, find out by the end of today! Unplug all electrical devices and move all those that are small enough away from the water, to remove the risk of electric shock. Move any people in your care away from the floodwaters.

After the water has receded:

* Make sure any electrical items have dried out before you turn them back on.

* Open the doors and windows to ventilate the building. Remember to unblock your airbricks and doorways.

* Watch out for any broken glass or nails while you're clearing up.

* Run taps for a few minutes before use.

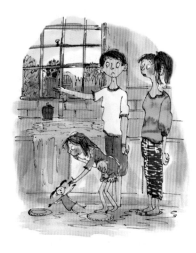

*Water, water everywhere and not a drop to drink.*

**Stopcock** The main tap or valve on the pipe bringing water from the mains into the building.

# Breach of security

A breach of security can take several forms. In your workplace you should receive security training for breaches in the following areas.

### An unauthorised person comes onto the premises

There will be many visitors to any care setting (e.g. friends and relatives of those being cared for, trades people and so on) and most workplaces have a policy on how they are dealt with. Visitors will be expected to make an appointment. They should sign in at reception on arrival and be given some form of badge to show that they are a visitor. If you see an unauthorised person on the premises, it is advisable to ask a colleague to go with you to challenge them, but if they are behaving in any way suspiciously do not hesitate to call security staff, if there are any, or the police.

### Stealing of data or valuables

All data should be backed up and copies kept elsewhere. All valuables should be kept in a secure place. In a school, for example, all computer rooms should have bars on the windows. In a setting such as a residential care home, clients should be able to have their valuables locked away for safekeeping.

You should immediately report any theft in the workplace to the manager and call the police.

### Missing person

A child wandering away from a nursery, an elderly person with dementia wandering away from a residential care home, a person escaping from a facility for those with severe mental illnesses or a prison: this should not be allowed to happen. All outside doors should be kept locked and only authorised visitors should be allowed in. In the event of such a breach of security, it is vital that managers, other staff, families and the police are alerted as soon as possible and the area searched for the missing person.

# Calling the emergency services

There are other types of emergencies that we have not discussed. In most these it will be necessary to call one of the emergency services. Dial 999 if you need the police, ambulance and/or fire service, but only in an emergency. If you need to report a crime, for example, but an immediate response is not necessary, you can ring the local police service using the number in the phone book.

If you do ring 999, you will be asked which service you require. You should answer as clearly and calmly as you can. You will be asked for various details, such as your name and phone number, and details about the incident you are calling for help with.

Other emergency services include the lifeguards and Mountain Rescue. Their numbers can be found in the front of the phone book.

## Activity

1 Look up all the local emergency numbers and produce a leaflet that explains clearly and briefly to school children what each service does, when they should be called out, how to contact them and any other information that you might feel would be useful. Use a computer to do this if you can.

2 What information would you expect parents to receive about dealing with emergencies when they are considering using a particular school or nursery? Find out what procedures are in place in your own school and produce an A4 poster summing up the information.

## Personal, learning and thinking skills

The activity should help towards PLTS: Independent enquirer; Creative thinker; Self-manager.

## Just checking

* Why does a worker in a care sector need to know what to do in the case of flooding?
* What should visitors be given after they have signed in at reception?
* Why should you call the emergency services only in the case of a real emergency?

# 3.7 How infectious!

This topic looks at the main causes of infection and how infection can be passed on. It is important to understand these so you realise how infection can be prevented and controlled.

## What causes infection?

Bacteria, viruses and fungi are all examples of **microorganisms**. Some, such as yeast, are very useful to us, but others cause infections.

### Bacteria

Bacteria are single-cell organisms, most of which are harmless, but some cause disease. They attack body tissue or release poisons, making you feel ill. They can reproduce very quickly; some can divide every 20 minutes. Some examples of illnesses they cause are food poisoning, tetanus, whooping cough and sore throats. Some useful microorganisms provide us with medicines such as antibiotics, which can be used to fight many illnesses caused by bacteria.

### Viruses

Viruses are the smallest microbes. They comprise a strand of genetic information with a protein coat. They invade living tissue and take over cells, making them produce millions of copies of the virus. When the cell is full of viruses it bursts open and those new viruses can attack even more cells. As well as destroying cells, viruses can release poisons that make you feel ill. However, antibiotics do not affect them, and so they cannot be used to treat the illnesses viruses produce. Examples of these are colds, influenza (flu), chicken pox, German measles and polio. Some of them are very dangerous. In 1918 a flu pandemic swept across Europe and killed many millions of people.

### Fungi

Another type of microorganism is a fungus. Unlike bacteria, a fungus cannot make its own food so has to feed on other things. Athlete's foot is a disease caused by a fungus. It grows on the soft damp tissue between a person's toes and feeds on the tissues of the foot. Thrush is another example of a fungus.

## How does infection spread?

Infections are spread when microorganisms, commonly called germs, are **transmitted**. This can be in a number of ways:

* *Direct contact*. Influenza is often spread by touch because a person blows their nose and then touches someone else.

* *Indirect contact*. Some diseases can be passed on by touching something that an infected person has used, such as clothing.

* *Inhalation*. Many infections are passed on by people breathing in infected droplets from a cough or sneeze, most commonly influenza.

* *Ingestion (eating)*. People get food poisoning, for example, when they eat something contaminated with certain kinds of bacteria, such as *Salmonella*.

* *Injection.* Infected blood can be accidentally passed from one person to another by injection. For example, when drug addicts share needles, HIV or the hepatitis C virus can be transmitted.

There is a chain of infection, as illustrated in the diagram. Infection control involves breaking the chain.

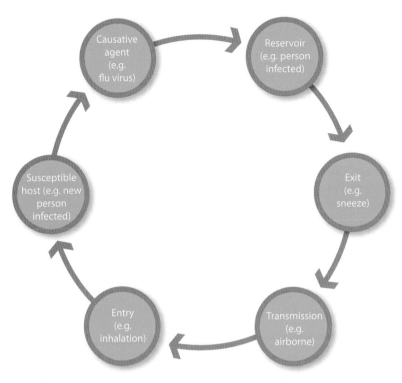

*The chain of infection.*

## Immunity

Some people are immune to certain infections, so either cannot catch them or develop only mild versions.

Natural **immunity** arises either when **antibodies** are passed on from a mother to her child via the placenta or breast milk, or when a person makes antibodies when microbes infect their body.

Artificial immunity arises in one of two ways. One way is by vaccination, when a harmless (dead or modified) microbe is injected into a person's blood. This causes antibodies to be made by the body, ready for when a real infection happens, and those antibodies can kill off the microbes before illness sets in. That is why young children have injections such as MMR (mumps, measles and rubella). The other way of acquiring artificial immunity is to have serum with antibodies injected directly.

### Activity

1 Draw up a table with two columns. In the left-hand one, list ways in which germs can be transferred. In the right-hand column, record the names of several infections that can be passed on by each method.

2 Do some research into the meaning of the term 'epidemic' and the causes of flu epidemics.

3 Find out why people who have flu jabs need a fresh one each year.

**Immunity** Resistance to a particular disease caused by infection.

**Antibodies** Proteins in the body that help to kill microbes.

### Just checking

* Name three types of microorganism that cause infection.
* Why can't antibiotics be used to fight the common cold?
* How can a person develop immunity to a particular microorganism?

## 3.8 The super bugs and others

In this topic we will look at the importance of infection prevention and control. There are standard procedures to follow to prevent infection and its spread, which include hand hygiene, personal protective equipment and general cleanliness.

### Why is infection control so important?

Preventing infection is important not only to stop people becoming ill and suffering physically, intellectually, emotionally and socially, and maybe even dying, but also to stop people who are already ill becoming more ill. Infection takes up staff, resources, money and time. Service providers in the care sectors often work very closely together and frequently touch the people in their care, or may sneeze or cough on them, which means the chance of passing on infection is high, unless precautions are taken.

Infection can also be spread by pests such as rats, cockroaches and other insects, especially in food preparation areas, so pest control precautions should also be taken.

#### Super bugs

When antibiotics were first discovered, starting with penicillin, they were seen as a cure for everything. They were given out very readily by doctors, including for the treatment of viral infections such as colds and flu. It is now known that antibiotics cannot cure viral illnesses and they are prescribed much more sparingly. However, because of the over-use of antibiotics, some bacteria adapted and developed resistance to them. Bacteria that have become resistant to several antibiotics are known as 'super bugs'.

MRSA, mentioned in topic 3.3, is resistant to most antibiotics but there are still some that will work, which are given by injection for several weeks. If someone becomes infected with MRSA in hospital, they will be moved to a separate room to stop the bug spreading. The bugs are on the person's skin, hair and the inside of the nose, and have to be removed by regular washing with a special lotion.

Another super bug is *Clostridium difficile* ('C. diff'). Infection often arises when antibiotics are used to treat other health conditions and interfere with the balance of good bacteria in the digestive system. It causes symptoms such as diarrhoea and fever in people who are already ill; most cases happen in health care settings such as hospitals or care homes. The number of cases of C. diff rose from 22,000 a year in 2002 to almost 45,000 in 2004. It is extremely **contagious**.

## WHY DO I NEED TO WASH MY HANDS AGAIN?

Microorganisms can quickly spread from surface to surface, from pets to people, from person to person, and so on. Imagine you go to visit someone in hospital. Think about everything you might touch (including parts of your own body!) between washing your hands before you leave home and arriving at the person's bedside. Make a list and imagine how many germs you might be transferring.

**Contagious** Spread very easily.

# Standard procedures to prevent infection

Advice given to visitors in a health care environment is that they should:

* wash their hands with soap and water when entering and leaving a ward
* also use an antimicrobial alcohol hand gel, which is now provided by the door of many health care settings
* avoid sitting on beds
* not visit if they have recently been unwell or had diarrhoea or a stomach upset
* wear protective clothing, such as disposable bootees and aprons, in some cases.

Service providers are expected:

* to wear disposable aprons and sometimes gloves
* to wash their hands regularly with soap and water, as well as to use alcohol gel
* to clean surfaces such as toilets, beds and bedpans thoroughly with water and disinfectant
* to be more cautious in prescribing antibiotics.

## Case study: Jan's story

Jan works in the baby room at Oak Trees Nursery. The nursery has in place a procedure for changing nappies that states, among other things, what Jan should wear when changing babies (including disposable gloves and apron), how to disinfect surfaces, and how to dispose of used nappies. Jan can't see the point in washing her hands when she has finished, which is what the procedure calls for, as she wears disposable gloves anyway, and so she no longer bothers.

1 What risks is Jan taking by not washing her hands, to herself and others, and by not following the nursery's official procedure?

2 Find a nursery's full detailed procedure for changing nappies. What elements relate to infection control? What else is covered in the procedure?

## Activity

1 Imagine a school canteen. List the ways in which germs could be spread. Then produce a poster suitable to put up in the school canteen on how to help prevent the spread of infection. Do one poster each for the common cold and food poisoning. You will have to do some research into safety precautions to be used when handling and cooking food to do the second poster properly.

2 Put up a display of the posters produced by the class. Make notes on the good and less good points of each one. Pick which poster you think is best and write down why you have chosen that one. This is called peer assessment.

3 Look at your poster again and decide what its good and less good points are. How do you think it compares with the others? This is called self-assessment.

4 Now repeat step 1 for a reception area in a residential care home for elderly people but this time for posters on C. diff and pneumonia.

## Personal, learning and thinking skills

The activity should help towards PLTS: Independent enquirer; Creative thinker; Reflective learner; Self-manager; Effective participator.

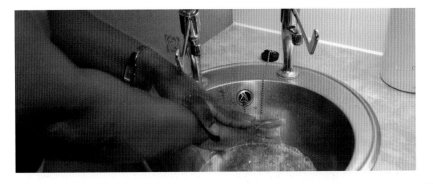

*You can't be too careful! Do you know how to wash your hands properly? There are recommended ways of doing so. They are easy to find on the Internet.*

## Just checking

* List three ways in which visitors in hospital can help with infection control.
* What is C. diff short for and how is it caused?
* Give three reasons why infection control is important.

# 3.9 A risky business

This topic looks at the need to be able to recognise hazards and the risk they could pose, in order to maintain a safe environment and working conditions.

### SPOT THE HAZARD

Look at the picture on the right, of a child playing happily in a nursery. Can you spot any hazards? What risks do they pose? How can the risks be reduced?

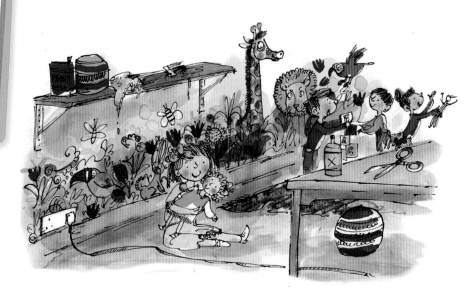

*How many hazards can you identify?*

## Risk assessment

Remember (see topic 3.4), risk is the chance or possibility of suffering harm, loss, injury, danger or some other bad consequence. A hazard is anything that has the potential to harm someone in some way.

In order to be able to minimise risk, we first need to analyse that risk using a process called risk assessment. We can then manage the risk by either reducing it or removing it altogether. There are five stages to carrying out a risk assessment.

### 1. Identifying the risk

This involves spotting hazards that could cause a risk, such as seeing that someone has left something at the top of a flight of stairs which could cause someone to trip and fall.

### 2. Estimating the risk

This means estimating the extent of the risk, that is, the likelihood of something happening. It is often done on a scale of 1 to 5, where: 1 is not very likely and so low risk, such as catching your foot on the leg of a large, obvious table and falling over; 3 means there is a moderate risk of something happening, such as tripping over wires training across an open floor; 5 means very possible or even probable, such as a volatile liquid bursting into flame if left by a fire.

### 3. Controlling the risk

This means deciding what to do to reduce or remove the risk. The moderate risk of tripping over wires can be reduced to a low risk of 1 simply by taping them down or by re-routing them around the edge of the room.

## 4. Monitoring how effectively the risk is being controlled

This means making sure the precautions taken to reduce the risk remain in place. This could involve, for example, having clear written instructions for service users and providers. **Monitoring** should be done at regular intervals, preferably by a person with specific responsibility for it. This might be a head of department or a health and safety officer.

**Monitoring** Making (and recording) regular checks on something.

## 5. Reassessing the risk

This is looking at the risk again to see if it can be reduced still further. In the example above it could be by removing the wires altogether, perhaps by repositioning the machine they come out of. This is part of the monitoring role of a health and safety officer. Reassessments need to be done regularly, to make sure any risks that have been reduced or removed stay this way, and to make sure no new risks appear.

### Activity

1 For each of the examples below, first decide what the nature of the hazard is. Then indicate on a scale of 1 to 5 what the risk is (as set out under 'Estimating the risk', on page 74). Then write down what can be done to reduce the risk.

* The possibility of a regularly checked fire alarm not working.

* A chair in a residential home left balanced on a broken leg.

* A sleeping cat curled up in a ball at the top of a flight of stairs.

* The chance of a care assistant falling over a ball when bringing a large load of washing in from the garden.

* A prison floor that has just been mopped.

* A chemist working with strong acid to make up drugs in a pharmacy without wearing goggles.

* Someone on crutches going up some steep steps at the entrance to a dental surgery.

2 Who should monitor the risk in each of these cases?

3 How often do you think each separate risk should be checked?

## Who oversees health and safety in the workplace?

The Health and Safety Commission (HSC) and the Health and Safety Executive (HSE) are responsible for regulating health and safety at work. The HSE supports the Health and Safety Commission by ensuring that the health and safety of people at work are not put at risk. The HSE does this via codes of practice for employers, which are intended to prevent illness and accidents at work by providing guidance and up-to-date information. Examples can be found at www.hse.gov.uk.

The HSE has the power to prosecute employers who fail to safeguard the health and safety of people who access and use their premises. As mentioned in the introduction to this unit, the Health and Safety at Work Act 1974 lays down the duties of employers and employees.

### For your project

When you are on work placement, find out who is responsible for health and safety. Complete a risk assessment for the area you are working in and write a summary of your findings. Then produce posters to put up to warn service users and providers of any hazards you have identified.

### Just checking

* What is the difference between a hazard and a risk?

* What are the five steps in carrying out a risk assessment?

* Who is responsible for overseeing health and safety in the UK and which Act helps support them in this?

# 3.10 Don't risk it

In this topic you will have the chance to have a go at conducting a risk assessment for yourself. You will then know how to carry out real ones when you go out into the workplace on a work placement. Remember, the risks can relate not just to physical harm but also to infectious disease or abuse.

## Your turn now

Look carefully at the picture and then carry out the *Diploma Daily* activity. Obviously, ambulances are really safe to travel in and save many lives – this is just an illustration to help you practise your risk assessment. You may need to look back at the last topic to remind yourself of some of the issues and to answer the 'Just checking' questions at the end.

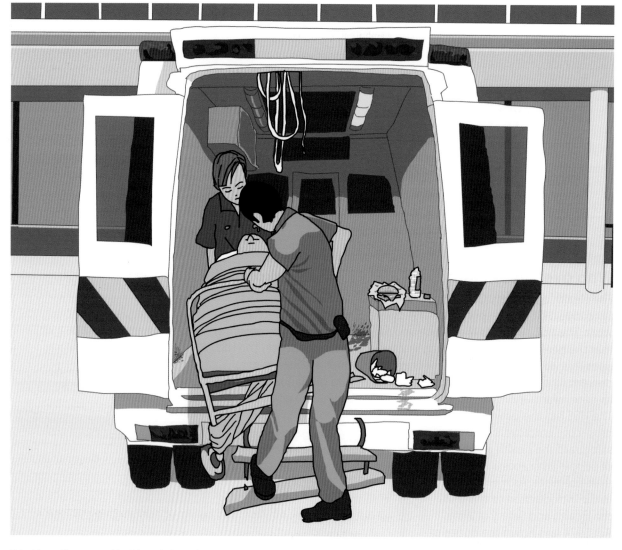

*Would you like to travel in this ambulance?*

# Diploma Daily

# Dirty ambulances put patients at risk

*Written by Stanley Sleuth*

Patients are being put at risk before they even reach hospital in one authority because they are being transported in dirty ambulances. Some crews are mopping out their own ambulances using only disinfectant and cold water. This is because despite more funding being provided to make hospitals cleaner, ambulances are being forgotten and left out of improvement programmes.

Spokeswoman Lindsey Hoyle said that although very clear guidance was available on how to deep clean an ambulance, more funding was needed to provide specialist equipment and cleaning staff. She said, 'Ambulances play an important role in the whole package of patient care and no one should have to travel in a dirty ambulance. Ambulance cleanliness is an important factor in the ongoing war against infection and the mandatory standards laid down by the NHS should be adhered to and monitored. In this authority crews are expected to clean out their own ambulances. This is not only inefficient because they are not trained to do it but is a waste of their time and specialist training.'

Ambulance crews claim that tough government targets, a lack of training and a lack of resources all contribute to the problem. One said, 'Our Trust has no specialised cleaning staff so we have to do it ourselves. My mate in a neighbouring Trust has a dedicated cleaning crew who clean his ambulance overnight, deep clean regularly to kill off any of these super bugs and then restock it with fresh supplies. All I've got is a mop and bucket.' Another said, 'If the paramedics say a patient has C. diff we simply mop it out when they have been moved into the hospital.'

Health Minister Owen Noser said last night that there was no evidence to suggest that ambulances are a major source of infection and that the whole of the NHS had to tackle the problem of super bugs and other infections.

1 You are now going to carry out a risk assessment of the ambulance in the picture opposite. The patient has a *Clostridium difficile* infection. Remember to look for as many risks as possible, of many different kinds.

Draw up a table using the headings below:

| Hazard | Risk (1 to 5) | Action taken to reduce it | Risk when reassessed | How often it should be checked |
|--------|---------------|---------------------------|----------------------|-------------------------------|
|        |               |                           |                      |                               |

2 In pairs, carry out a risk assessment on a room or a block of your school or college. Your teacher will tell you which one. Use a similar table to the one you have just used.

3 With your partner, prepare a health and safety report for your school or college governors, making recommendations to reduce any risks you may identify.

4 Plan a presentation of your findings and recommendations to the governors. Include a visual aid such as a set of photographs or a table. Practise it. Your teacher may pick you and your partner to present your talk to the rest of the group.

## Personal, learning and thinking skills

The activity should help towards PLTS: Independent enquirer; Creative thinker; Reflective learner; Team worker; Self-manager; Effective participant.

## Just checking

✳ How do you score risk?

✳ Why do you score it again when you have taken action to reduce the risk?

✳ Why does risk need to be reassessed on a regular basis?

# 3.11 The signs of abuse

Safeguarding and protecting an individual means not only from accidents or infection but also abuse. This topic looks at how to recognise the signs that an individual is at risk of harm or abuse.

## The signs of abuse

As you can see from the figure of 32,000 given in the Thinking Point, which includes only children, the number of individuals at risk is huge. It is not only young children who are abused: adolescents, those with disabilities or special needs and older people are particularly **vulnerable** to abuse when other people are caring for them, be it in their own home or in some other care setting. The types of abuse were discussed in topic 1.7 and some examples are listed in the table opposite. But how can we recognise abuse and what can we do when we do see it? Abuse may be carried out deliberately or be unintentional. Both are distressing to the individual concerned and appropriate action needs to be taken. Some people may even abuse themselves – it is not always something that is done by others.

There are certain signs to look out for, as shown in the table, but it is important not to assume that just because you see one of these signs the person is being abused, as discussed in topic 1.5. There may or may not be a perfectly good reason for it.

**Vulnerable** A state in which being physically or emotionally hurt is more likely.

### Emotional harm

The signs of emotional harm may be present in individuals who are being physically or sexually abused; they may also be seen in children who suffer perhaps lesser types of abuse, such as children who have over-critical parents, individuals who are being isolated, avoided or verbally abused. These signs are:

* excessive behaviour, for example excessive bedwetting, overeating, rocking, head banging
* self-harming (e.g. cutting or scratching, drug overdose)
* suicide attempts
* persistent running away from home
* high levels of anxiety, unhappiness or withdrawal
* seeking out or avoiding affection.

*Would you recognise the signs?*

### Child abuse link to future health
Children who suffer abuse have an increased risk of physical ill health in adulthood, results suggest…

### Revealed: patients abused and assaulted in 'woeful' wards
Mentally ill patients are being physically assaulted, verbally abused and sexually harassed on hospital psychiatric wards, according to a damning new investigation…

### 'Witch child' abuse spreads in Britain
An official inquiry into the abuse of African children branded as witches is expected to conclude that there have been at least 50 such cases over five years in London alone…

### Gym teacher abused pupils
A former Olympic gymnastics judge has been jailed for sex abuse after a private detective used the Internet to trace his victims…

### Abuse victim's fury at judges
A woman who was sexually abused as a child has hit out at judges for the 'laughable' sentences they have given to paedophiles…

*Signs of different types of abuse*

| Type of abuse | Possible signs |
|---|---|
| Physical | Any bruising to a baby (i.e. a child who cannot yet walk) |
| | Multiple bruising to different parts of the body |
| | Bruising of different colours (this indicates repeated injuries) |
| | Fingertip bruising to the chest, back, arms or legs |
| | Burns of any shape or size |
| | An injury for which there is no adequate explanation |
| Sexual | Something a person has told you or someone else |
| | Worrying sexualised behaviour in the child's play |
| | Sexual knowledge inappropriate for their age |
| | Child visiting or being looked after by a known or suspected sexual offender |
| Neglect | Squalid, unhygienic or dangerous living conditions |
| | Parents failing to attend to the child's health or development needs (e.g. attending clinics, parents' evenings etc.) |
| | Child persistently undersized or underweight |
| | Child continually tired or lacking in energy |
| | Frequent injuries due to lack of supervision |

## What do I do?

If you are a family member or friend of someone who you suspect is being abused in some way you should:

✱ try talking to the individual if you think they are likely to respond to you, but do not promise to keep anything they tell you confidential

✱ ask advice from a helpline such as the NSPCC's free 24-hour helpline on 0808 800 5000, or Action on Elder Abuse on 0808 808 8141

✱ report your suspicions to someone you trust, such as social services.

If you are a care worker and you see something happening that you are not comfortable with, tell someone who is in a position to do something about it, such as your manager. If it is your manager you suspect and there is no one else you can turn to, use some of the suggestions above.

In both these cases you should write down exactly what you have seen or been told, with details such as the date and time and names of any other witnesses, if there were any. It is important to be completely factual and accurate, avoiding personal opinions, in case the information is later needed in a court case or a case conference.

**Activity**

1 In a group, discuss how it would feel as a parent if your son hurt himself several times because he was clumsy and you were accused of abusing him.

2 Now in your group imagine how it would feel if you were in a caring profession, suspected that someone in your care was being abused but did nothing about it and they ended up being really badly hurt.

3 Write a piece of imaginative writing, maybe a story or a poem, based on one of these situations.

**Functional skills**

This activity will help towards FS: English – writing.

**Just checking**

✱ Which sorts of people are more vulnerable to being abused?

✱ List five signs that someone may be being abused in some way.

✱ Write down three things you should do if you suspect someone is being abused.

The final topic in this unit looks at the importance of establishing and maintaining a trusting relationship with individuals. Without such a relationship it is much harder not only to help service users but also to protect and safeguard them.

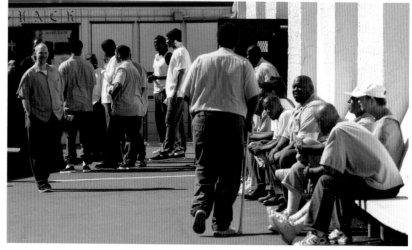

*Who could you trust? How do you make that judgement? How could you gain their trust?*

### What is important in establishing and maintaining a trusting relationship?

#### Boundaries

It is important in any relationship to establish boundaries. For example, a teacher may chat and joke with her students but there is a line beyond which students are not allowed to go, such as not call the teacher by her first name, be over-familiar and ask personal questions or invade her personal space. It is important the students know what these boundaries are, not only so that they do not get into trouble by exceeding them but also so that the teacher feels comfortable. If students know what to expect from a teacher and vice versa they can then build on the relationship and the teacher is able to teach the students without wasting time telling them off. By establishing boundaries and building good relationships the teacher enables her students to talk to her when they have problems. She will also be in a position to notice signs of abuse in her students.

#### Promoting independence

No relationship should be such that it stifles independence, which is crucial to a person's well-being and self-esteem. For example, if a care worker ignores the wishes of an elderly resident, not allowing him any choice in his meals, what he watches on television and so on, he will feel unvalued and resentful, and is unlikely to confide in that care worker or ask for help. If, however, the care worker asks his opinion and allows him choice within the boundaries of the rules and the wishes of the other residents, he will feel cared for and feel as though his views still matter; he will be more likely to trust the care worker.

### Supporting individuals with good communication

Less than 10 per cent of our communication is spoken (see topic 2.1). Good communication is not only about people understanding you clearly but also about you allowing them to make their feelings and views clear. This is important, because the information and ideas you are trying to communicate could be misinterpreted and trust can break down. A nurse working in a hospital, for example, has to be able to understand what a patient is trying to convey. Patients are more likely to trust and communicate with the nurse if the nurse not only keeps them fully informed about what is happening to them and what will happen to them but does it in a warm, approachable way, using eye contact, bending down to the same level, using friendly body language and speaking clearly using words they can understand. If a patient does not speak English there should be an interpreter on call to help communication and information leaflets available written in the relevant language. Communication is covered more thoroughly in Unit 2.

### Consistency and reliability

It is crucial to be both consistent and reliable, as this will help to establish and maintain trust. A woman with learning difficulties living on her own in sheltered accommodation needs to know that whenever she rings the bell for help, the warden will not only come to help straight away but is always pleasant and fair in his dealings with her. This will make her feel supported and safe and so help build up a relationship of trust. Similarly, if a judge gives more lenient sentences on a day when she is in a particularly good mood and vice versa, the lawyers will not know what to expect and will be less well placed to help their clients.

### Helping and enabling

Any relationship, and particularly when one person has to trust another to look after them, will be more successful if those concerned try to be as helpful as possible. If you go the doctor and the doctor does not offer any ideas as to the illness or its remedy but simply hands over a prescription, you will come away feeling that he has been less than helpful and you will be unable to stop the problem occurring again because you have not been helped to understand what caused the illness. If, on the other hand, he is helpful and shares information with you, this is **enabling** you to look after yourself better.

### Others factors underlying trusting relationships

These include:

* promoting rights, covered in topic 1.3
* being non-judgemental, covered in topic 1.6
* maintaining both privacy, and confidentiality (within limits), covered in topics 1.2 and 1.7.

**For your project**

When you are on work placement, think about the relationships you are building with your fellow workers and the people who use the service you are working in. Think of someone you feel you do not relate to as easily as others and make a determined effort to build a trusting relationship with them. If this succeeds, write down the steps you took to make it happen. If it doesn't succeed, try to work out why and decide the consequences of either accepting things as they are or trying again.

**Enabling** Supplying with the means, knowledge or opportunity to do something; giving a person the ability to do a certain task.

**Just checking**

* Why is it important to build up trusting relationships if you are to look after an individual?
* List eight factors that are important in establishing and maintaining a trusting relationship.
* For three of the factors, give examples of a care setting where the factor is especially important and explain why.

# Unit 3 Assessment guide

This unit is assessed by an assignment which will be marked by your teacher. You need to produce a training pack for new workers that explains how important health, safety and security are for staff and individuals who receive services. You will investigate how two organisations provide a safe environment and carry out a risk assessment, identifying hazards and risks within each organisation, and make suggestions for how these can be reduced. Some of these will include: the risk of infection and how to reduce it, the risk of abuse and how to recognise and prevent it, and the hazards seen within the environment. You will also need to show that you understand how legislation is designed to help us be safe, and how organisations devise their own policies to tell their employees exactly what they should do to keep themselves and the people they look after safe. Professionals such as nurses and social workers often have their own codes of practice to ensure their safety and the safety of others. Throughout this assignment you will carry out primary and secondary research and you will need to show your teacher what research you did.

## Time management

* Manage your time well and participate in all class activities. This will help you carry out the research that you need to do, for example carrying out a risk assessment in your school or college. It will also show that you are an independent enquirer, which is one of the personal, learning and thinking skills.

* Be well organised and keep any information that you are given in a folder where you can easily find it. This will include copies of health and safety laws – for example, the Health and Safety at Work Act 1974 or COSHH (Control of Substances Hazardous to Health) Regulations 2002. You may also be given copies of organisations' policy that sets out how they will provide a safe environment for everyone.

* Be prepared with a list of questions that you could ask if your teacher arranges for a speaker to come and talk to your class or if you visit an organisation. For example, you may want to ask a nursery nurse how small children's safety and security are maintained. You may want to ask how staff know who is collecting the children or the measures in place to ensure only authorised people are allowed on the premises. These could contribute towards your primary research.

* When you visit an organisation, try to observe how infection is controlled. Ask if the organisation has a policy about cross-infection. You may want to look at one area such as the dining room, and observe if everyone washes their hands before eating or serving food or if staff are wearing clean uniforms.

## Useful links

* There are lots of useful websites that will help with your investigation of legislation relating to health, safety and security. This includes the Health and Safety Executive (www.hse.gov.uk), which tells you about health and safety law, or Childline (www.childline.org.uk), which tells you how to recognise signs of abuse.

* Work experience will also be useful, as this will enable you to talk to members of staff about the policies and procedures that are used to ensure a safe working environment for all and you will also be able to carry out a risk assessment. You may choose to base your assessment in a children's nursery or a day centre for older people. Both organisations will have a policy telling staff how to keep people safe but there may be different hazards and risks. Try to find out where the health and safety law poster is displayed – this should be where people can see and read it, for example in the staff room.

* You may be given the opportunity to do a first aid, food hygiene, or an infection control course. Although these are not compulsory for this unit, they are very useful and will give you a great deal of knowledge which you can use in your training pack. They are also valued by employers.

## Things you might need

* The relevant forms with which to carry out a risk assessment; your teacher will provide these but you will need to complete them and keep them safely.

* Craft materials or use of ICT to produce your training pack for new workers. A training pack should be colourful and easy to read, but should contain lots of factual information that is useful.

# How you will be assessed

| You must show that you *know*: | Guidance | To gain higher marks you must *explain*: |
|---|---|---|
| How to use primary and secondary research. | ✳ Primary research is research you have carried out yourself in the form of two risk assessments and by talking to people about health and safety in their workplace. Secondary research is research that other people have conducted that you access via books or the Internet. | ✳ How you have used both primary and secondary research in your investigation into the health, safety and security of individuals in organisations. Include any information that you have collected from people you have interviewed and your risk assessment form in your work. |
| How legislation, regulations, codes of practice, policies and procedures help protect health, safety and security in organisations.<br><br>How emergency situations are dealt with. These may include fire, flood, intruder and first-aid emergencies. | ✳ Investigate how health and safety and security are maintained and protected in an organisation. For example, what precautions are taken when a floor is wet.<br><br>✳ Choose two organisations to investigate from the four sectors.<br><br>✳ All organisations will have a policy on fire evacuation and how to deal with other emergencies, including first-aid emergencies. | ✳ How three pieces of legislation, regulations or codes of practice are used in two organisations, and how three policies related to these are used. You may decide to look at the code of conduct for workers who provide social care (see www.gscc.org.uk).<br><br>✳ The correct action to take in six emergency situations within the organisations that you are investigating. |
| How infection is controlled in organisations.<br><br>You need to show that you know what bacteria and viruses are, how they are spread and how this can be prevented. | ✳ Investigate how viral and bacterial infections can occur and how they are prevented in your two chosen organisations.<br><br>✳ Prevention methods include hand washing and good personal hygiene, and good kitchen hygiene. | ✳ How the infections are caused, transmitted and controlled in particular areas of the two organisations – for example, in the dining room, reception or lounge area of an organisation. |
| How to carry out a risk assessment.<br><br>You will need to identify any risks to people's health, safety and security. These may include fire risks, risks of people falling over objects or incorrect lifting due to poor technique or a lack of equipment to help. | ✳ Your teacher will give you a form that will enable you to carry out risk assessments in two organisations. One of these organisations could be your school or college. | ✳ What the role is of risk assessment in both organisations.<br><br>✳ How you planned, carried out and evaluated your risk assessment. This will contribute to your primary research.<br><br>✳ How hazards are minimised and offer reasons for these. For example, you might see a fire exit with a sign that tells people to 'keep the exit clear'. What might be the hazard if it is not clear? |
| Why it is important to develop trusting relationships with individuals.<br><br>Be able to recognise the signs of abuse; these may include physical, emotional, sexual, or financial abuse. | ✳ Staff and individuals receiving services need to develop good relationships with each other. It is important that both parties are aware of professional boundaries that protect them against abuse.<br><br>✳ Signs of abuse may include physical signs, a change in an individual's behaviour (they may become withdrawn or angry) or a complaint against someone else. | ✳ How staff enable individuals to be independent while still maintaining professional responsibilities in your two organisations. For example, staff should not take gifts or money from people they work with, as it may lead to complaints of favouritism or financial abuse.<br><br>✳ What the signs are of potential harm or abuse that might occur in organisations. |

## Introduction

This topic looks at the needs of a person specific to each life stage (general needs are covered in Unit 5). It includes the key changes that take place across the life span and the impact of life events and lifestyles. You will learn how the sectors support and monitor key developments and be introduced to methods of assessment of an individual's health and lifestyle.

### LIFE STAGES

How would you divide the human life span into stages? That is, how many distinct stages are there? What are they, and what ages do they apply to?

**Conception**
When an egg is fertilised and pregnancy starts

**Prenatal**
From conception to birth

**Birth and infancy**
From birth to the age of 3 years

**Childhood**
From 4 to 10 years

*That's life.*

### Health and well-being

Many modern ideas regarding **health** and **well-being** are based on the hierarchy of **needs** set out by the psychologist Abraham Maslow in the 1930s (see topic 5.1).

A **holistic** definition of health and well-being accounts for the whole combination of **physical**, **intellectual** and **emotional** and **social factors**. If you take the first letter of each of these words they spell the word PIES (see diagram on page 85).

* Physical needs are those that keep our bodies working, and include food, water, shelter, sleep, exercise and personal hygiene.
* Intellectual needs are those which develop our brains, such as mental stimulation, education and employment.
* Emotional needs are those that make us happy and relaxed, and include feeling loved, respected and secure.
* Social needs include good relationships and to live in an appropriate environment.

### Growth and development

People grow because:

* the total number of body cells increases
* each cell gets larger
* the body cells become more specialised in the jobs they do.

The term 'development' means the gradual change and increase in abilities, emotions and skills. Both growth and development

**Health** The state of being sound or whole, in body, mind and soul.

**Well-being** People feeling good about themselves.

**Needs** Requirements or things felt to be necessary.

**Holistic** Looking at a person or issue as a whole, rather than as a sum of parts.

**Factors** Things that contribute to, or affect, something else.

**Physical** To do with the body.

**Intellectual** To do with the brain.

**Emotional** To do with the emotions.

**Social** To do with life with other people.

happen most rapidly until a person is about 19 years of age. PIES is a useful way of thinking about human development.

## Life events

Some life events are expected or predictable, such as starting school, while others are unexpected or unpredictable, such as serious injury, disability and illness. Life events may affect our growth, development, health and well-being, as well as our opportunities and lifestyle choices.

## Lifestyle choices

Some lifestyle choices relate to diet, exercise, substance abuse, smoking and sexual practices. Some key influences on these choices are **socio-economic** factors, physical factors, culture and beliefs.

## Assessment of health, well-being and lifestyle

Assessments are made by looking at the positive and negatives aspects of our lifestyles. This may be by observation, interview, notes and written reports and physical measures of health, such as blood pressure. Recommendations for improvement can then be made if necessary.

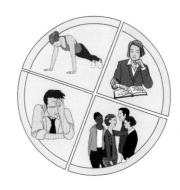

*PIES: physical, intellectual, emotional, social. You need to take all four aspects of development and health into account.*

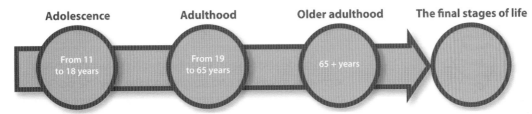

Adolescence — From 11 to 18 years

Adulthood — From 19 to 65 years

Older adulthood — 65 + years

The final stages of life

## How you will be assessed

For this unit you will be assessed by an externally set short-answer paper consisting of approximately seven questions, each made up of a number of smaller parts. As part of this paper you will be asked to interpret a case study, similar to those you have been using in other units. You will be required to respond to issues in relation to growth, development and healthy living raised in the case study. The paper will be sat under controlled conditions and you will have two hours to complete it.

**Socio-economic** To do with a mix of social/class considerations and money.

## What you will learn in this unit

You will:

* Know the key physical, emotional, social and intellectual changes and developments that take place across the life span
* Know how the sectors support and monitor these key changes and developments
* Understand how life events across the life span may impact on growth, development, health and well-being
* Understand how disability and illness might impact on physical, emotional, social and intellectual changes and development, lifestyle choices and opportunities for an individual
* Know the influence of different conditions, religions, beliefs and cultures on lifestyles
* Understand the impact of lifestyle choices on health, well-being and life opportunities
* Be able to assess an individual's health, well-being and lifestyle, and make recommendations for improvement

### Activity

1 With a partner, write down in rough as many physical features for each life stage as you can think of. For example, a feature of adolescence is puberty, when periods start and bodies change shape ready for adulthood.

2 Use your joint ideas to construct a table to show how physical features change as a person passes through the life stages. What other types of features are there besides ones to do with the physical part of our bodies?

## PIES FOR INFANTS

Look at the needs of a baby as set out in the spider diagram. Divide these into physical, intellectual, emotional and social (PIES) needs.

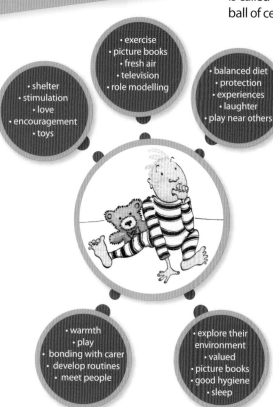

- exercise
- picture books
- fresh air
- television
- role modelling

- balanced diet
- protection
- experiences
- laughter
- play near others

- shelter
- stimulation
- love
- encouragement
- toys

- warmth
- play
- bonding with carer
- develop routines
- meet people

- explore their environment
- valued
- picture books
- good hygiene
- sleep

*Babies have specific needs.*

**Physical reflexes** Automatic, responses to a physical change, such as moving away from something sharp that causes pain.

**Gross motor skills** Control of the larger muscles, typically those in the arms and legs (e.g. kicking a ball).

**Fine motor skills** Control of the smaller muscles, such as those in the fingers (e.g. holding a pencil). These skills are more difficult to acquire than gross motor skills.

# 4.1 Starting out

This topic briefly describes what happens at conception and then looks at infancy.

## Conception, prenatal development and birth

The fertilisation of an egg by a sperm followed by implantation in the uterus is called conception. The fertilised egg divides many times to become a ball of cells called an embryo. Two months later it looks like a tiny baby and is now called a foetus. The foetus absorbs oxygen and food from the mother's blood and passes carbon dioxide and waste products into the mother's blood. About nine months after conception, the mother goes into labour, when contractions of the muscles in the wall of the uterus push the foetus down and out through the widened entrance to the uterus. This is the moment of birth.

## Infancy (0–3 years)

Growth and development are particularly rapid during infancy.

### Physical development

Physical development describes both the way the body increases in weight and height and the way the body gradually changes as a person gets older. Babies are born with a number of **physical reflexes**, some of which are lost as they get older. They learn **gross motor skills** and **fine motor skills** (see table, but note that the ages shown are rough averages, and there is wide variation in the acquisition of some these skills).

The primitive reflexes of a newborn baby are as follows:

* Rooting reflex: the baby turns its head in the direction of the touch, enabling it to find the nipple of its mother's breast to obtain food.

* Moro reflex: when startled, a baby throws out its arms and legs, then pulls them back with fingers curved.

* Grasp reflex: a baby will grasp an object placed in its hand.

* Walking reflex: when a baby is held with its feet touching the ground its legs make forward movements, as if walking.

### Intellectual development

Intellectual development describes the way in which an individual acquires the ability to use language, to develop concepts and to think. It is sometimes called cognitive development. The infant most importantly develops the ability to use language. Babies understand simple words such as 'bye-bye' at 6–9 months old and will be able to say about three words at the age of 1 year. By the age of 2 years most children have started using two-word phrases such as 'Ben wants'.

### Emotional development

Emotional development means we understand our feelings and those of others, and can form successful relationships. For this to happen, it is vital that the infant develops an 'attachment relationship' (bonding) with the main

## Infant development of motor skills

| Age | Gross motor skills | Fine motor skills |
| --- | --- | --- |
| Newborn | Primitive reflexes (see page 86) | |
| 1 month | Lifts up chin. Has some control of head | |
| 3 months | Reaches towards objects. Lifts head when laid on the stomach | Holds rattle for a few seconds. Moves hands towards a bottle |
| 4/5 months | Sits supported | |
| 6 months | Sits unsupported. Rolls over. Can kick strongly. Lifts head and chest when lying on the stomach | Can move objects from one hand to another. Picks up dropped toys if they are in sight |
| 9 months | Stands alone, holding on to something. Tries to crawl. Active movement of all limbs. Can lean forward without falling over | Begins to have 'pincer' movement between finger and thumb. Stretches out for held toy. Can release toy to drop it |
| 12 months | Pulls to stand. May walk alone or holding on to furniture. May crawl upstairs. Sits upright well | Good pincer movement. Bangs things together. Throws toys deliberately |
| 15 months | Can walk without help | |
| 18 months | Runs | Holds small objects. Can hold a pencil to 'draw' |
| 2 years old | Picks things up without falling over. Kicks a ball | Eats competently with a spoon. Can build a tower of six bricks |
| 2/3 years old | Stands on toes, jumps off a step. Can ride a tricycle | Can use crayons competently |

## Case study: Chyou's story

Chyou is two years old. Her parents have moved to England from China and have set up their own business. Chyou is their first child and is very precious to them. Until she was 12 months old her parents took it in turns to work during the day so that one of them could always be with her. When she was awake they sang to her, showed her picture books and fed and changed her. They cuddled her when she cried or was tired and wrapped her up well and put her in her pram outside to sleep when it was warm enough, so she would get lots of fresh air. They always stayed within sight of the pram so they could see she was safe. One or both of them took her for a walk in her buggy every day and pointed things out to her. As the business became more successful, both her parents had to work during the day but they continued to look after her the rest of the time. Now Chyou's grandparents come to the house to look after her when her parents are working. They take her out every day if possible, sometimes for a walk and at other times to their house or that of family and friends, all of whom adore Chyou, who is a cheerful, pretty infant. They play with her, helping her build towers with her building bricks, and sometimes watch a children's television programme with her, encouraging her to join in and sing or clap along.

1 Identify ways in which Chyou's PIES are being met.

2 Describe ways in which Chyou's parents and grandparents are making sure that she is able to form good relationships later in life.

carers (usually the mother and father). This happens during the first 18 months of life. It is the quality of love and care that matters most; even if the main carers are not present all the time, a strong attachment bond can still form.

### Social development

As children develop, they learn to socialise. Their first relationship is with their parents or main carers. As they get a little older, they become interested in other children. However, up until about two years of age they will play alone next to other children, not with them (this is called 'parallel play').

## Just checking

* What is meant by: (a) physical reflex; (b) gross motor skill; (c) fine motor skill?

* How does play help: (a) physical development; (b) intellectual development; (c) emotional development; (d) social development?

* Why is it important for an infant to develop an attachment relationship?

## THE IMPORTANCE OF PLAY

Identify with a partner what children can gain developmentally by climbing trees.

In what other ways could these same needs be met?

## 4.2 What a lovely child

In this topic you will learn about needs during childhood (4–10 years) and the developments that take place.

### Childhood (4–10 years)

There is very little difference in the physical needs of infants and children, more in their intellectual and social needs, and the most difference in their emotional needs.

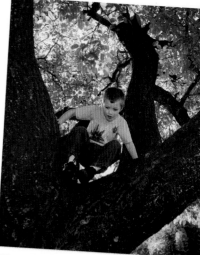

*Why do children like to climb trees?*

*PIES for children aged 4–10 years*

| Physical needs | Intellectual needs | Emotional needs | Social needs |
| --- | --- | --- | --- |
| Warmth | Play | Respect | Development of routines |
| Shelter | Stimulation | Love | Meeting other people |
| Balanced diet | More advanced toys | Encouragement | Playing and learning with others |
| Protection | New experiences | Laughter | Opportunity to explore the environment |
| Good hygiene | Books | Feeling valued | Taking part in social activities |
| Sleep | Television | Dignity | |
| Exercise | Education | Some independence | |
| Fresh air | Role modelling | Self-esteem | |

### For your project

You could explain how a child grows and develops from infancy to the end of 10 years. You could include pictures for each stage of development.

**Modelling** The demonstration of a type of behaviour in order for it to be copied.

## Growth and development

### Physical development

As children get older their physical appearance starts to change. They lose their baby shape. Their balance becomes good, so they can now run, climb and jump. They do not grow as quickly as when they were infants.

### Intellectual development

The brain and the mind continue to develop. Children at this age learn to count, communicate, make decisions based on logic rather than just feelings, recognise words, become more creative and understand better. They are interested in everything and ask many questions such as 'Why are those curtains red?' and 'Where did I come from?' By asking such questions and listening to honest answers children develop intellectually and learn about their culture and environment. They also learn by watching others, in a process called **modelling**. Children will often repeat something their parents have said without knowing what it means, sometimes embarrassing their parents in the process! They will also copy the things they do and the way they do things. They watch and learn what other people do, including bad behaviour. Children need to learn what is bad behaviour by having it explained to them, so that they will not repeat it.

As children get older they begin to learn to carry out a range of more complex activities, such as dressing themselves, writing, reading and arithmetic, and learning and understanding the rules of games. They complete more complicated tasks by using a mixture of skills. They play team games and learn not only new skills but also rules of behaviour, how to communicate with team-mates and how to cope when they win or lose.

### Emotional development

As children get older they have to learn how to cope with their own feelings, many of which they will be experiencing for the first time. Some of these are love, fear, anger, jealousy and respect. Younger children are sometimes confused by their feelings. They will have temper tantrums, as a way of expressing themselves and trying to get what they want when they don't get it straight away. They become less prone to these as they get older. By the age of 5 they are wanting to be in the company of other children and by the age of 10 have begun to learn how to cope with their feelings. Children are very sensitive and don't like being told off, especially in front of others, so they also start to learn how to take criticism.

### Social development

When children are about 4 they start to play properly with others. This is called cooperative play. The way children play changes as they get older. However, at any age play helps the child to develop, as shown in the figure.

Play can involve practising skills and abilities, such as making things. Physical practice encourages muscle development and coordination. Exploring through play can involve seeing what happens with things are touched or dropped. Pretend play stimulates the imagination and play can also promote social learning, through role-playing and cooperating.

Children learn to make friends with others in a variety of settings, be it at home, school or at an activity they take part in away from both, such as a sport or dance classes. The way we develop relationships depends on the culture we are born into. A person from a culture that does not approve of males and females mixing together outside the home may find it harder to make friends with someone of the opposite sex or may prefer friends of the same sex.

| Types of play | Type of development |
|---|---|
| Practising | Skills<br>Abilities<br>Activities<br>Actions<br>Making things<br>Muscles<br>Coordination |
| Exploring | An object<br>A situation<br>What happpens when something is touched<br>What happens when something is dropped<br>How something works |
| Pretending | Use imagination<br>Copying actions of others |
| Social learning | Role-playing<br>Cooperating |

### Activity

1 Look through old magazines or catalogues. Cut out pictures of activities children are taking part in, such as eating a meal with their family, horse riding, dancing, sports, playing games and with toys. Stick each picture in your work book and identify which one or more of the PIES are being met by the activity, for example stimulation as an aspect of intellectual development. Write this by the picture. Remember, childhood is from 4 to 10 years old, so do not use pictures of infants or adolescents!

2 By each picture describe how the activity is helping the child's physical, intellectual, emotional and/or social development.

### Just checking

* Why do children ask lots of questions?
* Why do younger children have temper tantrums?
* How does living in a culture that does not approve of males and females mixing together outside the home affect social development?

# 4.3 Teenagers

This topic looks at the key physical, intellectual, emotional and social changes and developments that take place during adolescence. Individuals enter this stage of life as children and leave it as young adults. You will have the chance to reflect on your own PIES.

### Diploma Daily

## High teenager truants school

A teenager was recently caught truanting from Smeston High School by the police and was found to be high on cocaine. When he was finally able to be interviewed Liam admitted that he had 'bunked off' school in order to shoplift to raise money to score drugs. He claimed that he gets picked on at school and that his teachers and parents don't understand him. He will appear in court for sentencing later today. As this is his second drugs offence it is expected that he will be sent to a Young Offender Institution.

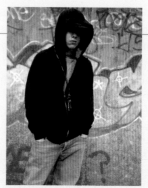

*Youth caught truanting to face Youth Offenders Board.*

1 What needs of the adolescent are currently not being met?

2 What might be the consequences of this situation on his PIES when he gets older?

## Adolescence (11–18 years)

Adolescence is one of the most difficult life stages for many individuals. It is the period which includes **puberty** and leads to adulthood. These changes are brought about by hormones, chemicals made in the endocrine glands and transported round the body in the blood system. It is also a life stage during which big changes in terms of body size, shape and functions, knowledge, experience and ability happen.

## Growth and development

Adolescents develop relationships with people of all ages and of both sexes, ready for more lasting relationships. They learn new skills ready for work and become much more independent. They also develop a set of values and morals, and become more aware of their social responsibilities and the consequences of their behaviour.

### Physical development

Puberty occurs during adolescence. The precise age at which it happens varies from person to person, but for most it is between the age of 12 and 14, and usually happens earlier in girls. Puberty is caused by hormones, oestrogen in girls and testosterone in boys.

## The major changes in puberty for boys and girls

| Girls | Boys |
|---|---|
| Gain weight | Gain weight |
| Grow body hair, mainly under-arm and pubic hair | Grow body hair, mainly under-arm, chest, face and pubic hair |
| Grow taller | Grow taller |
| Breasts develop | Penis develops |
| Hips widen ready for child bearing | Testicles drop |
| Periods start (menstruation) | Voice breaks |
| | Shoulders broaden |

### Intellectual development

While children are unable to plan and think ahead, because they cannot imagine and think about things they have never seen or done, adolescents *can* imagine the future and how they might achieve their dreams and ambitions. Where children might make guesses when they have to solve a problem, adolescents can apply logic instead.

### Emotional development

Adolescents are very affected by emotions. Mood swings can be caused by an imbalance of hormones while their bodies undergo the changes of puberty. This can lead to aggressive behaviour, weepiness and arguments with family and friends. Although this eventually settles down, it can be a frustrating and difficult time for both the adolescents and the adults who care for them, such as parents and teachers. It is therefore important that adolescents have someone to talk to about their problems, who can help with advice and explain why they are feeling as they are. Some, however, feel unable to talk to adults about things they feel sensitive about and therefore feel isolated, lack confidence and may even become depressed.

### Social development

During adolescence individuals become less dependent on families and more dependent on their **peer group** to provide support, advice and approval. They have a strong need to belong to, and be accepted by, their peers and this is apparent by their clothes, interests and behaviour. Some even go so far as to behave in a way they think is wrong deep down but do so because they are so desperate to be accepted by a group.

Adolescents start to experiment with relationships with the opposite sex and to test out sexual behaviour. As they take on more adult behaviour and try to assert their adult independence, conflict can arise with parents. Decision-making skills develop through life and depend on knowledge and experience of different situations; consequently, this is an area adolescents may have difficulties in.

> **Peer group** A group of people of the same age who are important to the individual. The peer group will influence the behaviour and attitude of the individual because they value their opinion.

### Just checking

* What causes the changes in males and females during puberty? State five changes in boys and five changes in girls associated with puberty.
* Explain why adolescents experience mood changes. What advice would you give to someone who is struggling to cope with this?
* Describe three problems adolescents might experience when making friends. Explain why these problems might arise.

# 4.4 All grown up

This topic covers the key physical, intellectual, emotional and social needs of adults and the changes and developments that take place during adulthood. This stage of life covers the largest range of ages.

## THEY THINK THEY KNOW IT ALL!

1 How many times have you thought this about your parents, teachers or other adults? They don't know it all but generally do know more, and can do more, than you! Think about an older adult at your place of work. Write down the skills (the things that they can do) that they have but you don't have yet.

2 How do you think they developed these skills?

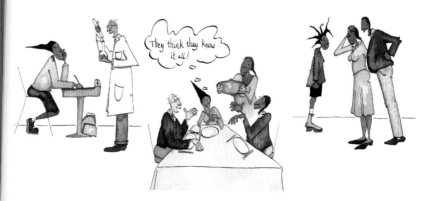

*They may not know it all, but do older adults know more?*

## Adulthood (19–65 years)

Adulthood is the stage of life when most people start to feel that they understand and accept themselves and begin to feel more settled. Although they never stop learning new skills and knowledge, this happens less quickly than for younger people. Adults tend to spend a great deal of time making decisions, such as what job to do, where and with whom to live, whether to have children, what to do for exercise, leisure activities … the list is endless! Because this is the longest life stage, adults have different needs within it.

*The PIES for adulthood*

| Physical needs | Intellectual needs | Emotional needs | Social needs |
|---|---|---|---|
| Warmth | Stimulating work | Respect | Money to access activities |
| Shelter | Learn new skills for home, work and leisure | Love | Opportunities to meet other people |
| Balanced diet | Conversation | Encouragement | Learning with others |
| Safe surroundings | New experiences | Laughter | Travel |
| Good hygiene | Books | Feeling valued | Leisure facilities |
| Sleep | Media | Dignity | Free time |
| Exercise | Education | Independence | Information about available activities |
| Fresh air | Role models | Self-esteem and self-awareness | |
| Health facilities | Job security | Stable relationships | |
| | | Preparation for parenthood, children leaving home, retirement, death of loved ones | |
| | | Financial security | |

# Growth and development

## Physical development

Adults are at the height of their physical powers and most able to have children in their 20s and 30s. The body begins to age discernibly as people reach their 40s and 50s:

* Men may lose hair.
* The hair often starts to grey.
* Eyesight may deteriorate.
* The skin loses elasticity and wrinkles appear.
* Female fertility decreases and ends with the start of **menopause**.
* Sperm production decreases.

## Intellectual development

If adults continue to exercise their intellectual skills and abilities, these will continue to increase. Although adults learn and react slightly more slowly as they get older, they are compensated by greater knowledge and experience on which to draw. This **wisdom** helps adults make better-informed decisions.

## Emotional development

Adulthood is a time when many adults look to form a steady relationship with another person which results in marriage or **co-habitation**. Often couples have children. As adults get older they might find their own parents need help as they become older and frailer. Other adults live alone, through choice or because they have not met a person with whom they feel they can have a lasting relationship, or because a relationship has broken up. All of these arouse a wide range of emotions that adults have to learn to cope with.

## Social development

Young adults often have no responsibilities and can go out whenever they like, money permitting. Many things can happen to affect this, such as having children. Social activities often change from going out for a meal to staying in with friends. Most adults have to work to earn enough money to support themselves and, later, a family. They have to cope with trying to balance work commitments with the demands of their home life, and their social life can be affected. As the children become older and less dependent on their parents, even though they may still live at home, parents become freer to enjoy the sort of social activities to which they were accustomed or to explore new possibilities with their friends. They may have more money to themselves by then and be able to afford better holidays, maybe on a cruise or in a nice hotel, where they will meet new people.

## Activity

1 Look at the table on page 92. Pick three needs that did not appear on the list of PIES for children (topic 4.2) and explain why they become needs for adults.

2 Why do you think the list of emotional needs is the longest?

3 Pick one emotional need that could also be a physical, intellectual and social need and explain why this is so.

**Menopause** The natural and permanent stopping of menstruation, occurring usually between the ages of 45 and 55.

**Wisdom** The ability to discern or judge what is true, right, or lasting; insight.

**Co-habitation** An emotional and physical intimate relationship which includes a common living place and which exists without legal or religious sanction.

## For your project

Describe what needs are met by forming a lasting relationship with another person. Include marriage or co-habitation, having children, looking after parents and coping with difficult times.

## Just checking

* List at least five decisions that adults have to make.
* What effect do you think gradual changes to the body will have on people's well-being as they go from their 30s to their 40s? How will these affect an adult's PIES?
* What are the benefits for an older couple of meeting new people?

# 4.5 Nothing to prove

In this topic you will learn about the key physical, intellectual, emotional and social needs in later adulthood and the final stages of life, as well as the changes and developments that take place at this time.

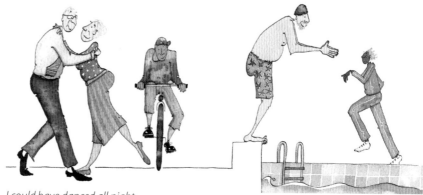

*I could have danced all night.*

## Later adulthood (65 years and over)

Inevitably, with age, people's bodies gradually change and start to let them down a little. However, many older people, especially those who have kept active and fit, continue to do many of the same activities as when they were younger. They may need to adapt them a little – for example, a runner may swap to running on grass rather than roads because it is kinder to the joints.

Getting older is often looked on as a negative thing, but many people look forward to this time of life, especially now that life expectancy is so much longer than it used to be. They can retire from work and their children have usually moved out. These older adults can therefore spend their days doing whatever they want. Those who have saved for their retirement and with pensions will have money and time to go away on holiday several times a year and take up new activities, without having to balance work and family commitments, although they may decide to help look after grandchildren. Other adults are not as lucky. They may not enjoy their retirement as much because of ill-health or the loss of loved ones, or money problems.

## Growth and development

### Physical development

The ageing process is usually very slow, so that people tend to notice the changes only in their 60s. These changes can include:

* thinner, less sensitive and less elastic skin
* wrinkles
* bones more brittle
* stiffer joints
* reduced height and some bending
* weaker muscles
* balance less good
* hearing, eyesight, smell and taste deteriorate
* breathing less efficient
* higher blood pressure
* less insulin production
* less hormone production

* men may lose hair
* eyesight may deteriorate
* female menopause starts
* female fertility decreases
* sperm production decreases

Although older people may suffer from more than one of these problems, they can still lead happy and fulfilled lives, with the right support.

### Intellectual development

People do not become less intelligent as they get older, but may need help gaining new skills and may find their memory deteriorating. Those who have good health and who continue to exercise their minds – maybe completing a crossword or Sudoku puzzle every day – generally keep their mental abilities better.

### Emotional development

As people get older their **self-concept** continues to change. When they retire they may feel they no longer know their role in life; ill-health can also mean they view themselves less positively. Older people suffer **stereotyping**, which can also have a negative effect on their self-concept. The death of partners or friends can leave some feeling lonely.

Others, though, relish the chance to give up work and keep themselves so busy that they wonder how they found the time to work. With the love and support of family and friends, many older people develop a more positive self-concept, feeling at ease with the person they have become and no longer feeling stressed by having to compete in the workplace.

### Social development

Most older people have established networks of family and friends, from different periods of their lives. In addition, they now have the time to lead a varied life and to make new friends. Others may be unable to take up such opportunities because of their own or their partner's ill-health, or lack of money. **Social isolation** becomes more common with increasing age.

## Final stages of life

People are often at peace and ready to accept death if they have lived a full and happy life. Others may be in pain or missing loved ones and so feel they have lived long enough. Such acceptance of death is much less likely in the case of a person younger than 65, or one who has missed out on the joys of having children, for example.

People who are dying have specific needs, such as pain relief, and having their loved ones with them to say goodbye to and to reassure them that they are loved and won't be forgotten. If their loved ones cannot be there, another person, perhaps a nurse or someone representing their religion, should give support.

Near the very end of life, a person's breath becomes slower and the organs and senses start to shut down. The skin becomes cool. The last sense to keep working is the hearing. At death itself, the chest no longer rises and the person stops breathing.

**Self-concept** This is a combination of our self-esteem, which is how highly we think about ourselves, and our self-image, which is how we think others think of us.

**Stereotyping** Thinking a group of people will all have the same attributes, for example, that all older people will be deaf and have memory problems.

**Social isolation** Living without regular contact with other people, especially friends and family.

### Just checking

* Why do you think people who are over 65 are properly called 'older people' rather than 'old' or 'elderly'?
* Why do people only really notice the changes in their bodies due to ageing in their 60s?
* How do health issues affect the intellectual, social and emotional development of older adults?

## THINKING POINT

Parents suspect their young child has a life-threatening illness. They ring their GP surgery.

1 Write down step by step which health care workers the family are likely to come into contact with from now until the end of the child's treatment and which health care services they may be referred to.

2 Think about what various professionals will need to do to diagnose the illness and what they will do for the child once the diagnosis has been confirmed.

**Ultrasound examination** A harmless, non-invasive and painless technique that generates images ('scans', produced by high-frequency sound waves) of the baby and its organs.

**Amniocentesis** A test where a little fluid is taken from the amniotic sac that surrounds the baby, and analysed. It can detect foetal conditions such as spina bifida (a defect of the spinal cord).

**Immunisation** The administration of a substance (usually by injection) to help the body fight infectious disease.

# 4.6 The health sector and settings

The health sector monitors and supports people throughout their lives. This topic explains how and why it does this throughout the early years.

## Monitoring and support

The aim of health monitoring is to make sure everything is as it should be and to detect any problems as early as possible, to give the best chance of correcting them. Problems that do arise are monitored during treatment. Support is given to help the person cope with the physical, intellectual, emotional and social aspects of the problem.

## The early years

### Prenatal

Pregnant women receive regular support and monitoring from an obstetrician or midwife. This is called antenatal care. A woman's GP will arrange her first antenatal appointment between 11 and 13 weeks of pregnancy. She will usually be seen by a midwife and will be asked about herself and her medical history. She will have her blood pressure, heart and lungs checked, be asked to give a blood sample (to test for blood type, immunities and infections) and a urine sample (to test for sugar and protein levels), and have her height and weight measured. Her belly will be examined to assess the size of her womb. The information gathered will be used to estimate when the baby will be born.

In the months leading up to the birth, the woman will regularly visit the antenatal clinic. She will have at least two **ultrasound examinations**. These are used to monitor the size, movement and position of the growing baby, as well as to confirm the expected date of birth. They can also show what sex the baby is and detect risks such as Down's syndrome. If any problems are detected, the woman may be offered further tests, such as **amniocentesis**.

During pregnancy, the woman and her partner will be offered antenatal classes that cover all aspects of birth and the care of a newborn baby.

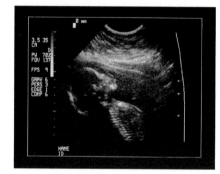

*Ultrasound scan of an unborn baby.*

### Birth

As soon as the baby is born, its length and weight are measured and it is given an Apgar score (see table). This gives a quick indication of the baby's physical condition. It is repeated five minutes after birth. Babies with a total score of 7 or above are considered to be in good health; babies with lower scores are often easily treated, for example with a little oxygen.

*The Apgar score*

| Apgar sign | Score 0 | Score 1 | Score 2 |
|---|---|---|---|
| **A**ppearance (skin colour) | Blue all over | Blue at extremities, body pink | Normal pink all over |
| **P**ulse (heart rate) | Absent | Below 100 beats a minute | Above 100 beats per minute |
| **G**rimace (reflex irritability) | No response to stimulation | Grimace/feeble cry when stimulated | Sneezes/coughs/pulls away when stimulated |
| **A**ctivity (muscle tone) | None | Some flexing of arms and legs | Active movement |
| **R**espiration (breathing) | Absent | Weak or irregular | Strong |

Nurses monitor the mother and baby for about 24 hours after birth and give any support needed, such as help with breast-feeding technique.

## Postnatal

Every family with children under 5 years has a health visitor, who will visit the home to advise on issues such as feeding and sleeping. Mothers are also encouraged to attend postnatal clinics for further monitoring.

## Infancy, childhood and beyond

Children's height and weight continue to be monitored throughout their early years; they will also have their eyes and teeth checked regularly. Children with conditions such as asthma can attend specialist clinics, where they will be monitored and treated.

Health visitors will continue to give support if needed, sometimes on common difficulties such as teething and behaviour. They can advise on where to find additional support, such as toddler and playgroups and day nurseries. They also give advice on **immunisation**. Through immunisation, diseases such as tetanus, diphtheria and polio have practically disappeared in the UK. They could come back, however, so it is important that children are immunised; this is usually done by practice nurses or school nurses. The table shows the UK's immunisation schedule.

### Activity

1 Look at the immunisation schedule. Research three of the diseases that you know least about. Use the information to make a leaflet to inform parents of the dangers of these diseases.

2 Find out why some parents don't allow their children to be immunised against certain diseases. Discuss with a partner your views on this. What do you think the consequences of such a decision might be both for the child and for society?

*The UK immunisation schedule*

| Age group | Immunisation against: |
|---|---|
| Babies up to 15 months | Polio; diphtheria; tetanus; whooping cough; meningitis; measles, mumps and rubella (MMR); tuberculosis (BCG vaccine) for babies at high risk |
| Children aged 3–5 years | Polio; diphtheria; tetanus; whooping cough; MMR |
| Children aged 10–14 years | BCG immunity test; those at high risk have injection |
| Young people aged 13–18 years | Tetanus; diphtheria; polio |
| All under 25 | Meningitis C for all those who were not vaccinated as babies |

### Just checking

✳ Name the five factors that determine an Apgar score.

✳ Why are pregnant women offered ultrasound examinations?

✳ Why are children monitored throughout their early years?

# 4.7 The Children and Young People sector

The Children and Young People sector provides monitoring and support in all areas of life. This topic will tell you about the support and monitoring of key changes and development in learning.

## The local authority's CYPS

Some services are used by nearly all children and young people, such as education or health, whereas others are needed by only a few, such as children's social services. Children and young people's services (CYPS) are council departments which have formed partnerships to bring together all agencies that work to improve the lives of children and young people. These partnerships cover issues ranging from dental health to mental health to teenage conceptions. All have visions for their children and young people based on the five aims of the government's 2003 Green Paper *Every Child Matters* (which is discussed further in topic 7.6):

* being healthy
* staying safe
* enjoying and achieving
* making a positive contribution
* achieving economic well-being.

The CYPS monitor the overall health and well-being of all children and young people in the **borough** and gather annual statistics on a wide range of issues, firstly to give an overall picture within the borough, and secondly to provide data for comparison each year, in order to monitor whether there has been any improvement or deterioration. This enables them to allocate support as soon as it is needed.

### Diet

One example of monitoring and support undertaken by the CYPS concerns the diet of children and young people. An unbalanced diet affects development in many ways:

* physically, by not providing the nutrients needed for body repair and growth
* intellectually, by not providing the food needed to maintain an active, alert brain
* emotionally, because they will feel tired and depressed because they are over- or underweight
* socially, because they will feel less attractive and will be less likely to enjoy going out if they have no energy and are unhappy about their appearance.

The CYPS will have a whole range of information, such as the percentage of children who go to school in the morning without any breakfast or the numbers on free school meals. They then target support where it will be most effective. Sometimes it is targeted at every child and young person, via schools and colleges.

### BEHAVE!

Jasmeen is usually a hard-working, well behaved student who has recently started to behave differently, answering teachers back and not bothering to complete any of the work set. Her parents have contacted school as they are concerned about her, because her behaviour has changed at home as well. They have asked the school for help and advice. The head of pastoral care interviews her and she breaks down and tells her that…

1 Think of three different things that could account for this change in Jasmeen's behaviour.

2 For each of these reasons write down the services, either within the school or in the wider community, that will be involved in helping Jasmeen solve her problem.

3 For each of the three reasons, write down the support you think Jasmeen will need.

**Borough** An area run by a council or local authority.

For example, the CYPS may actively encourage every school to apply for 'National Healthy Schools' status, as this will mean that school meals will be looked at by the assessors to make sure they are healthy. The assessors will also look at the provision for exercise, the availability of free drinking water, the quality of teaching children about a balanced diet and the whole issue of personal, social and health education. They not only talk to those who work in the school but all other **stakeholders** as well. In order to gain this status, schools have to communicate with parents to encourage healthy eating, including asking parents to think carefully about what they put in a child's packed lunch.

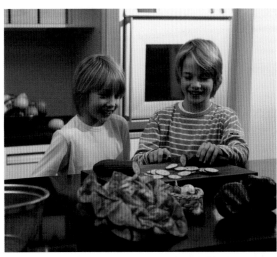

*Encouraging a balanced diet.*

Other support may be aimed at more specific groups of children and young people. For example, continuing on the balanced diet theme, CYPS promote the government's national fruit scheme. All 4- to 6-year-old children are entitled to a free piece of fruit or vegetable every day. This is to help them towards the target of eating five portions a day.

### CYPS in education

An example of a large specific group being targeted in education is boys. There is a gap between the attainment of girls and boys overall, so the CYPS will ensure that schools review the curriculum to ensure it encourages boys to raise their attainment and aspirations. They also encourage the engagement of more young people between the ages of 14 and 19 by increasing the diversity of courses and providing appropriate pathways into further learning.

### CYPS in social care

Also targeted are smaller, vulnerable groups such as looked after children or those most likely to be excluded from school. They support these by putting in extra help and guidance, in the form of education welfare officers and behaviour support workers, and by providing alternative teaching and learning methods for them. Another group is those with special educational needs. CYPS put strategies and funding in place to improve teaching and learning opportunities for such students. They also ensure that those who are gifted and talented are supported and encouraged, as there is a danger they will become bored because they are not being stretched.

> **Stakeholder** Someone who has a share in or an interest in an organisation.

> **Personal, learning and thinking skills**
>
> The activity will help towards PLTS: Independent enquirer; Creative thinker; Self-manager.

> **Activity**
>
> 1 Write down any examples of where teachers in your school collect information and data about you, for example examination results. For each of these, write down how you think the teachers or other adults in the school use this information to help and support you.
>
> 2 Can you think of any groups of children or young people who you feel need extra help and support, not necessarily those in your school, but perhaps those in a young offender institution? With a friend discuss and research how the CYPS might be monitoring them and setting up support for them.

> **Just checking**
>
> \* Give three examples of the kind of information the CYPS collect about children and young people. Why do they collect this information?
>
> \* How does collecting data about all children and young people help CYPS target support?
>
> \* Explain how encouraging schools to support an initiative such as increasing the number and range of different types of courses helps the development of children and young people.

# 4.8 The social care sector

The two other sectors, social care and community justice, also monitor and support people throughout their lives. This topic will tell you how the social care sector monitors and supports older people. It also looks at rehabilitation and early interventions. The community justice sector is covered in detail in Unit 6.

**WHO CARES?**

Who do you think the care assistant in the picture below should involve? In which order should she contact what services? Why do you think she should do this?

## Older people

The main role of the social care sector is to assess need and provide access to the services required, for people of all ages. If, for example, an older person decides that he can no longer manage to live on his own and would prefer to move into a residential care home with people of his own age, he or his family would contact social services. A social worker would visit him to find out how mobile he is, his general state of health, family details and so on. The social worker will also find out how much money he has available to contribute to his care if together they decide that he should find a place in a home. The social worker would then help him find a home that both he and his family felt was right for him and help him apply for a place and for any grants he is entitled to in order to help him pay for his care. The interview process is an aspect of monitoring; helping him get a suitable place and making sure he can afford it are aspects of support.

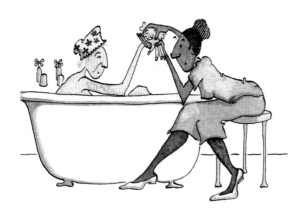

*To whom should she go for help?*

**Intervention** Any specific action a service provider takes on becoming involved in a case.

**Remedial** Working with existing problems to lessen them.

**Preventive** Working to stop problems arising.

## Additional support

People who require support include those who are:

* recovering from a serious injury
* recovering from a condition such as a stroke or brain tumour
* suffering from a life-threatening illness that is gradually reducing their mobility or communication
* losing their sight or hearing
* recovering from a mental illness and who need help to live in the community again.

People of all ages may need support from the social care sector at some stage of their lives. One example is people who have been left damaged in some way and need rehabilitation to help them regain their independence. Rehabilitation aims to:

* rebuild skills such as walking
* rebuild confidence
* teach new skills to help a person manage around the home
* keep the person out of hospital or any other permanent residential care unless this is proved to be right for that person.

This process starts in hospital, while the person is still being treated for their condition, but will be continued when the time comes to leave the hospital, when the medical staff have done all they can. A care manager from the social care sector will assess the needs of the person, in consultation with the medical team, and will decide what type and level of services the person will need. The local authority social services department will then organise access to these for the person. Rehabilitation may be based in a specially built unit that offers residential care for a short time, where service users can recover at their own pace and practise daily skills for living, such as washing, dressing and preparing meals. Specially trained carers work with the person under the instructions of occupational therapists and physiotherapists. They will give advice on how to cope with the illness or disability, providing aids and equipment to help the person do things more easily. They will be following a written care plan, which alters as a person improves. When the person is considered able to cope at home, rehabilitation continues either in a day centre or in the home.

## Early intervention

Early **intervention** is the introduction of a support system as soon as a problem is detected, to try to ensure it does not worsen over time. Early intervention can be **remedial** or **preventive**.

For example, if a child experiences a developmental delay, such as learning to talk at a late age, early intervention will be in the form of appropriate therapies to help the child catch up and reach each subsequent normal step of development. As well as therapy services, early childhood intervention includes special education and help for the whole family, through the provision of information, advocacy and emotional support.

Early childhood intervention is provided by a team which is usually made up of special-needs teachers, speech and language therapists, physiotherapists, occupational therapists and other support staff, such as music therapists and counsellors. The key to success is this multidisciplinary way of working: that is, different services work together to discuss and tackle each case. Services range from those that identify the problem, such as screening in hospital or a school setting, to the actual intervention, such as therapy.

Other examples of early intervention include early therapy for those who will need rehabilitation, such as starting simple exercises on a paralysed hand for someone who has had a brain injury while medical staff are still trying to find out the cause of the injury. Another is those who have a family history of a condition such as breast cancer and take action to prevent developing the condition themselves, such as having their breasts scanned regularly or removed.

### Activity

1 Put one hand behind your back. Try to do some everyday tasks, such as getting a big item out of your bag or typing on a computer keyboard. Practise until you can do it better. Note down your feelings as you tried to do these tasks. Write a list of everyday activities you would have trouble doing at home if you could use only one hand. Some people suffer far worse setbacks than the loss of the use of one arm.

2 Role-play with a partner. Pretend you are talking with a close friend who has lost the use of both an arm and a leg and is very depressed, feeling they are a burden and have nothing left to offer. After your partner has played the close friend, swap roles.

### Personal, learning and thinking skills

The activity should help towards PLTS: Reflective learner; Creative thinker; Team worker; Effective participator.

### Functional skills

It will also help towards FS: English – reading, speaking and listening.

### Just checking

* Give three examples of what social services will do (a) to monitor and (b) to support an older person.
* Give five reasons why a person might need rehabilitation. For each one describe: (a) the monitoring and (b) the support they will need from the social care sector.
* Why might a child who is exceptionally bright need early intervention?

# 4.9 Life events

This topic looks at some of the important things that happen to people during their lifetime, and their impact on growth, development, health and well-being.

## The nature of life events

Life events are important experiences that can have a major impact on growth, development, health and well-being. They can be classified as expected or unexpected, or as predictable and unpredictable. Even those that are expected are, of course, not guaranteed to happen. Unexpected ones are those that are not planned.

### Expected and unexpected life events

Expected life events might include: starting nursery and school; puberty; starting work/employment; leaving home; getting married; parenthood; retirement; or menopause. Unexpected life events could include: the birth of a sibling; moving house; redundancy; serious injury or illness; getting divorced or breakdown of a serious relationship; bereavement; abuse; or winning the lottery. Life events involve change, which usually produces some level of stress, even when the life event is a positive one.

Marriage and divorce are good examples to show how such life events can affect growth, development, health and well-being.

Many life events cannot neatly be categorised as positive or negative. For example, marriage may bring some initial sense of loss if it involves, say, leaving the family home, and it may produce some stress, with the taking on of new responsibilities. Nonetheless, a supportive relationship contributes to our health and well-being by helping us to achieve and maintain physical fitness and intellectual, emotional and social stability (see table).

Similarly, divorce may bring some positive effects, such as a feeling of relief from no longer living in an unhappy situation, although it is, of course, overall, a negative event for almost everyone. When people get married they believe it is for life, so divorce will bring a sense of failure, guilt or blame, and low self-esteem. The associated stress will undermine physical fitness and lead to a poor intellectual, emotional and social state. This will affect growth and development. For example, a loss of appetite due to stress will mean a person is not getting the right nutrients to build and repair body cells.

## Impact of disability and illness

Disability is covered in detail in Unit 9. Disabled people have to adapt their lifestyle to cope with everyday situations that able-bodied people deal with automatically. A disability or illness may affect physical fitness, hinder access to learning activities, cause emotional distress

## Contrasting effects of life events on growth and development

| Aspect of growth and development | Marriage (expected and positive) | Divorce (unexpected and negative) |
|---|---|---|
| Physical | Physical health; healthy sex life; someone to do activities with such as exercise; married couples tend to live longer and are less ill | Short-term and long-term effects of stress |
| Intellectual | Conversation and activities; advice | Lack of concentration on other matters; travel and visits may be cancelled due to lack of money or a companion |
| Emotional | High self-esteem; support in times of stress; happiness; good humour; caring relationship; high self-confidence | Sense of failure; disbelief; sadness; depression; anger; guilt; unhappiness; disappointment; low self-esteem |
| Social | Good relationship; sense of belonging; best friend | Friends often have to choose between divorcing couple; loss of activities the couple used to do together; harder to go out on own |

and remove some social opportunities, thus affecting health and well-being. It will also affect growth and physical development of the body; for example, a paralysed arm will lose muscle due to lack of use. Disability or illness also affects the development of new abilities and skills, as well as emotional development.

Whatever the condition, the needs of a disabled person include all those of an able-bodied person but they have important additional needs, especially in relation to access (to both places and services). If these are met through the provision of an enabling environment, the impact of the disability or illness will be decreased. This is discussed in Unit 9.

**Acute** Sharp or severe in effect; intense.

**Chronic** Having had a disease, habit, weakness for a long time

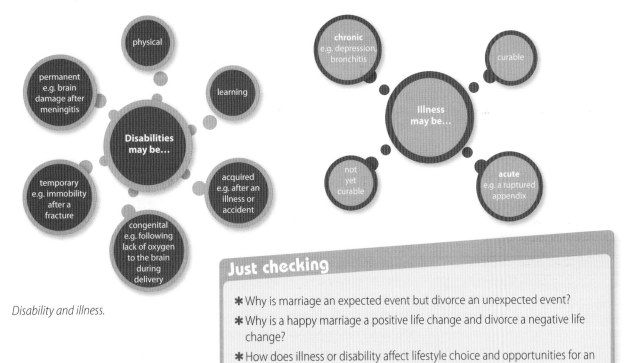

*Disability and illness.*

## Diploma Daily

### Burkha banned

A couple will not allow their daughter to go to school unless she is allowed to wear a burkha. The governors of the school are backing the school staff, who are refusing to teach anyone wearing the burkha because it is not correct uniform and it would make it hard for them to communicate with her.

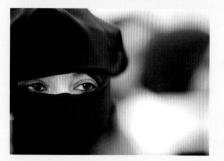

*Burkha banned.*

1 What effect are her parents' actions having on their daughter?

2 What do you think about this issue?

3 How should this problem be resolved?

4 Why does the burkha hinder communication?

---

## Activity

1 Find out (a) why the majority of Hindus believe the cow to be sacred; (b) what is meant by 'halal'; (c) why Jewish people consider some meats to be unclean.

2 Research, and construct a similar table to show, how religion can influence (a) dress and (b) hospital care. Add another religion, such as Jehovah's witnesses.

---

## Personal, learning and thinking skills

The activity should help towards PLTS: Independent enquirer; Self-manager.

---

# 4.10 Under the influence

In this topic you will learn about the influence on lifestyles of different conditions, including socio-economic and physical factors, and religions, beliefs and cultures.

## Influences on lifestyles

### Socio-economic factors

These include employment, housing, income, education and access to services. Employment is important to most adults because it gives them an **income** and income has a major impact on the way they lead their life. For example, people who can afford to buy high-quality food are more likely to be physically healthy, less likely to be ill and so be able to exercise more. They will also be able to afford to go to a variety of places and take part in a variety of activities, have more opportunities to learn and to meet new people or have a good time with their friends. Another advantage is being able to afford good housing, close to schools that provide high-quality education. Similarly, high-income families are usually able to access any other services they need. When a family has an adequate income there will be less stress because they are not worrying about financial problems and so fewer arguments and less chance of relationships failing.

An adequate income is important because it allows us to…

* live in a house with a garden
* afford leisure activities
* pay the rent or mortgage
* afford nice clothes
* socialise with friends
* eat a balanced diet
* live in the suburbs of a town or in the countryside
* travel to make use of NHS and community health facilities
* buy luxuries
* heat our homes
* afford a car and holidays.

### Physical factors

This group of factors includes inheritance, environment and also things that we do to our bodies (discussed in the next topic). Some diseases are inherited. One example is haemophilia, a condition in which the blood does not clot, and which affects only males. A haemophiliac would have to ensure that he didn't cut himself because he could bleed to death; he may therefore decide to avoid tackling do-it-yourself jobs in the home, taking part in contact sports or having a job that involves knives or spades.

The environment also influences people's lifestyles in many ways. For instance, a person living in a city is more likely to develop a respiratory condition such as asthma or have an already existing condition made worse because of increased amounts of pollution from vehicles and factories. City dwellers will also be more affected by noise and light pollution, which will affect quality of life. People who live in the country or in bigger, better spaced houses with a garden are more likely to get fresh air and exercise and so be healthier and less likely to succumb to illness.

## Religions and other beliefs

Religions influence the way people live, such as their diet (shown in the table below), dress and medical care.

### Religion and diet

| Religion | Influence on diet |
|---|---|
| Buddhism | Mahayana Buddhists are actively encouraged to be vegetarian but it is not compulsory and many eat meat; Theravada Buddhist monks are not allowed to eat the meat of an animal killed specifically for them |
| Christianity | The Christian faith does not forbid any type of food |
| Hinduism | The majority of the world's vegetarians are Hindus and those Hindus who do eat meat almost never eat beef, as they believe the cow to be sacred |
| Islam | Muslims may not eat any food containing pork, and other meats have to be from animals killed in the halal way |
| Judaism | Certain foods such as pork or shellfish are considered to be unclean by Jewish people and food that is acceptable to eat is called 'kosher' |

Diet may also be determined by non-religious beliefs. For example, many people choose to be vegetarian because they believe it is wrong to eat meat, for moral reasons.

Beliefs other than religious ones may be cultural. For example, travellers mainly live in caravans, sometimes without running water and electricity, because that way of life is their **custom**. Frequent moving about can result in apparent poor education but in fact some groups of travellers have advanced vocabulary and social skills because of their strong verbal and musical traditions.

**Rituals** are carried out in almost all known human societies and vary from hand shaking and saying hello to the various religious and cultural worship rites such as marriages, funerals and many more. Many people celebrate Christmas but in different countries and between different cultures Christmas rituals vary. Other cultures and religions do not celebrate Christmas at all.

Health and medical beliefs also affect lifestyles. For example, a Muslim woman would find being examined by a male doctor or nurse very traumatic because strict Muslims forbid any physical contact between males and females unless they are married. This means Muslims need to be able to be seen by a doctor of their own gender. If this is not possible, a Muslim woman finds it less shameful to be seen by a non-Muslim male doctor. Also, tradition dictates that the left hand is used to wash the genital area, so most Muslims use the right hand for everything else.

**Income** The amount of money that goes into a household, generally from earnings from work but also from sources such as welfare benefits, pensions and investments.

**Custom** A practice or way of living that is traditional, or a habit.

**Rituals** Prescribed or set ways of behaving in certain circumstances or of conducting a ceremony, proceeding or service.

## Just checking

* How does having an adequate income affect a person's lifestyle?
* How does the environment a person lives in affect their health?
* Explain the difference between doing something for moral religious reasons and doing something through personal choice. Give at least three examples.

## WHAT DOES THE FUTURE HOLD?

What effect do you think this choice of lifestyle will have on this young person's future (a) health, (b) well-being and (c) life opportunities?

*Our lifestyle choices affect our future opportunities.*

# 4.11 Lifestyle choices

Our lifestyles are influenced not only by factors such as those that affect us as members of a culture or group, or those conditions into which individuals are born, such as poverty or a poor environment, but also by our own choices, the things we do to our own bodies. This topic looks at some of these lifestyle choices and how they affect health, well-being and life opportunities.

## Diet and weight

If we make lifestyle choices that make us less healthy and feel less good about ourselves we will not be able to take all the opportunities life has to offer. For example, people who are overweight will be more prone to illnesses and conditions such as heart disease, will be less able to exercise and will feel less confident about their appearance in social situations. Obesity is certainly associated with a shorter life expectancy and ill-health. Very overweight people are less able to take up many life opportunities, such as hill walking, dancing or skiing, and are less likely to be successful at job interviews.

A balanced diet is one that contains the correct nutrients in the right proportions to keep our bodies and minds healthy. The essential parts of a healthy diet are fats (saturated and unsaturated), carbohydrates (sugars and starches), minerals, vitamins, water and proteins. The food we eat affects the way we feel and look and is very important to our health, well-being and life opportunities. Our dietary needs vary throughout life. If we eat more than we need, the body stores fat, which can lead to obesity, heart disease and high blood pressure, strokes, tooth decay and cancer. Eating less than we need can lead to anaemia, stunted bone growth, heart failure, depression, tiredness, cancer, mouth sores, scurvy and many other conditions. Both over- and under-eating can eventually result in death.

It is not just diet that affects health, well-being and life opportunities. Other lifestyle choices that have profound effects concern all of the following:

* exercise
* substance abuse (including smoking and alcohol)
* sexual practices
* personal relationships
* education
* use of leisure facilities
* use of health monitoring
* personal hygiene.

## Exercise

Exercise improves our **strength**, **stamina** and **suppleness** as well as our muscle and body tone. It also relieves stress, relaxes us, is enjoyable, makes us feel good, gives us a chance to meet others and

## Activity

1 Discuss with a partner the possible effects on (a) health, (b) well-being, (c) future life opportunities of having an unwanted pregnancy. Think in terms of PIES. Present your conclusions on a large piece of paper.

2 Research the signs, symptoms and long-term effects of three of the sexually transmitted diseases.

gives us personal satisfaction. Lack of exercise can lead to stiffening of the joints, poor stamina, decreased strength and suppleness, obesity, stroke, coronary heart disease, poorly developed heart and skeletal muscles, heart attack, sluggish blood flow, osteoporosis and other conditions. If our health and well-being suffer in this way, we will be less able to take life opportunities.

## Substance abuse

In addition to the unsafe use of solvents or the taking of illicit drugs, substance abuse can also involve too much use of alcohol, smoking, and the overuse of prescription drugs. Some of the effects are shown in the table.

**Strength** The body's physical power.

**Stamina** The heart's ability to work under strain.

**Suppleness** The body's ability to bend without damage.

*Effects of substance abuse*

| Solvents | Alcohol | Drugs | Cigarettes |
|---|---|---|---|
| Hallucinations | Obesity | Anxiety | Cancers of the nose, throat, tongue, lungs, stomach and bladder |
| Headaches | Reddened skin | Disorientation and depression | Heart disease and poor circulation |
| Liver damage | Liver damage (cirrhosis) | Blood infection | Stroke |
| Lack of concentration | Stomach problems (e.g. ulcers, gastritis) | Heart and lung disorder | Gum disease |
| Kidney damage | Brain disturbance | Nausea, headache, giddiness | Thrombosis |
| Heart failure | Heart disease | Raised body temperature | Bronchitis |
| Suffocation | High blood pressure and strokes | High blood pressure and strokes | Emphysema |
| Vomiting | Cancers of mouth, throat, bowel and stomach | Organ damage | Asthma |
| | Depression | Suffocation | Exposure in pregnancies causes smaller babies, more stillbirths and more miscarriages |
| | Insomnia | Vomiting | Exposure in childhood means that children are prone to chest infections and asthma, tend to be smaller and weaker, and do less well at school |
| | Reduced sexual function | Mental illness | |

## Sexual practices

Unprotected sex can result in unwanted pregnancies and the possibility of contracting sexually transmitted disease. These include gonorrhoea, syphilis, HIV/AIDS, genital herpes, pubic lice and chlamydia. The long-term effects of these diseases can include mental illness and even death.

### Just checking

* Name three short-term and three long-term effects of lack of exercise.
* Why are people who are overweight less likely to be successful in job interviews? Give at least three reasons.
* How do you think smoking affects (a) health care, (b) workplaces, (c) the health of a smoker?

What effect would stopping drinking and smoking have on the health of the man shown in the picture? What else could he do to make himself healthier?

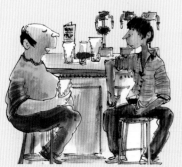

*Measures of health.*

# 4.12 Lifestyle assessment

This topic looks at the ways in which an individual's health, well-being and lifestyle can be assessed and improved.

## Assessment of physical health, mental well-being and lifestyle

In order to make recommendations and set targets to make improvements to health, well-being and lifestyle, it is important to conduct a thorough assessment of the person. Many aspects of a person's physical health can be easily measured. These include pulse rate, peak flow, temperature, blood pressure, waist measurement, height and weight charts, and body mass index. These are all covered in more detail in Unit 8.

Other aspects of health, and especially of well-being and lifestyle, are not so easily measured. One way of assessing the positive and negative aspects of a person's lifestyle (see table) is to collect the information in a questionnaire or interview.

### Positive and negative aspects of lifestyle

| Positive | Negative |
|---|---|
| Balanced diet | The opposites of all the positive aspects (e.g. unbalanced diet) |
| Regular exercise | Inherited diseases and conditions |
| Supportive relationships | Substance abuse |
| Adequate financial resources | Smoking |
| Stimulating work | Alcohol |
| The use of health monitoring and illness prevention services | Too much stress |
| Risk management to promote safety | Unprotected sex |
| Education | Social isolation |
| Leisure activities | Poverty |
| Enough sleep | Inadequate housing |
| | Unemployment |
| | Environmental pollution |

### Observation/interview

Service providers will gain information by observation as well as interview. For example, a doctor may ask a patient for details of the **medical history** in an interview, at the same time as taking measurements. Through observation, the doctor will also decide whether a patient is pale or flushed, sweating, panting for breath, limping, behaving oddly and so on.

**Medical history** A complete description of a patient's physical and mental condition, past and present.

## Notes/written report

Service providers will make notes of their observations, along with the answers to their questions, and if need be compile the information in a report for other professionals. For example, a doctor might write a report to send on to a hospital department for a patient referral, or might write a report on a person's mental capability to stand trial after committing a serious crime. Such a report will often contain recommendations on further health assessment or treatment.

## Recommendations

When a person has been assessed, a health improvement plan can be drawn up. This will give advice on how to improve health, well-being and lifestyle. It is important that such a plan includes short-term targets, such as 'to lose 4 lbs (1.8 kg) in week 1, and 2 lbs (0.9 kg) each week after that'. The long-term target might be to lose 2 stones (12.7 kg) in 6 months. The plan should also provide *strategies* to help the person achieve their *targets* (e.g. cut out biscuits and chocolate and drink more water), as well as *alternatives* so they feel they have some choice, and *information* to explain each step.

Such a plan should also take into account the person's age, gender, level of fitness and free time. The role of the service provider is to be sensitive to the feelings of the person and work with them to devise the plan. In this way they will be less likely to feel they are being told what to do and more likely to want to try to follow the plan.

Health promotion information aims to help people take more responsibility for their own health by providing advice, information and support. It comes in many forms, such as leaflets, videos, CDs, campaigns on the television and posters.

### For your project

Pick a person you know who has two or three habits that will cause them health problems in the future, such as smoking, drinking, over-eating or working too hard. Produce a health plan to help that person improve their health and well-being.

### Personal, learning and thinking skills

The activity will help with PLTS: Reflective learner.

### Activity

1 Write a questionnaire using the table opposite to assess the positive and negative aspects of someone's lifestyle. The questionnaire should collect as much detail as possible. For example, if you have a question to ask if they smoke, have a follow-up question asking how many cigarettes are smoked, and of what strength. Then answer the questionnaire yourself. Be honest!

2 Draw a cartoon picture of yourself in the middle of a piece of paper. Use this as the centre of a mind map. Have branches coming off that say 'Positive aspects', 'Negative aspects' and 'Physical measures of health' and then branches off each of those showing details about yourself. Try to include as much detail as possible. Your teacher may have equipment such as scales and a blood pressure cuff that you can use. If you don't want to write down your weight decide whether you are underweight, average or overweight and simply write that. You can refer to Unit 8 for help with the physical measures of health.

3 Write down what you need to change in your life and what you are willing to try to change. Draw up a health plan for yourself on a timetable.

4 Look at the plan you have drawn up. Check that the targets you have set yourself are SMART: that is, Specific (not vague and woolly), Measurable, Achievable, Realistic and Time-related (there is a timetable for them). If they are not, improve them.

### Just checking

* Name five aspects of physical health that can actually be measured.
* Why is it important to collect as much information as possible about a person's health, well-being and lifestyle before making recommendations for improvement?
* Why is it important that targets set for improvement are SMART?

# Unit 4 Assessment guide

This unit is assessed by an external test that will use questions from a case study. The case studies will be about people of different ages and you will need to show how they cope physically, intellectually, emotionally and socially in their lives. The questions will include:

* how people grow from babies and develop into adults
* how the sectors that look after our health, social care, community justice and children and young people ensure that we are developing normally
* how the different changes that people experience in their lives affect their health and development
* how illness, disability, socio-economic factors and cultural beliefs affect people's lives
* how lifestyle choices affect health and well-being.

## Time management

* In order to prepare you for the test, your teacher will structure lessons and activities to ensure that you are taught everything you need to know and give you opportunity to develop your understanding. You should make sure that you participate in all of the activities that are organised by your teacher, to ensure you understand all aspects of this unit. This will help you to get good marks in your test.

* Take as many practice tests as you can in preparation for the final test of this unit. This will help you understand how questions will be linked to a case study and how you should structure your answers.

* Although there is no assignment to be produced for this unit, you should make sure that you are well organised, with all your information stored in a folder. This will help you to revise and save time trying to find out the information you are looking for. Revise for a few weeks before the exam, not the night before, as you will not be able to revise everything in a short space of time.

* Be prepared when you take the final test – arrive on time, bring pens and any other equipment you need with you.

## Useful links

* Work experience will be useful as you will be able to see how different sectors provide support for individuals at different stages of the life span. For example, you may visit a children's nursery and see children at different stages of growth and development; you may also see the school nurse visit them to check that they are growing and developing normally. Alternatively, you may visit a care home for older people, where you will see people experience physical change as they age.

* Your teacher may arrange a visit from a health worker, who may explain to you how lifestyle choices – for example, poor diet, lack of exercise, smoking or drug abuse or risky sexual practices – can affect people's health and well-being. If you have any questions about how people of different ages are affected by these factors, don't be afraid to ask. The information will be easy to remember if you have asked a question!

* Some television programmes look at different aspects of people's growth and development. These may range from serious documentaries, for example, *Child of Our Time*, in which Professor Winston follows a group of children as they grow up, looking at how different aspects of their lives are affecting them, or you could watch a soap opera like *Eastenders* and see how unpredictable life events like divorce or bereavement affect people's emotional and physical health.

## Things you might need

* ICT to investigate the work of different organisations that provide support or information about lifestyles. A useful website that provides information on smoking and a healthy diet is www.patient.co.uk. Another useful website that looks at issues that may affect teenagers is www.connexions-direct.com.

* You may need to interview people of different ages about their health and well-being and produce a plan to improve their health. This will help you familiarise yourself with the lifestyle and socio-economic issues that affect health and well-being. In your test you will be given a case study that will ask you to do this. Remember to maintain confidentiality and be sensitive to people's feelings when you carry out this interview.

# How you will be assessed

| You must show that you *know*: | Guidance | To gain higher marks you must *explain*: |
|---|---|---|
| What the physical, intellectual, emotional and social changes are across the lifespan.<br><br>Lifespan usually covers: conception, prenatal, birth–3 years, childhood (4–10 years), adolescence (11–18 years), adults (19–65 years), older adults (65+) and the final stages of life.<br><br>How are people monitored or supported? Think about all the people who make sure that we are fit and well. | ✱ You can remember physical, intellectual, emotional and social changes by the initials PIES. **Don't write PIES in your test** – use the full, correct words.<br><br>✱ An example of key changes that an adolescent may undergo would be:<br>• physical – puberty<br>• intellectual – developing moral values and thinking skills<br>• emotional – developing relationships and becoming independent from the family<br>• social – interacting with others and developing their own identity. | ✱ How the physical, intellectual, emotional and social changes that take place at various stages of life are monitored or supported in any of the four sectors.<br><br>✱ For example: you may be asked who are the people, apart from the family, who make sure an adolescent is developing and maturing normally. Your answer might include: school nurse or GP from the health sector, teachers or Connexions officers from the Children and Young People sector, a social worker from the social care sector or the youth offending team from the community justice sector. You would need to say exactly how they check on growth and development. |
| How life events, including disability or illness, affect people's lives.<br><br>Disability may cause problems not only for physical, intellectual, emotional or social development but may affect life opportunities. For example, a person who uses a wheelchair may find it difficult to get a job, leading to depression and isolation. | ✱ Life events can be predictable (going to school or work, having a relationship, becoming a parent and retiring from work) or unpredictable (suffering from serious illness or bereavement, abuse, divorce or redundancy). | ✱ How life events affect growth and development, and health and well-being at various stages of the life span. Be able to apply this knowledge to different case studies. |
| How different factors affect people's lives. Socio-economic factors include employment, housing, income, education and access to services. All of these factors will affect people's health, well-being and their life opportunities.<br><br>Cultural beliefs or religions also affect the way people live their lives. | ✱ You may be given a case study that describes an adult who is unemployed, living in a crowded house, poorly educated without access to a GP or a dentist. You will need to identify the effect of these factors on health, well-being and opportunities. Think about PIES to help you. | ✱ What are the socio-economic factors (e.g. employment, housing, income, education, access to services) and how they, along with people's beliefs, influence lifestyles. The case studies that you are given in the test will ask you to explain how these factors affect health, well-being and opportunities. |
| How lifestyle choices affect people's lives and how this could be improved.<br><br>For example, if someone stopped smoking, how might this improve their health and well-being? Could you help them by writing them a plan to help them stop smoking? | ✱ Lifestyle choices may include diet, exercise, drug abuse, smoking or unsafe sex.<br><br>✱ Assess your own level of health or another individuals – how could it be improved?<br><br>✱ Remember to maintain confidentiality. | ✱ The impact of lifestyle choices on people's health, well-being and life opportunities. You must make recommendations for how they might improve their lifestyle. |

# Introduction

In this unit you will learn about human needs – physical, intellectual, emotional, social and spiritual – and how those needs are addressed. It covers assessment, and how services are planned and delivered in this context, including the importance of **joint working** across organisations, as well as the involvement of carers and families. How information is gathered, from assessment through to reviewing services delivered, is addressed throughout the unit. The importance of confidentiality is consolidated in topic 5.12.

## Need

In this unit you will learn about human needs – physical, intellectual, emotional, social and spiritual – and how individuals' preferences and choices should influence how their needs are addressed. You will find out why good communication skills are important in working with individuals who often need support and reassurance to express what they think and feel about how their needs might be met, and to ensure appropriate services are provided.

## STREET SCENE

Look at the street scene pictured below and think what might be the needs of the people shown. They are all individuals across a range of ages and life situations. Are their needs all the same? What about you and your needs? Using pictures, notes or a spider diagram, identify what your needs are.

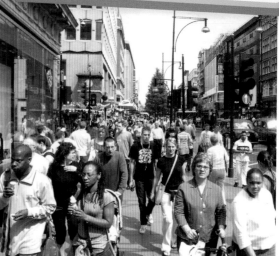

*And what about the needs of people you wouldn't see in the street?*

## Assessment and service delivery

You will learn about the assessment, planning, implementation and review process – how it is used to identify needs and then to plan how to meet needs, by delivering appropriate services. Any services provided are reviewed to check they are effective and meeting the individual's needs. This involves gathering and sharing information along the way from all those involved, through discussion, interviews and meetings.

## Working together

You will have the opportunity to look at case studies across child care, social care, health and criminal justice to help you understand the range of roles involved in the assessment process and how agencies use joint working to provide services. You will also discover how technology is being used to support people, meeting their needs and enabling them to be more independent, feel safer and hopefully have more fulfilling lives. These aspects are developed in topics 5.9 and 5.10.

**Joint working** Agencies working together.

## Diploma Daily

### PC Danny Brown to become Weston estate's new community officer

For the past two years PC Brown has been the community officer for Gladehill, where he was well known. He regularly visited the local primary and secondary schools and spent a morning each week at Gladehill Community Centre, where local residents would come in and talk about their concerns. He worked closely with the youth offending team and the Neighbourhood Watch Scheme. Through the use of interventions such as ASBOs and curfews, Gladehill saw a significant decrease in burglary, drug use and vandalism. He says he looks forward to moving to the Weston estate, where he hopes to repeat his Gladehill success.

1 What needs did the Gladehill community have, and what interventions were used to meet them?

2 Produce a list of ways or use a spider diagram to show how PC Brown could make contact with residents on the Weston estate – from children through to older people – to hear about what the community's needs are.

## How you will be assessed

For this unit you will be assessed by one assignment, which will involve an investigation into the breadth of individual needs and the role of the four sectors in supporting these, followed by the production of a report. In order to do this you need to understand how to carry out primary and secondary research, and then choose three individuals to investigate, with differing needs. Parts of your investigation could involve working in a small group, but the evidence you submit should be entirely your own work.

## What you will learn in this unit

You will:

* Know the breadth of individual needs in terms of emotional, intellectual, mental, physical, social and spiritual needs
* Understand the extent to which individuals' preferences and choices can determine how their needs are addressed
* Understand the importance of working with individuals receiving support and/or services and significant others
* Understand the role of assessment, planning, implementation and review in addressing need and delivering expected outcomes
* Know the information sources used to inform assessments
* Understand how interventions are designed to meet individual and, where relevant, community needs
* Be able to collect and collate information in relation to addressing the needs of individuals

# 5.1 What do we mean by human needs?

In this topic you will find out about basic human needs – including what we need to survive. Beyond survival, however, we also need to feel safe and secure, and to have social interactions and self-esteem.

## What people need

### Maslow's hierarchy of needs

Abraham Maslow (1908–1970) was a **psychologist** who described a pyramid of human needs (though he didn't include spiritual needs). Unless our physical needs are met (e.g. for food and water), we will not survive and so the most important or vital needs are at the bottom of the pyramid. Maslow believed that only when basic needs for shelter, food, water and warmth are met can people progress to the next level of the pyramid. Safety and security needs are the next most important. A small child left alone may feel frightened and insecure, especially if in unfamiliar surroundings. It will be necessary for adults to ensure that children and **vulnerable** adults are not exposed to danger. The next levels relate to social needs, self-esteem and finally, at the top, creativity or intellectual needs.

### Needs checklist

People's needs change. People at different life stages have their own ideas about what their needs are. Most people have clear ideas about how they would like their needs to be met. Some people really enjoy being on their own and seem to have little wish for the company of others. As mentioned above, Maslow did not include spiritual needs in his **hierarchy**; nonetheless, practising a religion can be a very important part of some people's lives.

* *Basic physical* – food and drink which is appropriate, meets dietary and religious requirements and reflects individual likes; accommodation, with heating, which enables people to move around and feel safe; clothing which is clean, comfortable and appropriate to the temperature, weather and activities

* *Safety and security* – living in accommodation which feels safe and secure, with chosen possessions around; sufficient money; privacy

* *Social* – being able to maintain relationships, feel cared for and loved, as well as opportunities to make new friends; having interests and keeping in contact

## THINKING POINT

Imagine a person selling the *Big Issue* outside the local supermarket.

1 What do you think that person's needs might be?

2 Design a poster highlighting some of the difficulties facing people who are homeless.

**Psychologist** Someone who studies the human mind and its functions.

**Vulnerable** A state in which being physically or emotionally hurt is more likely.

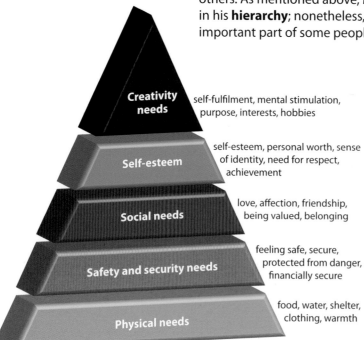

Creativity needs — self-fulfilment, mental stimulation, purpose, interests, hobbies

Self-esteem — self-esteem, personal worth, sense of identity, need for respect, achievement

Social needs — love, affection, friendship, being valued, belonging

Safety and security needs — feeling safe, secure, protected from danger, financially secure

Physical needs — food, water, shelter, clothing, warmth

*Maslow's 'hierarchy of needs' pyramid.*

with family and friends – through visits, telephone calls and email; the opportunity to join a group, try different activities and spend time with family and friends

* *Self-esteem* – feeling good about yourself and being treated with respect and dignity by other people; being treated as a person, with the right to make choices and express thoughts and feelings

* *Creativity* – opportunities to express yourself through words, music or art; the chance to learn and develop new skills and be mentally stimulated, perhaps through hobbies, interests and contact with other people

* *Spiritual* – this is not just about formal religious beliefs – Christianity, Hinduism, Judaism or Islam, among others – but reflects a **philosophy** of life (examples include a peace-loving person and an **environmentalist**).

> **Hierarchy** A system of persons or things arranged in a graded order.
>
> **Philosophy** An attitude that guides a person's behaviour.
>
> **Environmentalist** Someone who is concerned with the protection of the environment.
>
> **Alzheimer's disease** A degenerative disease marked by a loss of memory and decreasing ability to communicate, understand and function normally.

## Case study: Lisa's story

Lisa is 24 and lives in a two-bedroom rented house with her two sons, Sam, aged five years, and Kyle, aged nine months. She moved in three months ago, to live nearer to her mum and sister. Lisa and her partner often had rows and sometimes he hit her. She left after a scary incident when her partner physically assaulted her and neighbours called the police. Lisa and the boys then moved into a women's refuge, where they stayed for nearly three months.

Although Lisa is feeling more settled, she still worries her partner will turn up and demand to see the boys. Her family encouraged Lisa to have a dog. Lisa, with her boys, went to the local RSPCA and found Bruno, a friendly mongrel. Bruno is now part of the family and Lisa enjoys going for walks with the boys and Bruno. This is helping Lisa and her family to make new friends in the area.

Lisa has panic attacks now and again and relies quite a bit on her mum and sister for support. Her granddad, Harry, is, and always has been, special to Lisa. He has **Alzheimer's disease** and lives next door to her mum. Lisa spends as much time with him as she can. Her sister gets very embarrassed when Harry forgets who she is and talks about her granny as if she were still alive.

Lisa wishes she had finished the hairdressing course she started when she left school. She plans to find out about beauty therapy courses at the local college and hopes to get a job when Kyle is three years old.

**1** Draw a copy of Maslow's pyramid and place in it examples of Lisa's needs.

**2** Produce a chart listing Lisa's needs that also indicates whether these are being met or unmet. Include pictures or diagrams to illustrate your work.

## Just checking

* What are the five levels of need identified in Maslow's hierarchy?
* Give three examples of what might help individuals to feel safe and secure.
* Describe what self-esteem means.

# 5.2 Changing needs across the life span

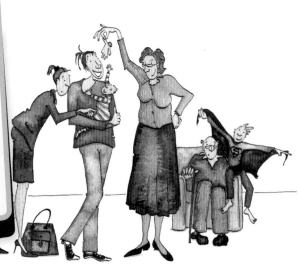

*Lisa's family of four generations. Will they all have different needs?*

In this topic you'll be finding out about changing needs and life stages. Although basic needs are common to us all, at different stages of life some needs may become more important than others and have to be met in a particular way.

## LET'S THINK ABOUT FAMILIES

Look at the picture of Lisa's family (see also Lisa's story from the previous topic) and write down what you think each of them may need in terms of different food requirements.

## Are needs the same for people of all ages?

### Basic physical needs

These are common to all ages but will be met differently:

* *Appropriate food and drink*. Babies need milk and soft foods. Health conditions at any time of life may mean certain foods have to be avoided.
* *Sleep*. The amount of sleep people need tends to decrease with age (babies need a lot of sleep).
* *Good hygiene*. Babies need *everything* doing for them. Most young people and adults can manage their own personal hygiene.

### Safety and security needs

* *Routines*. Babies and young children benefit from certainty and routine.
* *Danger*. Awareness of risks tends to increase with age.

### Social needs

* Babies and young children need attention and interaction with parents/carers to help them develop.
* Play is important for young children and helps them to learn and make friends.
* As children get older, particularly in adolescence, their friendship network usually expands and they form more intimate relationships associated with their sexual development.
* Friendships and supportive relationships are important for adults. When relationships break down or friends and partners become ill or die, loneliness and a sense of isolation may be experienced.

### Self-esteem

* Babies and young children need to be loved and cared for, preferably with some continuity by the same person or people.

## Activity

Talk to different people about what their experience of school, work and family life was like. You may have an opportunity to do this when you are on work placement. Many older people lived through the Second World War and may share with you what their lives were like then.

1 Produce a list of as many life changes and life events as you can, indicating which you think would be the most difficult to cope with.

2 Explain how four of these life changes/events might affect an individual's life or how a family might manage them.

* Children need to feel good about themselves, to be respected and to be encouraged to learn and develop independence.

* Adolescents continue to need support to develop increased independence. Self-esteem is often a problem at this age because of the effects of hormonal changes and body image.

* Adults also need to feel valued and respected, to feel they belong and to have a sense of achievement.

* Older adults have similar needs, but may be especially appreciative of being independent (having control over their lives).

## Effect of life events on needs and preferences

Some **life events** can happen at any time or **life stage**. Examples include the onset of a health condition or having an accident which results in a long-term disability, or the death of a relative or friend. Family break-up would affect all age groups.

### Examples of life events and their effects on needs and preferences

## Diploma Daily

### Older people deserve better care than this

Chief executive of large hospital resigns after reports of appalling neglect in the care of elderly patients. Wards were dirty and patients were left for several hours in soiled sheets and not given appropriate care and attention. An investigation is underway and changes are being introduced to improve the situation. We want to hear from you so please write or email with your comments.

1 Read the *Diploma Daily* headline and using a spider diagram write down your reactions.

2 Describe which human needs are not being met in these wards and explain why.

3 Write a letter to the newspaper expressing what you think about this situation and what needs to happen.

| Life stage | Typical life events | Examples of needs and preferences |
|---|---|---|
| Early childhood (birth to 10 years) | Starting at nursery or a new school, which involves being separated from main carer | Need for some familiar routines and certainty (e.g. food which they enjoy or maybe taking a favourite object or toy with them). These can help a very young child to feel more secure |
| Adolescence | Hormonal changes in puberty (see Unit 4) | Self-esteem and confidence are affected as adolescents may feel less attractive at the same time as they are becoming interested in forming intimate relationships |
| Adulthood | Losing a job through redundancy, retirement, or being unemployed for a long time<br><br>The breakdown of a close relationship, which affects the whole family | May affect how basic needs are met – accommodation, food and sense of security. Reduced income can mean having to move to a smaller house, no longer having a car, having a less active social life<br><br>Loss of self-esteem and confidence may also affect the individual's physical and mental health and put a strain on relationships |
| Older adulthood | Developing a health condition or experiencing the death of someone close | May result in loneliness, loss of confidence and feelings of insecurity. Often reduced income in old age results in basic needs not being fully met – not keeping warm, not eating well, not going out as much and so having less contact with friends |

**Life stage** A distinct period of growth or development in the life span.

**Life events** Any particularly important things which take place or happen during the life span.

### Just checking

* Describe four different life stages.
* Explain how safety and security needs change from early childhood to old age.
* Describe six life events which can make a difference to people's lives.

# 5.3 Individual preferences and choices

In this topic you will discover why it is important to find out about individuals' preferences (their likes and dislikes) and explore how this determines the ways in which their needs might be best addressed.

## Why is it important to find out what each person likes and dislikes?

* Asking someone about their likes and dislikes, and encouraging them to express their preferences, demonstrates respect and acknowledges that we are all unique individuals. Treating everyone the same rarely means that the individual's needs are met.

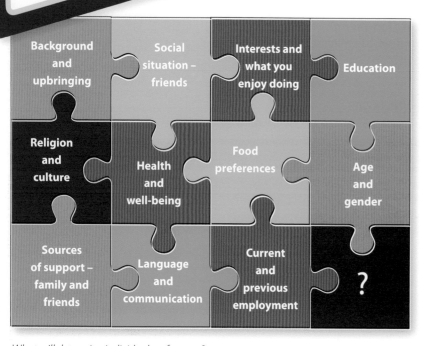

*What will determine individual preferences?*

* Making assumptions about individuals, whether it is about what activities they could get involved in or who they spend time with, may result in getting it wrong. Playing sport or being a spectator may be enjoyable for some, while others will have no interest whatsoever. In residential units, some people will spend most of the day in the communal space and use their room only at night. Others will enjoy the privacy of their own room and join other residents only at mealtimes.

* A person's beliefs, culture and upbringing matter too. Some religions have dietary restrictions; for example, Orthodox Jews, Muslims and Seventh-Day Adventists don't eat pork. And some people won't buy raffle tickets or go for a pub lunch because they think it isn't acceptable. This may also apply to clothing (e.g. Sikh males wearing a turban).

* Individual preferences in terms of food can vary enormously. Some people like spicy food, while others prefer very plain food; some people are vegetarian and so don't eat meat, while others seem to live on hamburgers.

* Individual choice of clothing is also important for most people. Some prefer to dress more formally, to wear a suit and tie, whereas others like to feel casual in jeans. Choice of fabric and colour may also matter.

* Lifestyle choices also influence a person's preferences about health care and treatment options. Rather than take medication prescribed by a doctor for anxiety, for example, an individual might choose to take up yoga and learn relaxation and meditation.

## Activity

1 Talk to three people across different life stages (child, adolescent, adult, older adult) about their likes, dislikes and preferences in terms of food, interests and what they enjoy doing. Write down their answers.

2 Devise a set of questions you could use in an interview for people across different life stages to determine their preferences. Design a grid on which to record their responses. Think about the methods you use to gather information – observation, types of questions (e.g. whether open or closed).

3 Find out when you are on work placement how notes from meetings and interviews are kept – as paper files or on computer?

**Cerebral palsy** A condition caused by brain damage before or at birth which causes difficulty in controlling or moving muscles.

**SCOPE** A disability organisation in England and Wales whose focus is people with cerebral palsy.

* Personal care and how it is managed, as well as who should be able to provide this care, may vary depending on someone's culture and beliefs.

* Feeling secure and comfortable is important too. Some people love meeting new people and going to different places, while others become anxious, often because they don't like change and uncertainty. Keeping windows locked might help someone to feel safe while another person might prefer fresh air and to hear the noise of traffic and people outside.

Remember that it can be difficult for some people to express their preferences. This may be because they are used to others making decisions for them. Empowerment is about providing encouragement and support to enable individuals to say what they like, dislike and what is important to them.

Sometimes health problems will limit the choices an individual can make. Some health factors may determine what individuals eat and what they are able to do. Taking certain medication sometimes means not driving a car, avoiding certain foods and restricting alcohol. Health conditions like diabetes or a food allergy require people to carefully monitor what they eat in order to avoid further problems.

### Personal, learning and thinking skills

This activity may provide evidence of PLTS: Independent enquirer; Reflective learner.

### Functional skills

It may also provide evidence for FS: English, writing.

## Case study: Ashley's story

I'm 12 and love my music – I've got loads of CDs and DVDs and I love watching football with my mates. I can't play as I've got CP – that's **cerebral palsy** – and I use a wheelchair. I live with my mum, dad and my brother, Gary. I go to a school run by **SCOPE**. I'm good with computers. Dad's a builder and he's made my room bigger downstairs so I can get myself around in my chair. I like going to Jamaica for holidays, as that's where my grandparents live and I just love Grandma's rice and peas – well, everything she makes really!

1 Produce a poster showing Ashley's family and interests.

2 Think about two young people you know and compare their likes and dislikes with what you know about Ashley's.

## Just checking

* Why is it important to check with people what their likes and dislikes are?

* Give three examples of how people's preferences in terms of lifestyle and health can affect how their needs are met.

* How might a person's religious beliefs affect their preferences?

# 5.4 Older people's preferences and choices

**THINKING POINT**

In a group, make a list of all the advantages and disadvantages of being an older person in Britain today. First you will need to discuss at what age a person becomes an older person. Can you agree?

In this topic you will find out more about why it is important to check with people what their preferences are and how this may influence ways of addressing their needs. This topic will focus on older people's needs.

## Attitudes towards older people in our society

Older people are very often not treated with respect because they are perceived to be a drain on society – needing lots of support and care from a range of services, including the National Health Service. Opinions like these are a form of **stereotyping**. Other stereotypes of older people include that they all enjoy playing bingo and will be a bit deaf, so that you need to raise your voice when talking to them. These beliefs are obviously inaccurate: each person is a unique individual and this applies to older people too.

The Employment Equality (Age) Regulations 2006 made it unlawful to discriminate against workers, employees, job applicants and trainees because of their age. They also made it unlawful to subject someone to harassment because of their age.

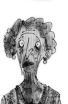
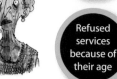

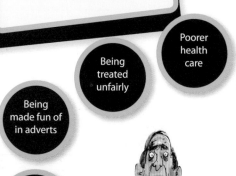

Poorer health care

Being treated unfairly

Pressurised into retiring from work

Being made fun of in adverts

Patronised, even ignored

Treated like children

Refused services because of their age

Feeling excluded, isolated

Made to feel unwelcome because of their age

Told their symptoms are due to getting old

Low confidence and self-esteem

*Age discrimination is a serious matter.*

## Case study: Harry's story

Do you remember Harry, Lisa's granddad? He has lived alone since his wife died five years ago and was independent until about a year ago. He was diagnosed with diabetes two years ago and then was found to have Alzheimer's disease. He had always kept himself fit, enjoyed his garden, gone for long walks with his dog, Nelson, and taken an active role in the local Methodist church. He is well known in the area, as he ran the local greengrocers for 30 years, until he retired. The **community support officer** knows Harry and often stops for a chat.

Mary lives in the house next to Harry and keeps telling his family that he shouldn't be living on his own. She's worried as he goes off for long walks, forgets to lock his door and leaves pans on the cooker. She's frightened that there will be a gas explosion. She has telephoned the RSPCA about his dog, and also the police when Harry wouldn't answer the door one day. Mary thinks Harry should be in a care home. But Harry wants to stay in his own home and his family is happy to help him.

Imagine you were from the local authority social services and were looking into Harry's case. You would first want to talk to him and listen carefully to what he says. You would also involve the family. This would allow you to find out what he enjoys doing, what is important to him, what he can do for himself, what things were proving difficult, and what kind of support might help. Now answer the following questions from the story above:

1 Who might already be helping Harry?

2 What specific things does Harry need help with?

3 Do you think Harry should now go into a residential care home? Give at least two reasons for your answer.

# Problems faced by some older people

## Dementia

There are estimated to be 700,000 people with dementia in Britain, of whom 15,000 are under 65. One in six people over 80 has dementia. Alzheimer's disease is the most common form.

There are no cures for dementia, although some drugs can slow the disease in some patients. The symptoms include loss of memory, increasing difficulty in communicating, reasoning and understanding, with a gradual loss of the skills needed to carry out activities of daily living. Older people without dementia can also face difficulties with these activities.

## Activities of daily living

These include:

* keeping safe
* communication (verbal and using equipment such as telephones, personal alarms)
* personal care (bathing, hair washing, brushing teeth, nail care and toileting)
* eating, drinking, preparing food, cooking
* household tasks such as washing and ironing clothes, cleaning
* managing money (paying bills, dealing with letters)
* getting around the home
* going out and using transport
* leisure activities (reading, keeping fit, going to the cinema, gardening, etc.).

It is important to remember that often a person can manage some aspects of daily living, and will need support with only one or two activities. And while it may take an individual a long time to do something, such as getting dressed, this does not mean they need help with it. Individuals need to be encouraged to identify what it is they can do for themselves and what they need assistance with. More important than anything else for some people can be having a clean, tidy home rather than a busy social life!

**Community support officer**
A uniformed member of the police service but without the powers of a full police officer.

**Stereotyping** Thinking a group of people will all have the same attributes, for example that all older people will be deaf and have memory problems.

### For your project

You could research dementia, and then describe how it affects individuals, explore attitudes to people with dementia, and say what medication and treatments are available.

### Personal, learning and thinking skills

The activity may provide evidence for PLTS: Independent enquirer.

### Activity

1 Make a collage showing how dementia can affect people. Remember to think about activities of daily living.

2 Find out about at least two organisations (one being a voluntary organisation) which provide support to people with dementia and their families.

3 Describe a range of ways to support those affected to continue living at home. If you can, interview a homecare worker or an informal carer who supports a person with dementia and include this in your report.

This activity gives you an opportunity to do research (both primary and secondary) into what support is available in your locality.

### Just checking

* Give three examples of age discrimination.
* List three facts you have learned about dementia.
* Describe how someone might feel as they realise they need others to support them with activities of daily living.

**Braille** A written language of raised dots, used by some blind people.

**Makaton** A system of communication designed for people with learning disability that uses speech together with signs (gestures) and symbols (pictures).

# 5.5 Speak to me, hear me: I matter!

This topic looks at the importance of putting the individual at the centre of any work undertaken with them. This process is often referred to as person-centred planning (PCP). You'll find out about ways of supporting people with a learning disability.

## Communicating and working with individuals

Those who work with people who need their support have to have particular skills. To make service users feel more comfortable in asking for help and advice, they must be the sort of people who:

* listen carefully, give people time to explain and don't tell them what to do
* check with clients that they understand exactly what they are saying
* use language and expressions that the clients are familiar with, and avoid complicated words
* know who to involve with specialist skills, if needed (e.g. translator, British Sign Language interpreter, **Makaton** user)
* provide information in a format clients can access (e.g. enlarged print, **Braille**, audio tape)
* ask clear questions and explain rights, options and where else to go for help
* are trustworthy and treat people with respect.

### Case study: Milly's story

Milly is 26 and has Down's syndrome. She says: 'I may not be able to use the right words, but I need you to listen to me. I can't understand the long words you use and I forget things. But if you take time, and explain things in simple words, then I can manage okay. Pictures help too and in our drama group we use Makaton. A friend of mine, someone I trust, helps me out sometimes too. I know other people are quicker than me. And because I'm slow, you think I can't speak up for myself. But I can and I do. It really matters that you listen to me and hear what I say. Okay?'

Milly recently moved into a house with three other people who also have a learning disability. They chose this house because they like having a garden, in which to grow flowers and have barbecues. Mencap, one of many organisations supporting people with a learning disability, provides workers to help these four young adults, in what is called **supported living**. Milly and her housemates pay rent and enjoy their independence. However, not everyone is as happy about this arrangement. Some of the neighbours have said things like 'They need looking after – they should be in a home', 'Since they moved in, it has reduced the value of our houses' and 'There's men and women in that house – who knows what goes on in there?'

1 What do you think about Milly and her housemates living independently in the community, which most of us assume is our right?

2 What do you think about the comments made by neighbours?

### Valuing People and person-centred planning (PCP)

A key part of the strategy document produced by the government entitled *Valuing People* is about enabling people with a learning disability to lead fulfilling lives. Many people with a learning disability are effectively excluded from the community in which they live. They may have few friends, very limited work opportunities and little choice of housing. They may be dependent on carers, often their family. What many of us take for granted – having a job, enjoying a range of interests as well as being able to form relationships – may not be options for people with a learning disability but *Valuing People* clearly states that these opportunities should be available for everyone.

Four key principles have been identified to tackle these problems:

1 *rights* – ensuring that all individuals are informed of their rights (this will empower them)

2 *independence* – promoting independence for everyone

3 *choice* – offering choice about what support, services and options are available

4 *inclusion* – to lead full and purposeful lives within the community and to develop a range of friendships, activities and relationships.

This approach can be used with all groups of people. It should improve the quality of people's lives.

**Person-centred planning** requires workers to place the individual with a learning disability at the centre, as the expert, involving and including them in any planning and decision making about their lives.

> **Person-centred planning**
> A process of helping people (usually with some form of disability) to find out what is most important to them and what they want from their lives.
>
> **Supported living**
> An arrangement whereby people with a disability can live within the community, with carefully tailored assistance.

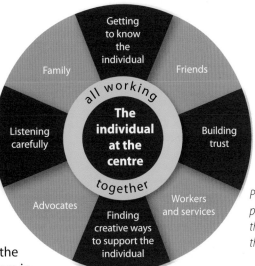

*Person-centred planning places the individual at the centre.*

---

### Activity

A new resource centre has been designed for adults with disabilities; it will offer a range of activities, including sports and drama.

1 Design a poster for young adults like Milly who find written information hard to understand. Use pictures and symbols as much as possible.

2 Do some research about how day centres for people with a disability are changing to become resource centres. Check out what is happening in your area. Produce information about the new centre in two formats – on tape and using pictures with easy-to-read text.

### Personal, learning and thinking skills

The activity may provide evidence of PLTS: Independent enquirers; Creative thinkers; Reflective learners.

### Functional skills

It may also provide evidence for FS: English, writing.

### Just checking

✳ Describe three different ways in which information should be made available so that it is accessible to everyone in the community.

✳ Explain what person-centred planning means.

✳ What is meant by the term 'supported living'?

# 5.6 Informal carers – who are they and what do they do?

In this topic you will discover what is meant by the term 'informal carers' and the important part they play in caring for and supporting individuals to continue living at home.

## Diploma Daily

Dear Dorothy

My wife was only 40 when she was diagnosed with **motor neurone disease**. Last year I gave up my job to look after her full time but it's tough. I hate to see her suffer and I'm exhausted caring for her 24/7. Can you help at all?

Terry

Dorothy's reply:

I suggest you contact the Carers Federation and the Motor Neurone Disease Association. Both organisations will give you useful information. The Carers Federation's adult carer support team listen to carers and explain their rights and where they can access information and services. They will also look at any benefits you might be entitled to. Try to take good care of yourself too.

1 What support might Terry need in caring for his wife?

2 Create a poster illustrating what support informal carers might need.

## Informal carers

Informal carers are people who provide unpaid care for family members, friends and neighbours or others who are sick, disabled or elderly. It is estimated there were six million informal carers in the UK in April 2001, although it is difficult to be certain of the actual number.

Caring for someone can have life-changing effects on the carer. For example, where people are caring for more than 50 hours per week, they are twice as likely not to be in good health as those who are not carers. Around 75 per cent of carers are financially worse off because of their caring responsibilities.

The things carers do include:

* giving medicine
* providing personal care
* helping with mobility
* reading and writing letters
* dealing with bills and other financial matters
* taking people out
* keeping them company
* and sometimes simply keeping an eye on someone.

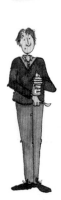
*'I love my mum but sometimes I wish someone would look after me.'*

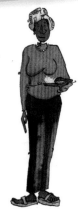
*'Nobody can look after my son as well as me. I'm his mum – it's my duty.'*

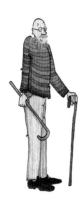
*'My wife looked after me when I was ill and so it's my turn now. It's not easy though when she doesn't know who I am.'*

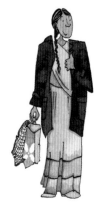
*'My son is very good – he comes to help his dad have a shower and he takes me shopping.'*

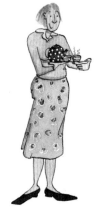
*'She's been my neighbour for 20 years and helped a lot when my children were at school.'*

*Informal carers and what they have to say.*

## Why do informal carers look after their relatives and friends?

* Carers are concerned about services not meeting the needs of the people they care for.

* There are no appropriate services available in the area or within easy access.

* They feel a sense of duty and responsibility to provide care for family members.

* Simply because supporting someone they love and care about matters to them and they want to do it.

* They can provide continuity of care and ensure the person is properly looked after on a one-to-one basis.

* They, and the people they care for, are worried about the quality of care provided by the NHS and other organisations following recent reports about infection rates and poor hygiene in some hospitals as well as other agencies providing care services.

## Young carers – some facts and figures

Not all informal carers are adults! The average age of a young carer is 12. The UK 2001 census found that there were 175,000 young carers, 13,000 of whom cared for over 50 hours per week. Over half of these young carers lived in one-parent families and almost a third cared for someone with a mental health problem.

> **Motor neurone disease**
> A progressive, incurable, degenerative disease that leads to weakness and wasting of muscles.
>
> **Epilepsy** A disorder of the nervous system that causes convulsions and/or periodic loss of consciousness.

> **Personal, learning and thinking skills**
>
> The case study questions may give evidence of PLTS: Independent enquirer; Reflective learner.

---

## Case study: Peter's story

Peter is 13 years old. This is a page from his diary:

7.30 a.m. Woke up, checked Mum was OK, got her tablets ready with a cup of tea and some toast.

8 a.m. Helped my little sister, Penny, get ready for school, made some tea and toast, checked Mum was all right.

8.45 a.m. Dropped Penny off at her school then ran for the bus but just missed it.

9.10 a.m. Late for school and told off again by the teacher.

Couldn't concentrate all morning as I'm worrying about how to pay the gas and phone bills.

Lunchtime: Rang to check Mum was OK and what to get from the shop for tea.

4 p.m. Collect Penny and go and buy food for tea – tins of beans and a loaf of bread and some ice cream.

5 p.m. Get home and start making tea, talk to mum, who is feeling pretty bad today and try hard to stop Penny hassling Mum.

7.30 p.m. Time to get Penny ready for bed – she's only 7. Read her a story but she won't settle, keeps calling me.

8.30 p.m. Mum went for a bath half an hour ago – need to check she is OK – she's got severe **epilepsy**.

9.30 p.m. Mum goes to bed, Penny is asleep at last and now I'm too shattered to do my homework... again.

1 Produce a collage or drawing which illustrates the demands on a young carer like Peter.

2 Research organisations which support young informal carers. Produce a fact sheet signposting where a young carer could go for help and advice. Reflect on what you have learned from this research, particularly about young carers, after reading about Peter's typical day.

---

## Just checking

* Why might informal carers provide support to their relatives, friends and neighbours?

* How many informal carers are there estimated to be in the UK?

* What is motor neurone disease?

# 5.7 Assessment, planning, implementation and review (APIR)

This topic looks at what the process of assessment, planning, implementation and review (APIR) involves. The focus here is on health care, but APIR can be applied across all sectors. The single assessment process is included here, as this is how information is gathered and used to plan effective ways of meeting an individual's needs and providing appropriate services. The monitoring of services to check whether they are meeting the individual's needs is dealt with in topic 5.11.

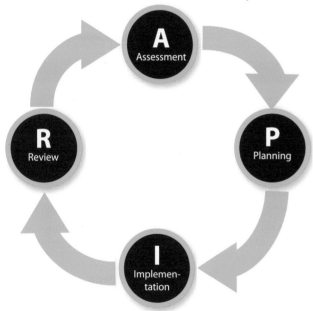

*The APIR cycle.*

**Assessment** The gathering and evaluation of information in order to be able to understand a particular situation.

**Planning** Setting out detailed proposals for doing or achieving something.

**Implementation** Putting a decision or plan into action.

**Review** To look at something again with a view to improving it.

## Assessing need and delivering outcomes

### APIR

What do you do when you don't feel well? Let's imagine you've been feeling sick and dizzy. Where or to whom do you go for help and advice? You decide to see your GP…

Your doctor will make an **assessment** of your health problem by both observing you and asking you questions. She may decide to examine you by looking at your ears, eyes or throat. She may also take your temperature or blood pressure.

When she has all the information she thinks she needs, she starts **planning** what action to take, including whether medication would help. Her plan is to prescribe some medication for vertigo, which she thinks may be the problem. She explains how you should take the medication and says to come back and see her if you don't improve within the next few days.

You follow your doctor's advice. This is the **implementation** of her plan.

You go back to see your doctor five days later as you still don't feel well. The doctor does a **review** of her original assessment (diagnosis) and treatment plan. She decides to refer you to a specialist and also writes out another prescription for different medication which she thinks may be more effective. She suggests you arrange to see an optician for an eye test too.

Note that the review involves further assessment and the production of a revised plan. The APIR process is in fact a cycle, as shown in the diagram.

## SAP

The single assessment process (SAP) aims to ensure a good understanding of all an individual's needs.

* **Eligibility criteria** are used to decide whether an individual qualifies for a service.

* Qualification for a service depends on the level of need.

* There is no charge for the actual assessment but there may be a charge for services provided.

### Case study: Karl's story

Karl is 84 and lives alone following his wife's sudden death last year. His daughter, Linda, lives in Canada and phones him every week. Peter, his son, is 49, has multiple sclerosis and lives in a residential home mile 15 miles away.

Eight years ago Karl had a stroke, which affected both his speech and his mobility. Speech therapy and physiotherapy really helped him but recently walking and going upstairs have become difficult. He says he knows he needs some help. Karl's niece visits weekly, does his shopping and takes Karl to see Peter when she can.

The district nurse, Jan, is visiting daily as Karl has developed leg ulcers, which need frequent changes of dressings. She observes that Karl often cries when talking about his wife and seems depressed. He says he is lonely and always tired as he doesn't sleep well on the settee and can't get upstairs to sleep in bed. He isn't eating much and is unsteady on his feet. Jan is concerned that Karl is at risk and suggests that the GP visits to check him over. She asks Karl if she can also refer him to social services so that someone, maybe either an occupational therapist or a social worker, can visit and assess his situation to see what services could be offered.

Karl agrees and the social worker, Amardeep, visits. He explains about the **single assessment process** (SAP), which he completes. The SAP aims to ensure a good all-round understanding of Karl's needs, including risk factors, such as, in his case, likelihood of falls, not eating properly and being depressed.

A plan is drawn up based on the assessment and the following services are provided:

* An occupational therapist will visit to assess which aids and possible adaptations will help with Karl's mobility, falls prevention and generally how to manage activities of daily living.

* Homecare workers will call every morning to check Karl is okay and to make his breakfast and prepare something for his lunch.

* The district nurse will call daily to do dressings and will monitor Karl's health and well-being and also whether the **care package** is working effectively.

1 List the services that have been offered to Karl.

2 Explain what the risk factors are in Karl's situation and how they are being addressed through the care package.

3 Why is Jan, the district nurse, monitoring Karl?

### Activity

1 Find out about a range of daily living aids which might benefit Karl and produce a poster with illustrations which could be displayed in a health centre, describing how these aids can be used.

2 Describe and explain with illustrations how six daily living aids can be used. Find out about the role of the occupational therapist and how they assess what aids would benefit people like Karl. This information could be produced as a booklet.

### Personal, learning and thinking skills

The activity tasks will provide evidence for PLTS: Independent enquirer; Creative thinker.

**Care package** A collection of services to be provided to help an individual to maintain their independence, living in their own home.

**Eligibility criteria** A set of conditions which, if met, means someone can receive a service.

**Single assessment process** Sharing information about an individual and their needs, with the aim of having a good all-round understanding of the individual's needs.

### Just checking

* Explain what assessment involves.
* What is the SAP?
* Explain what APIR means.

# 5.8 Practice with children and young people

In this topic you will find out more about the assessment part of the APIR process. Here, it is applied in addressing the needs of children and young people through the provision of appropriate services. This links with Units 6 and 7.

## Outcomes

The government paper *Every Child Matters* (see topic 7.6) stated that five outcomes are important for all children:

* being healthy – enjoying good physical and mental health and having a healthy lifestyle

* staying safe – being protected from harm and neglect and growing up able to look after themselves

* enjoying and achieving – getting the most out of life and developing broad skills for adulthood

* making a positive contribution – to the community and to society and not engaging in antisocial or offending behaviour

* economic well-being – not being prevented by economic disadvantage from achieving their full potential in life.

## The assessment process for children and young people

In children's services, several types of assessment are in use. *Every Child Matters* recommends the use of the Common Assessment Framework (CAF). It applies to services for children and young people, covering education, health and social services, youth offending teams and Connexions, as well as others. It offers several advantages:

* It provides a standardised approach to assessment across services.

* It gives a holistic view of a child's needs and strengths.

* It reduces the number of different assessments being done.

* It facilitates early intervention.

* It should improve service delivery.

## PARENTS NEED HELP

What do you think helps parents in bringing up their children? You could begin with a sheet of paper and draw a mind map with the parent in the centre and then write down all your thoughts. Compare your ideas with those of other students and see whether you have similar thoughts.

## For your project

Do research to find out more about projects like the 'one-stop shop' mentioned in the snapshot opposite. You could ask other students what they think about projects of this kind. Work placements will give you a chance to find out what is happening locally.

Labels around the triangle:

Health
Emotional and social development
Behavioural development
Identity
Family and social relationships
Self-care skills and independence
Learning

Basic care, ensuring safety and protection
Emotional warmth and stability
Guidance and boundaries

Development of the baby, child or young person
Parents and carers
Family and environment

**Child**

Family history, functioning and well-being
Wider family
Housing, employment and financial considerations
Social and community elements and resources

*Common Assessment Framework – the assessment triangle (adapted from Nottingham City Council website, http://www.nottinghamcity.gov.uk*

## Case study: Lisa's story

Let's look at the earlier part of Lisa's story from topic 5.1. Lisa and her partner had always had a stormy relationship. The health visitor was concerned about Lisa, who had depression after she had Sam. Lisa and Sam would often go and stay with her mum for several days at a time. This helped and gradually things improved with her partner until Lisa discovered she was pregnant again. They had a violent argument when Lisa was six months pregnant, and the police were called. Lisa's neighbour had rung 999. Lisa's partner was charged with assault.

The health visitor made a referral to social services and after an assessment Lisa's family was offered support, including access to a children's centre, a **Home-Start** volunteer and details about a local women's support group.

Kyle was a premature baby and weighed only 1.8 kg. Three months later Lisa and her boys moved into a women's refuge.

**1** List the services that had become involved with Lisa and her family.

**2** What do you think the assessment identified as Lisa and her children's needs, and how they might be met?

**3** Produce a poster showing what support a children's centre can offer to families like Lisa's and find out more about what an individual job role involves, for example a health visitor or play worker.

### How problems are identified and appropriate action taken

Once a referral to children's services (social services) is made in a situation such as Lisa's, a full assessment is then undertaken. This could be a new assessment or an addition to an existing CAF assessment that perhaps had been started by the health visitor after Sam was born and Lisa became depressed.

As the CAF assessment triangle shows, an assessment must look at the *child* at the centre. It should: examine the child's development; identify any areas of concern; and look at what needs to be put in place to support the family and address the unmet needs.

This assessment must also consider any child protection and safety issues. Most parents will recognise any difficulties they are having in caring for their child. They will work in partnership with social workers and any other agencies to put together a package of support. In serious cases the local authority can trigger court proceedings and apply for a care order with a view to removing the child from the parents' care. Early intervention is really important in such cases. However, the aim is, wherever possible, to keep children with their families, as long as this is safe. The welfare of the child is always **paramount**.

Legislation requires that the child's wishes and needs must be taken into consideration when making decisions. They won't always be followed, as, for example, a child may be too young to understand all the issues properly. When a child is identified as having more serious or special needs, then specialist assessments are arranged.

A wide range of services are available to children, young people and families: after-school clubs; children's centres; nurseries; speech and language therapy; Home-Start volunteers; Compass; teenage clinics; Parentline; Childline; Connexions; youth offending teams; CAMHS; interpreting and translation services; Citizens Advice Bureau; literacy classes; debt counselling; health visitors; women's groups.

**Home-Start** A charity that provides informal and friendly support for families with young children.

**Paramount** More important than anything else.

### Snapshot

New projects are being set up all the time and a key theme of *Every Child Matters* – integrated services – is reflected in a project within a school in Sunderland offering a 'one-stop shop'. This provides a 'healthy living' centre and a neighbourhood nursery for children between three months and three years. It plans also to provide a child and adolescent mental health service (CAMHS) and several community activities.

### Just checking

❋ What are the five outcomes listed in *Every Child Matters*?

❋ Describe the links between the five outcomes and Maslow's hierarchy of needs.

❋ List three of the advantages of the Common Assessment Framework.

**Diploma Daily**

Usha Khanna, a young Asian woman on the waiting list for a kidney transplant, was last night injured in a hit-and-run accident. Police are appealing for witnesses to contact them.

Who gets involved in situations like this?

# 5.9 How multidisciplinary working links to APIR: a health sector example

This topic looks at what happens when there is a health emergency and how different organisations work together to assess the level of need and risk, then plan, implement and deliver appropriate services.

## Care plans and interventions: the nursing example

Different services are involved in emergencies of the kind reported above in the *Diploma Daily* and each has its own approach and terminology. Care plans in a social care setting are the equivalent of the nursing plan: each identifies who will do what to support and enable the individual to achieve, maintain or recover their independence. It is important to stress that all staff involved should work together in the best interests of the individuals affected, including the community.

The Royal College of Nursing states that nursing interventions are concerned with empowering people, and helping them to achieve, maintain or recover independence. The nursing process has five stages:

* Assessment – collecting information about the patient from observation, interviews, reports and tests.
* Diagnosis – a statement of the actual or potential health problem.
* Planning – helping the patient to set goals, setting priorities and identifying the nursing tasks.
* Intervention/implementation – where the nursing plan is put into action.
* Evaluation of the intervention – including a reassessment.

As you can see, it is very similar to APIR.

## What is a care plan?

* It is a description of an individual's needs and indicates how these needs are to be met.
* It lists the services which need to be organised to meet these needs.
* It states what is to happen, who should do what, and when.
* It is an action plan in working with service users, as well as a written agreement and a legal document.
* It is written in a format that is easy to read, in order to be more helpful to the service user.

Care plans are generally used in the health and social care sectors. The other sectors have their own equivalents.

*An extract from Usha's care plan.*

| Name: USHA KHANNA | Date of birth: 14 May 1977 |
|---|---|
| Address and tel no: | |
| Next of kin: mother, Sunita Khanna | Tel no: |
| Client needs, abilities and wishes | Action/support required |
| Personal care, food preparation and meals<br>Assistance with medication | Needs support but her mother is prepared to provide this and Usha is pleased with this arrangement |
| Health needs – dialysis at the local hospital 3 times per week. Needs transport while her father and brother are away in India | Amordeep to contact the volunteer section to arrange for this |

The looked after children (LAC) system uses the term 'assessment and action record'. This focuses on aspects of development in a child or young person's life – health, identity, social presentation, emotional and behavioural development, education, family and social relationships and self-care skills.

Mental health assessment and support outside hospital uses the term 'care programme approach', which assesses the individual's health and social care needs. A key-worker is allocated as the main contact point. The individual's progress is monitored and regularly reviewed, and changes are made to the plan as agreed.

Person-centred planning (PCP) is from *Valuing People*, the government's plan for improving the lives of people with a learning disability, and of their families and carers (see topic 5.5). It applies only to England.

> **Appendicitis** Inflammation of the appendix, which is a small tube of tissue attached to the lower end of the large intestine.
>
> **Dialysis** The purifying of blood, as a substitute for the normal function of the kidney.

## Good practice and care plans

### The service user

The rights of the individual receiving a service include: being offered a choice of how the services are arranged; knowing how and when the services will be monitored and reviewed; and being informed how to complain if they are unhappy about any aspect of the service.

### The service provider

Health and social care workers should:

* follow the care plan, reading it carefully to check for any changes, remembering it is a legal document
* make notes on the care plan which are easy to read
* ensure any entries that they make have been signed and dated, and are legible
* report to their manager any changes in the individual's situation and any cause for concern.

> **Personal, learning and thinking skills**
>
> The case study questions may give you evidence towards PLTS: Creative thinker.

> **Functional skills**
>
> They may give you evidence for FS: English, writing; ICT, if you word-process your material.

## Case study: Usha's story

Let's take up Usha's story after the report in the *Diploma Daily*. As Usha's discharge from hospital approaches, a social worker, Jenny, discusses with her any support she thinks she might need on her return home, where she lives with her mum and dad and brother. This assessment is used to write the care plan. Usha needs a care package to enable her to manage at home and this is reviewed after an agreed period, and adjustments are made.

Two weeks later, the care plan was working well, but then, crisis! Usha's mother is rushed into hospital with acute **appendicitis**, which requires an operation. Usha's father and brother are in India visiting relatives and so Usha needs support urgently. Usha's care plan has to be adjusted. Her current needs are quite complex. They include support with personal care and other activities of daily living, such as food preparation, continuing support with transport to attend the hospital for **dialysis**, and assistance with medication.

The care plan will need to be reviewed again when her family returns home from India. Her mother's needs will also have to be considered when she is ready for discharge home.

1 Why is it important that Usha's care plan is reviewed?

2 Think of someone you know, or make up the case of an individual, who needs support and write what you think their needs are. Produce a simple care plan. Describe how you would check with the individual that the care plan is accurate.

3 If you are on a work placement, discuss with workers how care plans are used in their setting.

## Just checking

* Describe what a care plan is and how it is used.
* *Valuing People* was written to improve whose lives?
* Give two reasons why a care plan may need to be adjusted.

Lisa (from topic 5.8) was assaulted when she was six months pregnant and a neighbour called the police. Their **intervention** helped to control what was potentially a dangerous situation. Can you think of other interventions where the police provide support to people, individually or in groups, as well as protecting members of the community?

# 5.10 Service delivery and how this is designed to meet individual and community needs

The assessment of needs applies just as much to the justice sector as it does to the other sectors. This topic considers one such case and looks at the issue of community protection and how interventions with offenders are designed to meet individual needs and, wherever possible, community needs. This topic links with Unit 6.

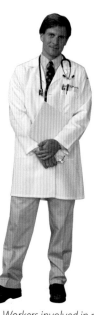 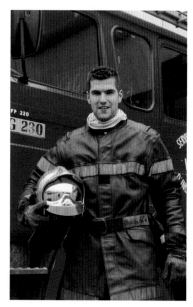 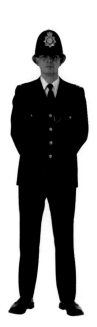

*Workers involved in protecting the community.*

**Intervention** Something done to prevent or improve or control a situation.

**Multidisciplinary** Made up of professionals of different types (often from different agencies) working together to deliver services.

## Case study: Chris's story

An elderly man, Mr Jones, hears the sound of breaking glass and realises his car is being broken into. He rushes out of his house, shouting, and a youth, whom he recognises, runs off. The police are called and a 15-year-old, Chris, is arrested later that evening. Chris is well known to the community protection service. Over the past few months he, along with four other local youths, has been involved in acts of vandalism, including damaging property on the estate and writing graffiti on garage doors.

Just as with service providers we have looked at in the health and social care sectors, the youth offending team (YOT) has to assess Chris's needs. The purpose here is to try to decide what will be the most appropriate action to take, given the nature of his offence.

Chris and his family are interviewed and assessed. The YOT worker, the police and the Youth Inclusion Support Panel (YISP) discuss whether an acceptable behaviour contract (ABC) would be a positive option to try to prevent Chris re-offending and committing further acts of antisocial behaviour. They decide that it is and that the ABC should cover four key points to which Chris must agree. These read as follows:

1 I will attend school.
2 I will write letters of apology to the victims.
3 I will not damage property.
4 I will not write graffiti.

Included in the ABC is the action to be taken if Chris does not comply. All involved, including Chris, sign the agreement and copies are given to all the agencies involved in monitoring Chris's behaviour. Monitoring and evaluating the ABC are important and require all agencies to communicate with each other, as they collect and share information in their **multidisciplinary** working. If Chris does not fulfil all the conditions he signed up to, it could result in a court appearance, where an application would be made for an antisocial behaviour order (ASBO) or a curfew. A curfew would impose restrictions on when Chris could be out in the community. It might state he could not go out between 7 p.m. and 7 a.m., as this is the time when he has offended.

The Community Protection Service applies for ASBOs for adults as well as young people. ASBOs are intended to protect the community and are used where an individual has been warned repeatedly and possibly convicted on numerous occasions for antisocial behaviour. Such behaviour can include being abusive, being drunk, begging, public order offences, criminal damage, assault and burglary. ASBOs are discussed in Unit 6.

1 Design a poster showing what you consider to be antisocial behaviour and how it affects the local community.

2 Describe four ways in which individuals might be supported in addressing their antisocial behaviour and how these interventions might also meet the needs of the community. Give examples indicating which organisations and workers are involved.

## Personal, learning and thinking skills

The case study tasks may provide evidence for PLTS: Creative thinker; Independent enquirer.

## Snapshot

Here are some examples from across the country of new ways of working and good practice.

* Parenting coordinators provide support for parents whose children are supervised by the local YOT.

* In the BUSTED project, run by Staffordshire YOT, young people who had committed burglaries work with volunteers from the local community to produce posters that are displayed on local buses, advising the community about things burglars look for when deciding which properties to target.

* The Blackpool YOT has a project that links the local community with young people on reparation orders. They have produced a mural on a warehouse wall, for example. Reparation orders are designed to help young offenders understand the consequences of their offending and take responsibility for their behaviour.

## Just checking

* Give three examples of how the police provide support and protection to the community.

* Describe what a curfew is.

* List three organisations involved in supporting young offenders.

**THINKING POINT**

Try to remember some of the comments teachers have made about you in a school report or during an open evening. Was that an opportunity to monitor and review your progress?

# 5.11 Keeping track of interventions

In this topic you will learn more about how services provided are monitored and reviewed to ensure they are effective and are meeting individuals' needs. It also looks at interventions based on assistive technology and how these are designed to meet individual needs.

A range of daily living aids which can make everyday tasks safer and more manageable. These include items such as:

* folding walking sticks
* walking frames with net bag to hold items or shopping
* swivel shower seats
* power lifting cushions
* long-handled shoehorns
* large pill dispensers
* sound magnifiers
* folding book and magazine stands
* magnifiers with light
* easyswitches
* handiplugs
* two-handled cups and saucers.

| Client's name: | Monitoring officer details | Date: |
|---|---|---|
| Any changes in needs or circumstances? | | |
| Health and well-being | | |
| Family support | | |
| Finances | | |
| Emotional needs | | |
| Client's feelings about services being received | | |

*A form for monitoring the delivery of the care package.*

## Monitoring and review of the services delivered

### Monitoring
Monitoring involves checking on progress, whether services provided are effective and meeting the service user's current needs. Sometimes an individual's situation alters and the care plan will need to be revised. If the situation improves greatly, it may result in the service being reduced; if the individual has recovered and is able to manage without this support it can even be withdrawn.

### Review
Monitoring is an ongoing process and should be done throughout the time a service is delivered. In contrast, reviews of the services delivered are held at regular intervals. They should include all the key people involved – service providers, carers and family members – and the service user. The aim of a review (usually a meeting) is to look at the overall situation and consider whether the service user's needs are being met in the most appropriate and effective way. Information presented at a review is recorded (e.g. minuted – see topic 2.6) and kept on file, to be referred to at the next review. Review meeting dates can be adjusted if there is a significant change in the service user's situation.

### How things can change
In topic 5.2 we looked at how things can happen which alter people's life situation. Harry and Lisa experienced changes which really made a

difference to their lives. The difficult and violent relationship between Lisa and her partner resulted in the family's needs being assessed and plans being made to provide appropriate support and services (topic 5.8). Harry's deteriorating health and the onset of dementia meant Harry found it difficult to continue living independently (topic 5.4). We can explore how his situation has been monitored and reviewed. Jane's story provides another example.

> **Residential home** A place where people (adults or children) live and are cared for and supported by staff with social care (not health) training.

## Case study: Harry's story one year on

While Harry was still in hospital following an operation to amputate his left leg below the knee (because of complications from his diabetes), his needs were assessed. It was apparent he needed to be placed in a **nursing home** rather than a **residential home**. His social worker, Angela, involved Harry in deciding on which nursing home he should move to. They chose one with a garden, near where he used to live.

A review was held six weeks after Harry's move to the nursing home; it was attended by Angela and nursing home staff. The care/nursing plan was reviewed and ways to improve Harry's quality of life were identified. The team agreed that Harry might need a wheelchair, to enable him to spend more time in communal areas and go into the garden. If Harry agrees, an appointment could be made for him to see an occupational therapist to assess whether appropriate equipment (**assistive technology**), including mobility aids such as a wheelchair, would help Harry to be as independent as possible.

They also agreed that Harry should remain in the nursing home and that a further review should take place in six months' time.

**1** Who should attend the further review in six months' time?

**2** How is Harry's care monitored and who does this during the six months before the next review?

## Case study: Jane's story

Jane, 52, became very distressed when she was told that her father is terminally ill. Her parents are in their late 70s and live nearby. Jane's mother is deaf, has severe rheumatoid arthritis, uses a wheelchair to get round the house and is very dependent on her husband, who is now so ill himself that he cannot provide her with the support she needs. She contacts her local social services department, which arranges for Jane's mother to attend an Age Concern day centre five days a week. Social services have a range of assistive technology equipment in the home to support Jane's mother and additional home-care support is arranged. Working in partnership with the health services, they also make arrangements for Jane's father to attend a local **hospice** day centre. When his health deteriorates and he needs to stay in bed most of the time, the hospice community care team provide further support at home. Jane's mother continues to attend the Age Concern day centre, but Jane worries about who will look after her mother now.

**1** Why is it important to monitor and regularly review the services delivered to support Jane's parents?

**2** Find out what hospice care can offer and how this service tries to meet individual needs and preferences.

## For your project

You could find out more about assistive technology (AT), including information about a range of products and services and the ways in which they can improve individuals' lives. If you enjoy ICT and want to learn more about how computer software is being used in AT, then this project idea may appeal to you.

> **Nursing home** A place where adults can live with medical care provided under the supervision of nursing staff.
>
> **Assistive technology** Any product or service designed to enable independence for disabled and older people. Examples include a Zimmer frame, grab rails, shower stool, pendant and sensor alerts in case of falls.
>
> **Hospice** A home or service providing care and support for people who are sick or terminally ill.

## Just checking

* Why is it important to monitor services?
* What is the purpose of a review?
* Give three examples of assistive technology.

# 5.12 What about all the information collected?

This topic explains how information is collated in relation to addressing individuals' needs, as well as how it is maintained and stored. You know from earlier topics that information is collected and built up over time by observing individuals in interviews, asking questions and recording their responses. This information is noted down and kept on file and may also be logged on computer. This topic has links with Unit 2.

### Collecting information to address needs

Much information can be collected by observing how people relate to and interact with others through verbal and non-verbal communication – their facial expressions, gestures, body posture, how at ease they are and whether they are attentive or easily distracted. This is especially true of children's play, and observation can be a key skill for those working with young children.

Interviews provide an opportunity to ask questions as well as to listen attentively to responses. Sometimes, what is not said in an interview is as significant as what is said. How interviews are arranged, timed and where they take place can affect how successful they are.

The use of questioning requires some skill. For example, different responses may be obtained when closed questions are asked as opposed to open questions. If you are patient and sensitive, the use of open questions can encourage the individual to share more information.

Research involves carrying out an investigation into a particular subject. Primary research involves the collection of data that doesn't already exist. Observation and asking questions are techniques used in primary research. Secondary research is where you use information that other people have gathered through primary research. It is usually done by reading up on a subject, in books, journals and on the Internet, and so on.

### Computers and their value in collating and storing information

Most large organisations now use computers for storage of information and this has become important in the sharing of information between

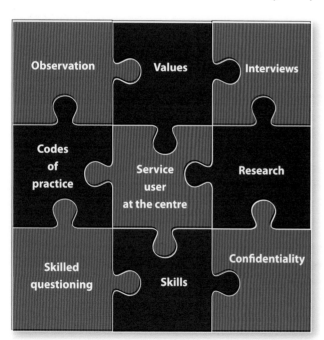

*How it all fits together.*

agencies. It is a critical aspect of working in partnership and in the best interests of service users.

Databases are used by organisations to maintain information about agencies providing services in their area. Surveys of service users' views about the service and treatment they receive, especially from large organisations such as a local authority and the health service, are also stored on computer and are used to assess the organisation's work practice. The Department of Health and other government departments collect statistics on service use.

ContactPoint is being developed and should be available to all local authorities in England during 2008. It will hold basic information about all children up to the age of 18 in England, including details of their parents or carers, contact details for other services involved and whether an assessment has been done under the Common Assessment Framework (see topic 5.8). Access to ContactPoint will be for **authorised users** only, and only when they need it for their work.

Workers who disclose information or break confidentiality may be in breach of the **codes of practice** which apply to their work as well as the Data Protection Act 1998.

## Snapshot

Before offering anyone a post where they will have substantial contact with children, young people or vulnerable adults, a **CRB** check must be done. This also applies to volunteers in these settings and individuals applying to become either foster carers or Adult Placement Scheme carers. Foster carers support children and young people in the foster carers' own home. In the Adult Placement Scheme, approved individuals are registered, like foster carers, to provide support in their own homes to adults with a learning disability.

## Activity

1 Produce a simple information sheet entitled 'Good Practice When Using a Computer'. The sheet should be for staff working in one of the four sectors – health, social care, children and young people or criminal justice.

2 Give three reasons why sharing information about individuals between agencies is important.

3 Devise a booklet entitled 'Good Practice in Sharing Information'. Make reference to the codes of practice on workers' responsibilities.

Work placement should provide an opportunity for you to find out how records are maintained and stored.

**Authorised users** People with official permission to use something, such as a computer database.

**CRB** The Criminal Records Bureau. The Bureau will search its files to identify job applicants who may be unsuitable for certain work, especially work involving children or vulnerable adults.

**Codes of practice** Sets of standards of conduct for workers and employers across the four care sectors.

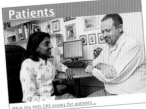

**NHS Connecting for Health**

Home | Accessibility

# NHS Care Records Service

Welcome to the NHS Care Records Service home page.

The NHS Care Records Service (NHS CRS) will improve the safety and quality of patient care.

It will give health care staff faster, easier access to reliable information about patients to help with their treatment.

Please follow the link below to the site you want to visit.

**Patients**

**NHS Staff**

What the NHS CRS means for patients …

© Crown C

Copyright WAI-A

*The National Health Service is in the process of developing a national database, the Care Records Service.*

## Just checking

✳ Give four examples of what you might observe when conducting an interview.

✳ Explain the difference between primary and secondary research.

✳ What are open-ended questions?

# Unit 5 Assessment guide

This unit will be assessed by an assignment, which is marked by your teacher. You will need to show that you understand that people have different needs. These needs will include physical, intellectual, emotional, social, spiritual and mental needs. You will also need to show how Maslow's hierarchy reflects these needs. Often, people have different preferences and choices about how their needs are met by organisations dealing with health, social care, community justice and children and young people. This might depend on their beliefs, their wish to be independent, the support they need and how much help they receive from their family and friends. You must show that you understand how important these preferences and choices are and how important it is to work with the individual and their family. You will be asked to look at the needs of three different individuals as part of your assignment; these could be in the form of a case study, following a character on the TV or by interviewing real people. When practitioners from the four sectors work with individuals, they write a care plan, based on different sources of information. You will need to do this for the three individuals you have studied. Sometimes services need to take action to ensure the well-being of the individual or the community. This is called an intervention and might include foster care for children, respite care for older people or antisocial behaviour orders for those who are a problem in their community. You will need to consider what possible interventions may be needed for the three individuals you have studied. You will also need to show how you have collected and collated all of the information you have used when studying the needs of the three individuals. You will have used both primary and secondary research and will have used a mixture of ICT and files in which to keep this information and use it to write your report.

## Time management

* Manage your time well as you have to assess the needs of three different people and show how these needs are met. For instance, you may investigate the needs of a small child, an older person, a victim of crime, or a teenager seeking contraceptive advice. You will need to find out what their needs are, how an individual's choice is respected and what type of information is required to design a care plan. You will also need to consider what interventions may be needed.

* Be well organised. This is your chance to show that you are an independent enquirer and a self-manager and therefore will contribute towards achievement of your personal, learning and thinking skills. Ensure that you keep any class work safely, for example interviews that you have carried out or notes that you have made about the needs of an individual. This research will need to be collated in a folder or in an electronic format, ready to be written up as a report.

* Be prepared with a list of questions that you could ask if your teacher arranges for a speaker to come and talk to your class. For example, you may be able to speak to a social worker who produces care plans for a variety of different people with different needs. They may explain how different people are involved in planning care, including the individual receiving services, their family, their carers and other professionals. This could contribute towards your primary research.

## Useful links

* There are lots of useful websites that will help with your investigation of the care and support that individuals can access. For example, voluntary organisations such as Age Concern or SCOPE explain what they do and what services they can offer.

* You can also get lots of information from your local council in the form of leaflets or via the Internet, describing the types of social care services they can help with. This is secondary research.

* Work experience will also be useful, as you will meet people who have different needs and require care or support from a variety of services. For example, if you visit a day centre attended by people who have a learning disability, you may see what other social care services they receive and be involved in devising a care plan for them. This might include transport arrangements to the centre, the care they need while at the centre and the care they receive when at home. Remember to be sensitive to others' feelings and to maintain confidentiality.

* You may have a relative who receives care or support who may be happy to be interviewed for your report. This would count as primary research.

# Things you might need

* ICT to investigate the support and services that are available for people who need them.
* A folder or filing system to help you organise the research you have collected.
* ICT to present your report. You do not have to type up your report, but it will look more professional and be easier to make changes to if you need to.
* Your school, college or local library to look up what Maslow's hierarchy of needs is about.

# How you will be assessed

| You must show that you *know*: | Guidance | To gain higher marks you must *explain*: |
|---|---|---|
| What an individual's needs are, how an individual's choice can determine how these needs are met and why it is important to work with the individual, their family and carers.<br><br>You need to consider three people who have different needs. | * Needs may be physical, intellectual, emotional, social, mental or spiritual. You need to think about how Maslow described needs in order of importance. Do you agree with this?<br>* People's preferences and choices about the types of care they receive may be based on their beliefs, their wish to be independent, the support they need and how much help they receive from their family and friends. It is important for professionals to work with individuals and their families to ensure they are involved in every aspect of their care. Imagine if you were receiving care and were never asked what you wanted or never told what was going to happen. You would probably feel angry or worthless. | * How the needs of all three individuals are met, describing how their preferences and choices may affect how these needs are met. You should choose people who have different needs, for example a small child at a nursery, an older person receiving day care at a centre and a teenager who is homeless.<br>* Why adopting an approach of respect and understanding by practitioners is important when working with individuals and their families or carers. You should consider issues such as self-esteem and respect. |
| How care plans are devised to meet the needs of individuals and the sources of information required when planning care. Use your three individuals that you have described to use as an example of how care plans are written.<br><br>Why interventions are sometimes needed. | * Practitioners have to assess, plan, implement (put the plan into action), monitor and review the care and support that individuals need. They need different types of information on which to base this care plan, e.g. information from the individual, their family or carers and other practitioners.<br>* Interventions used as examples should be relevant to the three people described in your report. | * How interventions are designed to meet individual needs.<br>* At least three sources of information used in the care planning process. You should make links to your chosen individuals and give examples. |
| How to collect and collate (examine the information you have collected and put it in order) your information when investigating the needs of three individuals. You should show how you collected and used the information about the three individuals you have studied. | * Primary research is research that you have carried out in the form of interviews, observations, and questioning of individuals/practitioners. Secondary research could be an investigation of local services and support using the Internet or the local paper. | * How your research has been collected and organised. You should discuss its use and evaluate its effectiveness during your investigation of the needs of three individuals. |

# 6 ANTISOCIAL AND OFFENDING BEHAVIOUR

## Introduction

The **justice sector** has to deal with all types of crime, find suitable punishment for wrongdoing and also try to ensure that people do not re-offend. At the same time, ways have to be found of cutting the crime rate. You will be looking at some ways in which offenders are dealt with, and what attempts are made to prevent criminals from re-offending. In this unit you will also find out about the ways in which individuals and communities are fighting crime without the need to use the 'heavy arm of the law'. It is in everyone's interest to live in a place where everyone feels safe and at ease with their neighbours. So, finally, you will be expected to suggest ways in which crime could be reduced in the area in which you live.

### THINKING POINT

A recent newspaper report told of the death of a 40-year-old man, killed by two boys, aged 13 and 15. The victim had been threatened by the youths when he visited a local shop. On leaving the shop, one youth had hit him so hard that a piece of the victim's tooth was stuck in his hand. The victim died three days after the attack, as a result of cracking his head on the pavement. The youths got sentences of three years and two and a half years, but would serve only half of that time in custody.

Do you feel that 'justice was done'? Was this an appropriate sentence? What feelings do you have about the justice sector and the way in which it dealt with this case? Can anything be done to prevent tragedies like this happening again? These are the types of issue that are covered in this unit.

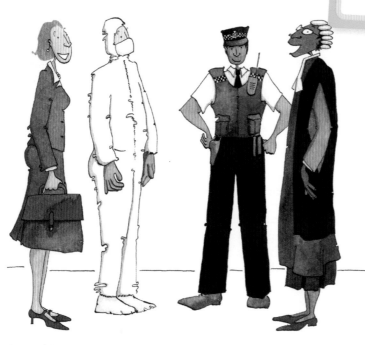

*Some of the individuals involved in the justice sector.*

**Justice sector** All the people and services involved in dealing with crime.

# Crime in the media and society

Crime is constantly talked about in the media. Particular groups of people are affected by crime in different ways. Young people are especially affected by 'street crime', whereas older people can be subjected to campaigns of bullying by small numbers of young people. Surprisingly, the highest rates of burglary are found not in wealthy areas of a town, but in its poorest. Most people do not experience crime on a regular basis, but fear of crime can be constant and almost as worrying as crime itself.

Perhaps you know someone who has been involved in crime. They may have committed one offence or many. Why do some people behave in a criminal way, while others, from very similar homes and backgrounds, do not? There are no simple answers to this, but studies have suggested what may lead a person into a life of crime and in this unit you will look at some of these factors.

# How you will be assessed

For assessment of this unit you will need to produce a display for your school/college or community centre concerned with all aspects of the justice sector. This will include the structure of the justice sector, penalties that can be given for wrongdoing, an explanation of antisocial behaviour and a survey of crime in your area.

You are to work in a group to do this. Sometimes when people work in a group, individuals decide what they want to do without considering what part everyone else can play. Some people tend to let others do the majority of the work, without making a fair contribution to the group effort. To avoid this happening, you are also to produce a report that explains exactly what you contributed to the display. You must include witness statements and peer assessments that will state what part you played in the project.

# What you will learn in this unit

You will:

* Know the purpose and overall structure of the justice sector
* Know different patterns of antisocial and offending behaviour and the factors affecting the likelihood of offending and re-offending
* Know the range of penalties that may be imposed as an alternative to court appearance
* Be able to evaluate information to recognise the consequences of behaviour for self and others
* Understand the impact of crime on victims and witnesses and their need for protection, respect, recognition, information and confidentiality
* Know the ways in which crime and disorder can be reduced in a community
* Be able to generate ideas to reduce crime and disorder in an area

## Activity

The press reported in November 2007 that only 1 in 20 offenders actually goes to court. The rest were let off, given cautions, fines, fixed-penalty notices or warnings. This included 25 per cent of burglars and 28 per cent of sex offenders, among whom were 24 rapists.

1 Discuss in a group whether you think this is an appropriate way to treat offenders. Do you think that all offenders should be brought to court?

2 Do some research to find out what cautions, fines, fixed-penalty notices and warnings are, and to whom they are given and why. Present your findings to others in the group.

# 6.1 Why do people behave like that?

This topic will help you to explore the reasons why some people become involved in crime. But remember that many people to whom these factors apply do not become involved in crime. Perhaps it would be interesting to find out why not!

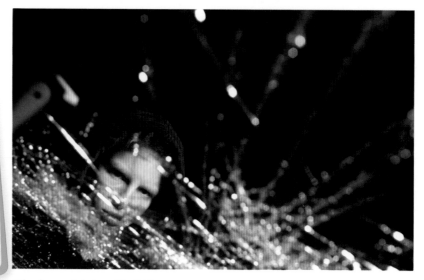

*Why do people behave like this?*

## Factors that may lead to antisocial and offending behaviour

### Lack of family support
The family provides the child with the first lessons in how to behave in society. This is as simple as teaching a child to say please and thank you. If the parents do not provide clear boundaries, the child grows up unclear as to how to behave. Instead, as the child grows older, they will look for other people to provide a role model.

### Peer pressure
In the teenage years, the influence of friends or the **peer group** is very important. If a child becomes involved with a group who are involved in criminal behaviour, then there is pressure on the child to join in. They will want to conform to the group so that they remain part of it. Younger members of the group may look on older members as role models and copy their behaviour.

**Peer group** A group of people of the same age who are important to the individual. The peer group will influence the behaviour and attitude of the individual because they value their opinion.

### Unemployment
Those who are unemployed generally live on benefits. The government decides the minimum amount of money a person needs to live on. There is just enough money for the essentials in life, such as food and heating bills. There is no money for treats, such as meals out or holidays. Unemployment can lead to crime, as people try to gain the things they want by criminal means rather than by working.

## Social exclusion

The government describes social exclusion as meaning 'what happens when people or places suffer from a number of problems such as unemployment, poor skills, low incomes, poor housing, high crime, ill-health and family breakdown'. It is often linked to poverty.

Offenders (and victims of crime) often suffer from one or more of the factors listed by the government. Multiple problems such as these can lead people into offending behaviour as a way of improving their circumstances. Statistics show that those who live in poorer areas of towns are more likely to be victims of crime than those who live in wealthier areas.

## Substance misuse

The misuse of alcohol and illicit drugs has a significant effect on the amount of criminal activity. Some 44 per cent of violent incidents and 54 per cent of violence committed against strangers is reported as being due to the influence of alcohol. Three-quarters of cocaine users admit committing crime, such as burglary and robbery, to feed their habit.

The government pays for programmes to help people beat their addictions to both drugs and alcohol, but breaking these addictions is not easy. Many addicts try to give up but do not succeed. This is because there are complicated personal reasons why people become addicted in the first place, and these have to be overcome before the addict can break the habit.

## Mental health

Mental health problems are increasing in young people. These problems include behaviour disorders, depression and hyperactivity. Some surveys report that up to 20 per cent of children aged between 5 and 15 years need help with their mental health. It is believed to be a significant cause of offending behaviour. Research has shown that 9 in 10 of young offenders between 16 and 20 years old showed some evidence of mental illness. Of young people in custody, 31 per cent have mental health problems, such as self-harming. However, it must be remembered that most of those with a mental health problem do not become offenders.

### For your project

You may want to investigate more fully the reasons why people become offenders. There is a lot of information available, both in textbooks and on the Internet. You could also look at different patterns of antisocial and offending behaviour, for example:

* in different areas
* between men and women
* among young people
* among prolific offenders.

### Activity

1 Make a poster to illustrate the type of person who might become a young offender. Use the information on these pages to help you.

2 Try to suggest why the factors you identify can lead to offending behaviour.

### Just checking

* Describe the influence of the family and peer group on the young person.
* What is social exclusion and why does it affect the possibility of offending?
* Why is unemployment often linked to offending behaviour?

# 6.2 Stephen, the ASBO kid

Having learned in the previous topic about some of the reasons why young people become involved with the court system, here is a fictional account of one of them.

## Diploma Daily

### Neighbours party as local tearaway is given custodial sentence

Neighbours of Stephen Walker, a 17-year-old local tearaway, celebrated at an impromptu party in the garden of Tracey Taylor, one of Walker's many victims. 'He has made the lives of people round here a misery,' she said. 'He would take drugs and swear in the street at the younger children. The old people round here were terrorised by him, because he would throw eggs at their houses and stones at their windows.' Walker was given a custodial sentence for the breaking of his ASBO, but was thought

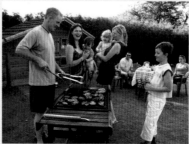

*Neighbours celebrate the imprisonment of local troublemaker.*

locally to be at the centre of a drug-dealing ring that had tried to get the younger residents on drugs so they would be his future customers.

A custodial sentence means that Stephen Walker would be locked up. Make a note of your initial reactions to this case. Then read the case study in this topic and see if you have further thoughts afterwards.

## Case study: Stephen's story

Stephen was born when his mother, Michelle, was only 16. His father, Dean, was 18 and already in trouble with the local police, mainly for offences involving cars. Michelle was nearly 18 when they got a small council flat. By then, Dean was largely absent, leaving Michelle to raise Stephen on her own.

At the age of five, Stephen started school. He did not enjoy it. He found reading difficult and Michelle, now busy with her new baby, found little time to help him. 'After all, that's what teachers are paid to do aren't they?' she often complained to her mother. She tried to spend some time with him, looking at picture books in an attempt to improve his reading, but it bored both of them, so she soon stopped. From an early age, he spent most of his time hanging around the rather rundown estate on which they lived, playing 'knock and run' and finding other ways to annoy the neighbours.

Secondary school proved to be no better than primary school. Stephen was in the bottom sets for most subjects and relieved the boredom he felt by causing disruption. His teachers despaired of him. Michelle got weary of the phone calls of complaint and the demands to visit the school to discuss her son's behaviour. She knew that, despite her promises to deal with her son, in reality she could do little to control Stephen's actions. She tried to encourage his father, Dean, to speak to their son, but Dean was too interested in his 'career' as a petty thief to be of any real help. Unfortunately, Stephen seemed very impressed by his father's ability to make some easy cash while claiming benefits. This was not the type of help Michelle had wanted!

By the age of 15 Stephen was permanently excluded from school. He was supposed to receive a few hours of education each week, but he refused to turn up for that. His days were spent hanging round the local shopping centre with a group of older boys, many with a similar history to him. He tried using cannabis and later, looking for greater feelings of excitement, he tried ecstasy. Needing to fund his by now increasing drug habit, he began stealing from local shops. Bored by his daily routine, he made himself feel more powerful by bullying his more vulnerable neighbours, like the elderly couple at the end of his street. The neighbours got together and after some months (and despite threats from Stephen), they collected enough evidence to have him served with an **ASBO**.

Unfortunately, this did not have the effect it was supposed to have. Stephen was now seen as 'hard' by the other young troublemakers on the estate. He liked this – at last he was being admired for something he had done. This was not what the neighbours had hoped for. Some months later, after they had again compiled pages of evidence, Stephen was taken to court and received the maximum penalty, a six-month **custodial sentence**.

1 Stephen found school difficult. How would that make him feel?

2 How could Stephen's parents have provided more support for him?

3 How would his father's lifestyle have affected Stephen?

4 Describe the effect of the 'peer group' on Stephen.

5 Why do young offenders such as Stephen often misuse alcohol and drugs?

6 Imagine you are Stephen. Why do you think he needed to feel 'more powerful'?

7 What do you think could have been done to help Stephen as he grew up?

8 Stephen is an example of someone who is 'socially excluded'. Use the information in topic 6.1 to explain why he can be described in this way.

**Antisocial behaviour order (ASBO)** A court order given for general antisocial behaviour (see topic 6.3) or as part of a sentence if a person has been involved in criminal behaviour. It states exactly what the person can and cannot do, depending on the reasons why it was given. For example, an offender who has been harassing someone may be forbidden to visit the street the person lives in.

**Custodial sentence** A sentence given by the court where the criminal is locked up in a prison or, for young offenders, a secure training centre, a secure children's home or a young offender institution.

## Activity

Stephen is coming to the end of his sentence. He will be released to return home. You are a social worker who visits Stephen in prison.

1 Can you suggest reasons why Stephen became an offender?

2 What advice and practical help would you give him to ensure that he does not re-offend? You could present your ideas as a role-play between the two or write a letter to Stephen setting out your ideas.

## Functional skills

This activity will help towards FS: English – literacy.

## Just checking

✳ How are success in school and unemployment linked?

✳ How are substance misuse and mental health linked?

✳ List the things that could have been done to prevent Stephen becoming an offender.

**Antisocial behaviour**
Repeatedly acting in a way that is likely to cause alarm, harassment or distress to people who do not live in the same house as the person carrying out the behaviour.

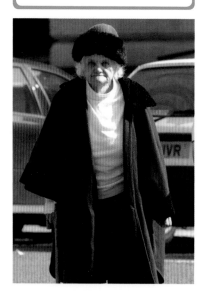

*Some surprising people have received an ASBO. Dorothy Evans from Abergavenny was 79 years old when she got hers. She received a lot of press attention because of her age. Use the Internet to find out more about her case. Start with www. bbc.co.uk and use the search to find articles about her.*

# 6.3 Antisocial and offending behaviour – what's the difference?

Antisocial and offending behaviour cause great distress for other people. This unit looks at the difference between the two. It also examines the type of person who may become involved in such behaviour.

## Antisocial behaviour

**Antisocial behaviour** in itself may not be against the law. It can even include things like playing music – but at a volume loud enough to cause alarm, harassment or distress. If the behaviour is repeated and causes annoyance to others, then it can be called antisocial.

Antisocial behaviour can be divided into three groups:

* *Street problems.* Such behaviours as public drug dealing, begging and riding mini-motorbikes come under this heading.
* *Nuisance neighbours.* One or two families can have a huge effect on the quality of life of other people (remember in topic 6.2?). Trouble caused by such people includes loud music, rowdiness and uncontrolled dogs.
* *Environmental behaviour.* Dumping rubbish, graffiti and vandalism are examples of this category.

The sorts of behaviour described above have become more common during recent years. While single events can be a nuisance (e.g. a noisy birthday party), nuisance behaviour is not considered 'antisocial' unless it happens repeatedly.

### Who engages in antisocial behaviour?

It is often thought that it is only the young who engage in antisocial behaviour, as this is the group that gets the most publicity. However, people of different ages and of both sexes have been shown to behave in this way. Sometimes whole families are involved, as the parents behave in an antisocial way themselves and make no effort to control the behaviour of their children, who follow their parents' example. There have been instances of very elderly people who have behaved badly, particularly towards their neighbours, and they have been convicted of behaving in an antisocial manner.

## Offending behaviour

Offending behaviour is a single act that breaks the criminal law. It could include stealing, shoplifting, assault or one of many other acts of criminal behaviour.

### Who offends?

Again, people of all ages and both sexes carry out offences, although 80 per cent are male and the tendency is for people to stop offending as they get older.

**Patterns of re-offending**

In topic 6.1 you looked at some of the reasons why people offend. Some people commit one crime, are punished in some way and never commit a crime again. However, it is more common for people to commit offences time after time, and be punished again and again, before they stop behaving in a criminal way.

So why do some individuals continue to commit crimes? Sociologists have looked into this and have come up with the factors shown in the diagram as being particularly relevant to the likelihood of re-offending.

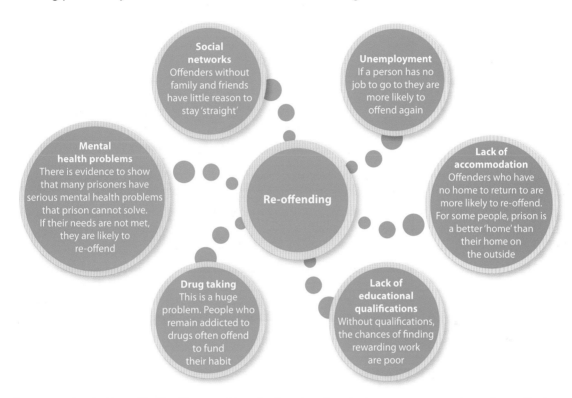

*Factors associated with re-offending. These are things that have been found to be common among those who re-offend.*

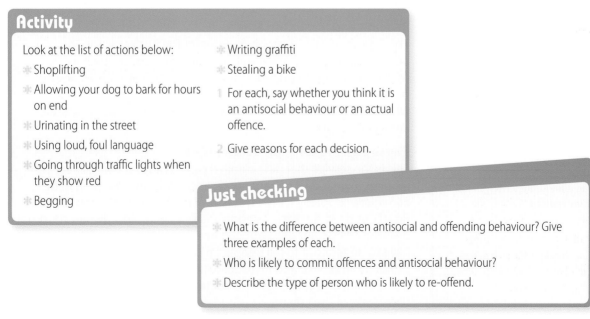

## Activity

Look at the list of actions below:

* Shoplifting
* Allowing your dog to bark for hours on end
* Urinating in the street
* Using loud, foul language
* Going through traffic lights when they show red
* Begging
* Writing graffiti
* Stealing a bike

1 For each, say whether you think it is an antisocial behaviour or an actual offence.

2 Give reasons for each decision.

## Just checking

* What is the difference between antisocial and offending behaviour? Give three examples of each.
* Who is likely to commit offences and antisocial behaviour?
* Describe the type of person who is likely to re-offend.

# 6.4 What is the justice sector?

**THINKING POINT**

What do you think is meant by 'the justice sector'? Write a list of the people you think are involved and for each state what you think they do. Start with the police.

Imagine your house has been burgled. There will be a great variety of people who will try and catch the burglars, bring them to justice, decide their punishment and supervise them until the punishment has been carried out. This topic considers who these people are.

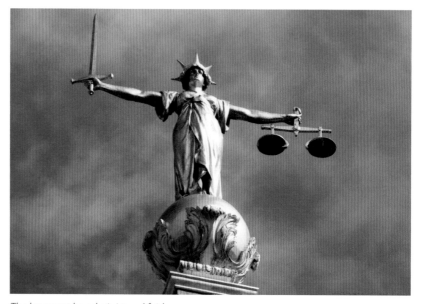

*The law must be administered fairly.*

## The justice sector

This is a term used to describe the work of over half a million people in the UK who are involved in one or more of the following different areas. Below is the explanation of the work they do.

### Policing and law enforcement

This is probably the most obvious job of the justice sector. The police, supported by office staff and support services such as fingerprint experts and forensic scientists, carry out this work. The police investigate crimes, catch suspects, collect evidence and deal with suspects up to the point when the courts have decided their innocence or guilt.

### The Crown Prosecution Service (CPS)

This is the service that gets criminal cases ready for court. Every case requires a great deal of paperwork, as the law must be seen to be administered totally fairly. (This is why the figure on the top of the Royal Courts of Justice in London wears a blindfold – the law must not be affected by someone's appearance, status or manner.) **Summonses** have to be sent out to tell people on **bail** when to attend court. The prosecution service also investigates all deaths that are 'suspicious'; this is defined as those where a doctor has not seen the person within two weeks of their death.

**Summonses** Written orders to attend court at a stated time.

**Bail** A sum of money paid by or for a defendant so that they can await trial in the community, rather than in prison.

## Court services

There are many types of court. They are all concerned with administering justice in some way. The criminal courts deal with offending behaviour of all sorts, whereas the civil courts deal with matters where people are in disagreement, for instance divorce cases or arguments between neighbours. Adoption cases have to be dealt with in the courts. Decisions are made by paid professionals such as judges, or by volunteers, such as magistrates. There are also people involved in the day-to-day organisation of the courts, such as ushers and secretaries.

## Custodial care

A person in custody is someone who is being held against their will. Suspects in police cells as well as people in prison are in custodial care. Prisoners and suspects have to be moved from the police station to court and from court to prison or another place where they can be held for imprisonment or treatment.

## Community justice

This is a wide-ranging aspect of the justice sector's work. It covers crime prevention and all aspects of community safety. This includes:

* support for the victim and witnesses who have to attend a trial
* community safety and crime prevention
* supervision of offenders when they have been released from prison or a young offender institution, to ensure they do not re-offend.

### Snapshot

Did you know that people who are given a 'life sentence' are rarely kept in prison until they die? They are supervised for the rest of their life after release. If they do anything thought to be suspicious, they can be recalled immediately to prison. This supervision is carried out by the community justice sector.

### Activity

There has been a burglary and the burglars have been caught. They are taken to court and sentenced.

1 Try to list all the different people who might have been involved in the case. Don't forget support staff, such as fingerprint experts or drivers.

2 Explain what part they would have played in bringing the offenders to justice.

## Who works in the justice sector?

The organisations involved include:

* the police
* the prison service and other places where offenders are held in custodial care
* the probation service
* the courts
* the local authority
* various charities that help both offenders and victims, such as Victim Support and NACRO (the National Association for the Care and Resettlement of Offenders).

You will find out more about some of these in the next topic.

### Just checking

* What is meant by the 'justice sector'?
* Explain the different aspects of the community justice team.
* Who works in the justice sector?

# 6.5 People who work in the justice sector

Now you know what the different aspects of the justice sector are, this topic looks at some of the groups of people who work within it.

## The different bodies involved

### The police

There are 140,000 police officers in Britain. Their main role is to catch offenders, but they have many other roles too. They are principally there to uphold the law, but are also the first people to be called upon in many crises, such as when a child is lost or when there is a disaster, for example a flood.

Nowadays, they also try to become involved in the community in which they are based, so that the relationship between the public and the police is improved. This is to help both the police and the public. If the public have confidence in the police, they are more likely to provide information when a crime occurs. This is called community or neighbourhood policing.

Some officers are also involved in crime prevention. You may be able to ask police officers to visit your home, so that they can advise about home security.

### The Crown Prosecution Service

The Crown Prosecution Service (CPS) advises the police as to whether they have enough evidence to be able to send a suspect to court. It may decide that the offender should be given a caution or an official warning. In those cases, the offender will not go to court. However, if the case does go to court, the CPS will decide what the charge is to be. Once the case comes to court, the CPS **barristers** will present the evidence. Many people who work for the CPS are **solicitors**.

### The magistrates' court

All cases involving adults begin in the magistrates' court. Justice is administered by three magistrates (or justices of the peace – 'JPs'). They deal with three types of case:

* less serious offences, like speeding or shoplifting, where they can decide the punishment if they find the defendant guilty
* 'either-way' offences, which could be dealt with either by the magistrates or by the Crown Court (if the suspect pleads not guilty or the magistrates believe that the offender, if found guilty, should receive a heavier sentence than they can give, then the case must be heard at Crown Court)
* serious offences, although these are referred almost immediately to the Crown Court.

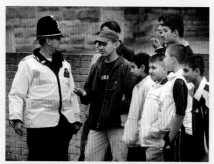

## The youth court

If suspects are aged 10–17 years, they will be sent to the youth court. Here justice is administered by one magistrate or a district judge. The public are not allowed in, although relatives of the suspect may attend.

## The Crown Court

This is the court that many of us are familiar with, because it is the scene of so many dramas on television. The judge and barristers wear wigs. The jury of 12 people decide whether the suspect is innocent or guilty. These courts are used mainly for the most serious of crimes, such as murder, rape or robbery.

## The probation service

The probation service supervises 175,000 offenders each year, 90 per cent of whom are male. If offenders are sentenced to some sort of community service, they will be supervised by the probation service. They also supervise those prisoners who are coming to the end of their prison sentence. Another part of their work is to provide reports on prisoners before they are released to try to decide if they are still a risk to the public.

## Local authorities

The local authority or 'the council' is responsible for linking together different services to try to reduce crime in its area. For example, the youth offending team will work for the local authority and will liaise closely with members of the community police.

## The prison service

Offenders who have committed a serious crime or who persistently break the law may receive a prison sentence. The prison service protects the public by holding prisoners securely. It also attempts to reduce the chance of re-offending by improving the prisoners' skills.

> **Barristers** Lawyers who defend or prosecute suspects in court.
>
> **Solicitors** Lawyers who give legal advice and draft documents. Some appear in court for defendants.

> I try to help the inmates stop offending. We can do this by giving them the skills to get a job when they come out. We should also try to help them see why they offend. If we don't help them in this way, then there is no point in prison.

> I think prison does its job because it stops criminals from committing crime. This protects the public. I think prison works and we should build more.

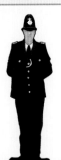
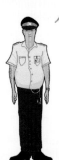

## Activity

1 Whom do you agree with in the cartoon?

2 Why do you agree with them?

3 When the prisons were full, the government tried to persuade the judges to send fewer people to prison. Were they right to do this? Give reasons for your answer.

## Just checking

❋ Describe the different aspects of the work of the police.

❋ Explain the differences between the three types of court.

❋ How is the work of the prison and probation service linked?

# 6.6 Outcomes of offending

There are many different outcomes for young people who offend. Court appearances and custodial sentences are generally seen only as a last resort. This topic illustrates the outcomes with three stories.

In recent years, attempts have been made to devise different, more imaginative ways of dealing with young offenders, without just using the court system. At the same time, attempts are made to discover why the young person is behaving in an antisocial manner. Strategies can then be put in place to try to change their behaviour. For example, help may be given with drug or alcohol misuse or finding a suitable college course.

Let's look at the stories of two young offenders.

## WHAT DO YOU THINK OF ASBOS?

ASBOs are just one of the ways in which the police try to deal with antisocial behaviour. What do you know about them? Do you think they are successful? If so, say why you think that. If you believe they are not successful, say why. Be prepared to share your ideas with other members of the group.

---

**Anti-social Behaviour Order on Conviction**
(Crime and Disorder Act 1999 s1C)

**Bolton Magistrates' Court (1731)**

the Magistrates' Court sitting at Bolton convicted
1. On the

Name:             *Defendant*
Address:

Date of Birth:
Of the following offence:
(i)

And imposed the following sentence(s)

2. The court found that
(i) the Defendant had acted in the following anti-social manner, which caused or was likely to cause harassment, alarm or distress to one or more persons not of the same household as himself:

1. *[insert details of offending behaviour]*
And that:
(ii) an order was necessary to protect persons in England and Wales from further anti-social acts by him.

3. It is ordered that the Defendant is prohibited from:

(i)   Behaving in an anti-social manner so as to cause harassment, alarm, or distress to any person, not of the same household as himself (any person);
(ii)  Using, demonstrating or threatening violence towards any person;
(iii) Damaging, taking or interfering with the property of any person except with their express permission;
(iv)  Using threatening, abusive, insulting, racist or intimidating language towards any person;
(v)   Consuming or being in possession of alcohol in a public place;
(vi)  Entering Merehall Close, Bolton.

**Until and including** *[date]*

**Justice of the Peace**

NOTE: If without reasonable excuse the Defendant does anything which he is prohibited from doing by this order he shall be liable on conviction to a term of imprisonment not exceeding five years or a fine or both

*An ASBO ready for completion.*

---

## Case study: Mark's story

Mark lived in a detached house, in an affluent area of town. His parents both had good jobs and worked hard. After leaving school, he started at college but soon dropped out. He became the ringleader of a group of young people who spent most evenings hanging around the local shopping precinct. There they drank heavily and verbally abused the shopkeepers and their customers. Their behaviour became intimidating and the shopkeepers became concerned because the residents would not use the shops if Mark and his friends were around.

The local community police officer issued Mark with an antisocial behaviour warning. His parents were shocked, but defensive of their son, refusing to believe that he was the leader of the group. Mark took little notice of his warning and was issued with an **acceptable behaviour contract** (ABC). This also had no effect and Mark was soon issued with an ASBO, keeping him away from the shops. The group, now effectively leaderless, soon broke up and the shops soon started seeing takings go up as residents returned to shop there.

## Case study: Jimmy's story

Jimmy is currently serving a life sentence for a particularly horrific murder of a young girl. The reasons why he has behaved in this way are always of interest to psychologists and all those people involved in the justice sector. If reasons can be found as to why people behave in this destructive manner, perhaps steps can be taken to minimise the chances of this happening to others.

Jimmy was born in London. His parents divorced when he was only 18 months old and he never saw his father again. When he was 10, his mother remarried. Jimmy had a very poor relationship with his stepfather, who beat him regularly. Two years after the marriage, his mother took him to a children's home and left him on the doorstep. She never made contact with him again. At the age of 14, he was found guilty of a series of muggings in his local area. He also began smoking cannabis, something he would continue to do through the rest of his life.

At the age of 15 he was expelled from school for assaulting a teacher. The children's home were extremely worried about his psychological state, as they believed that he had serious emotional problems. They were also concerned that the cannabis was aggravating his emotional instability.

Jimmy formed a relationship with a fellow resident of the home called Melanie and they moved in together when he was 17. He was later found guilty of assaulting her and of exposing himself to two women.

He then emigrated to Australia with Melanie. She had two children with him, but the relationship did not last and he lost contact with both Melanie and his children. He moved back to Britain, where police now think he is responsible for several unsolved attacks on women who were out alone at night. Throughout the next 10 years, his drug-taking increased. He had several relationships with women, but none lasted, probably from the stress of his drug habit and mood swings, which often led to violence. At one point, he saw a doctor about his mental state, as he was suffering from insomnia, severe depression, mood swings and violent, uncontrollable temper tantrums. Unfortunately, he did not take the medication given nor attend follow-up appointments, so the medical problems remained unsolved.

One evening, when he had taken a particularly large quantity of both drugs and alcohol, Jimmy encountered a young girl, alone at night. He sexually assaulted her and then killed her. He was sent to the Crown Court and was found guilty. He will remain in prison for the rest of his life.

### Acceptable behaviour contract (ABC)
An informal procedure aimed at stopping antisocial behaviour; it is a voluntary contract and so has greater flexibility than an ASBO. Breaking an ABC may be a reason for serving an ASBO.

### Activity

Look at copies of your local paper. You will need to look at more than one edition of it.

1 What sort of crime seems to occur regularly? What types of people carry out these offences? Are they young or old, male or female? Do they come from all over the town or only from certain areas? If the offenders are caught, how are they dealt with?

2 Write a report based on your findings.

### For your project

It is up to each local authority to decide in what way it will tackle antisocial behaviour and young offenders. You may want to investigate how this problem is tackled in your home town.

### Activity

Read topic 6.1 again. Identify the features of Jimmy's story that indicate the chances of him becoming an offender were very high.

What do you think could have been done to try to prevent Jimmy's life from turning out in this way? Identify the different occasions in his life when perhaps something could have been done to try to help him overcome his problems.

### Just checking

* How are young offenders helped to change their behaviour?
* Why do you think Mark's parents did not think he was the ringleader?
* What is an ABC and how does it differ from an ASBO?

Offenders aged 10–17 are dealt with in the youth court. Under the age of 10, the offender cannot be brought to a court, as they are not thought to be old enough to understand that their behaviour is wrong. The youth court is not open to the public, although adults such as parents or carers can attend.

Why do you think young offenders are dealt with separately? Why are the courts not open to the public? Do you think that offenders aged less than 10 understand that their behaviour is wrong?

# 6.7 Sanctions the justice sector can impose

In the last decade there has been an increase in antisocial behaviour. In response to this, the justice sector has had to devise a variety of different ways of trying to deal with offenders. This topic presents the sanctions that can be imposed as alternatives to a court appearance when a person offends.

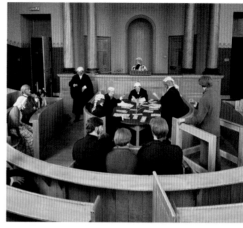

*The magistrates' court is used to deal with less serious offences. Youth courts may be held in the same building as the magistrates' court.*

*Sanctions available within different parts of the justice sector before a person is sent to court*

| Sanctions that can be given | Who can be subject to the order | Who supervises the offender | Conditions of the sanction | Additional comments |
|---|---|---|---|---|
| Caution | Adults (young offenders cannot receive cautions, only reprimands or final warnings) | Police | The offender must agree to receive the caution after admitting their guilt on tape. The offender may have to pay compensation if there is a victim involved | If there is a victim they may have to agree with this action being taken as a way of punishing the offender |
| Fines | Any offender | Police, **police community support officers (PCSOs)**, local council officers | There are two types of penalty. A fixed penalty notice (FPN) is used mainly with offences that affect the environment such as dog fouling or litter. A penalty notice for disorder (PND) is issued for more serious offences, such as throwing fireworks or being drunk and disorderly | |
| Acceptable behaviour warnings | Young people aged 11–18 | Youth offending team (YOT) | This is a letter sent to warn the individual that if their behaviour does not change immediately, then an application will be made for an acceptable behaviour contract | This can be effective in stopping poor behaviour without having to take further steps |

| | | | | |
|---|---|---|---|---|
| Acceptable behaviour contracts (ABCs) | Young people aged 11–18 | YOT | An agreement is made between the offender, their parents or carers and the YOT that the young person will stop causing a nuisance | |
| Eviction | All offenders | Landlords, backed by the court | This is not done lightly. The tenants are always given warnings about their antisocial behaviour so they have a chance to change | Unfortunately, evicted tenants often behave as badly in their new address |
| Injunction | All offenders | Landlords, backed by the court | This is a type of official warning to tenants to change their behaviour. It is usually linked to a particular type of behaviour that is causing the nuisance, such as a barking dog or playing loud music | These are issued to try to make offenders change their behaviour rather than evict them |
| Mediation | Individuals or the whole family | YOT | The offender may meet with the victim of the offending behaviour to offer an apology and gain some understanding of the effect of their behaviour on others | This is sometimes referred to as restorative justice. The offender can find this very difficult. It can be done only with the agreement of the victim |

## Activity

Read the examples of offending behaviour described below.

* There have been several complaints to the council about the behaviour of the Jackson family. They have recently bought two dogs that bark continuously and their middle son has been heard shouting and using foul language to the young couple who live next door. This is the first time there have been complaints about the family.

* A young man has previously been warned about his use of racist language with his neighbours. He has not changed his behaviour and is continuing to cause them distress.

* A 14-year-old girl has admitted to being drunk and shouting at some small children in a nearby playground. The offence is her first.

1 Use the table to decide what sanction you would impose on the offender(s) in each case.

2 Why do you think that some offenders find mediation (or restorative justice) very difficult?

**Police community support officers (PCSOs)** Uniformed police support staff. They do some of the tasks that do not require the experience or powers held by regular police officers.

## Just checking

* Can a 10-year-old be given an ABC?
* Who supervises a parenting order?
* Can you be cautioned for an offence you say you didn't commit?

**Criminal record** A police file of someone's history as an offender. The record is deleted after a period of time, depending on the seriousness of the offence.

# 6.8 How does crime affect people?

Crime has an impact on people in different ways. The main sufferer is the victim but others may be affected too. For example, witnesses to crime can be upset by what they see. In this topic, you will look at how crime affects the victim and others, including the offender.

## Effect of crime on the offender

If people commit offences and are caught then punished, it can have long-term effects on their future. Firstly, they will have a **criminal record**. If anyone applies for a job, they have to reveal any convictions within the last two and a half years (unless the sentence was longer than six months, in which case it will stay on the record for longer). Employers are less likely to employ a person who has a criminal record. People with criminal records are more likely to be unemployed, which means they will have a low income. This has an effect on all aspects of their life.

Secondly, other people are likely to form poor opinions about them, because they have a criminal record. This is what many potential employers do and other people who meet the person socially may do the same. This can lead to the person mixing mainly with others with a criminal record. You saw in topic 6.1 that the peer group can have a huge influence on the individual. If the peer group are involved in crime, then there is a greater chance that the individual will commit further criminal acts and become 'socially excluded'.

## Effect of crime on other people

The effect on other people of crime can vary greatly. The experience will differ for different groups of people. After being robbed in the street, for example, a young male victim may feel differently from an elderly lady. A wealthy person will probably be insured if their house is burgled, so goods can easily be replaced. People who are less well-off may not be able to afford insurance.

### Effect on the physical and mental health of victims

Crime can have physical effects on its victims. They may be injured or in the case of a sexual assault catch a sexually transmitted disease. The effects may be temporary or long term. There may also be psychological effects, such as a lack of confidence, fear or feelings of helplessness; these are just as unpleasant and damaging as physical effects, and sometimes harder to deal with. Long-term mental health problems can even occur, although this is rare.

### Effect on relationships and employment

Studies show that being a victim or witness to crime may affect relationships. In families who distrust the police, coming forth as a witness may be seen as a betrayal of the family's values. In some cases, witnesses may be asked to give evidence about a relative. It is easy to see that this will make family relationships difficult.

Being a witness or victim may mean taking time off work. This can result in loss of wages or holidays. If the court case is a long one (some can last weeks) this may even result in the loss of the job (e.g. if the person had just taken up the position). The anxiety of being involved in a court case can cause people to become distracted and lose concentration, which a boss may find difficult to tolerate.

## Safety and security

If you have experienced a street robbery or a burglary, it is inevitable that you will feel less secure. Sensible people will take steps to overcome the fear, perhaps by not parking their car in a dark side street. Women particularly can be upset by burglary, as their feelings of security in their home will have been challenged. Practical steps such as fitting better locks may help, but some people find that they prefer to move house rather than continue to live in the house that has been burgled. Such reactions may seem extreme, but seem to offer some sort of solution to the person concerned. The fear of crime can be as unpleasant as crime itself.

### Functional Skills

The activity will help towards FS: English – literacy.

### Activity

1  How might the following individuals be affected by being a victim of crime? In each case, describe how their behaviour may change and their feelings of personal security be affected.

a) A young woman has her phone stolen as she walks down the street.

b) An elderly man is knocked to the ground and has his wallet stolen.

c) A professional man is assaulted as he walks home after work.

d) An elderly lady who lives alone is burgled.

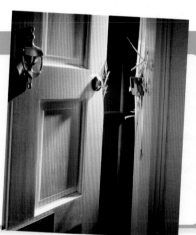

*What would you think if you returned home to find a scene like this?*

## 𝕯𝖎𝖕𝖑𝖔𝖒𝖆 𝕯𝖆𝖎𝖑𝖞

Dear Dorothy

I am 38 years old. I live on my own in a terraced house. Last year I was burgled. The burglar went through all my cupboards and drawers. Some jewellery and electrical items were stolen. I claimed on my insurance and replaced the items, but I still feel very upset about what happened. The burglar has not been caught. What can I do to try to get over this?

Jane

1  List the ways in which Jane might be affected by the burglary.

2  Write an answer to Jane, giving suggestions as to how she can come to terms with this event.

### Just checking

* How does crime affect the offender?
* How does crime affect the health and self-esteem of victims and witnesses?
* Why can fear of crime be almost as unpleasant as crime itself?

# 6.9 What does crime do to others?

What do you think Terry Smith will be feeling? If you were a witness to this crime, how would it affect you? Imagine you are either Terry or a witness to this incident. Either write a description of your feelings or devise a short speech to deliver to the group about how you would feel.

**Victim Support** An independent charitable organisation which helps people cope with the effects of crime. It provides free and confidential support and information, and works to advance the rights of victims and witnesses.

So far this unit has chiefly looked at the actions of offenders. However, crime creates both victims and witnesses. You will now look at how criminal activity affects these groups of people.

## Victims and witnesses

### Confidentiality and anonymity?

Without the evidence of the victim and witnesses, the police have great difficulty in bringing a case to trial. Witnesses to a crime and relatives of the suspect used to wait near to each other in the court building. However, in recent years, there have been attempts by suspects and their families to intimidate witnesses. This has focused the justice sector's attention on the needs of victims and witnesses, and has changed the ways in which both are treated. There is now more understanding about the confidentiality of both the victim and witnesses.

In sensitive cases, the faces and names of witnesses can be kept out of the media. In a recent murder case, witnesses were allowed to speak to the court from another building, via video-link, with their voices disguised and their faces hidden. In these ways, both victims and witnesses are encouraged to have more confidence in the legal proceedings, so that the police can gain their full cooperation and perhaps receive new evidence.

The conviction rate for rape has always been low. In an attempt to improve the rate, women who are victims of rape are kept anonymous. This means that their name or face is never printed in the papers. In contrast, the name and picture of the suspect can be printed. Sometimes the suspect is found not guilty, but by then he has been identified as a possible rapist. Do you think this is right? Should the woman's name be revealed if the man is found not guilty? In an age where we are very aware of sex discrimination, are men and women being treated equally?

### Helping victims

Being a victim of crime is a very unpleasant experience. Sometimes, the feelings of the victim can seem 'over the top'. This happens because although the actual crime may not be too serious, the victim has fears that if it happens again, it could be much worse. Their feelings of personal safety have been threatened.

**Victim Support** aims to help the victim cope with the unpleasant experience they have endured, in the ways shown in the diagram on the next page. It tries to get in touch with a victim within four days of a crime occurring, even if the criminal has not been caught.

### Helping witnesses

Victim Support has now increased the work it does by running the Witness Service in the criminal courts. Being a witness can be a worrying experience. The witness may be providing crucial evidence, without which the case could collapse. This is a great responsibility to carry.

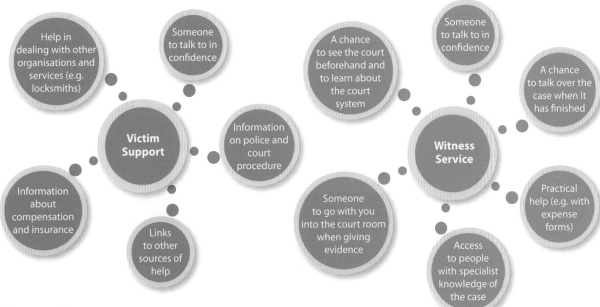

The diagram shows the following:

**Victim Support**
- Help in dealing with other organisations and services (e.g. locksmiths)
- Someone to talk to in confidence
- Information on police and court procedure
- Information about compensation and insurance
- Links to other sources of help

**Witness Service**
- A chance to see the court beforehand and to learn about the court system
- Someone to talk to in confidence
- A chance to talk over the case when it has finished
- Someone to go with you into the court room when giving evidence
- Practical help (e.g. with expense forms)
- Access to people with specialist knowledge of the case

## Young witnesses

Children and young people can be called as witnesses. Everything possible is done to make the experience as pleasant as possible. Children get restless when they are kept waiting, so they are provided with activities to keep them occupied. They do not have to wait with adult witnesses and are kept away from public view.

Courts can feel intimidating, especially to children and young people. There is now more effort to make the court seem less frightening. This is done by keeping the witnesses fully informed of what is going on and by the use of video-links to give evidence. Sometimes they are able to meet the lawyers and the judge before the case. The lawyers make their language and questions suitable for the age of the witness, which helps to increase their confidence.

*The help offered by Victim Support and the Witness Service it runs. You can find out more on the website www. victimsupport.org.uk.*

## Activity

A recent change in court procedure is that the victim can make a personal statement. Sometimes it is called an impact statement. This is a chance for victims to say how the crime has affected them. It is read to the court before the judge passes sentence.

1 Do you think this is a good idea? Give reasons for your answer.
2 How do you think it might help victims recover from crime?
3 Imagine you are Terry Smith in the case reported in the *Diploma Daily*. Write a personal statement to be read to the court about the theft of your phone.

## Personal, learning and thinking skills

The activity should help towards PLTS: Reflective learner.

## Functional skills

It will also help towards FS: ICT – find and select information; English – literacy.

## Just checking

* What are the main difficulties people experience in being a witness or a victim of crime?
* How does Victim Support help both victims and witnesses?
* How are child witnesses helped to give evidence in court confidently?

Think about your own home or car if you have one. What have you or your carers done to ensure you are not a victim of crime? How aware are you of the risk of crime at home? Have you recently fitted a burglar alarm or window locks? Do you or members of your family have a fear of crime that affects your daily life? Be prepared to discuss your ideas with others.

# 6.10 Cutting crime – what's being done?

An area with a high rate of crime and disorder is not thought of as desirable to live in. In this topic, you will look at the simple things that are being done to cut crime and antisocial behaviour, in order to make areas better places to live.

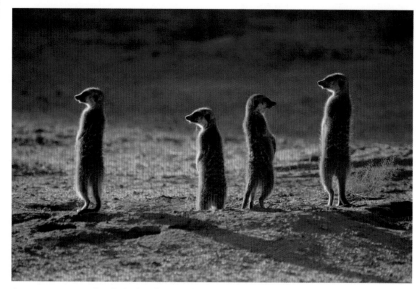

*A community is safer if it looks after itself.*

## Working in partnership

There are many simple things that can be done to reduce crime and disorder. People used to think that this was solely the job of the police. Recently there have been more attempts by local people to become involved in crime reduction in their own areas. Groups such as the local authority, fire service and community groups are now expected to play a part too. The youth offending teams (YOTs) and drug treatment teams are also involved. These different groups are brought together as crime and disorder reduction partnerships (CDRPs). You can find out more about your local partnership on the Internet at www.crimereduction.gov.uk.

## Who does what to reduce crime?

### The police

The police are seen as the main way that law is enforced in Britain. Police community support officers (PCSOs) and **special constables** are there to provide a visible uniformed presence in an area, directly helping the police to fight crime. The PCSOs are particularly good at getting to know a small area well, as they have contacts with local residents. They can gather evidence, provide reassurance and deal with low-level crime such as dog-fouling and littering. Issues such as these seem small, but they cause major irritation for local residents. The police can then focus their energy and time on detection of crime, presentation of evidence and catching criminals.

**Special constables** Uniformed volunteers who give a few hours each week to support the police in enforcing the law.

**Audit** Systematic check and assessment on a situation. Councils are required to conduct regular audits of crime in their localities.

### The council and local councillors

Your local council has responsibility for all aspects of your local area. It collects information about crime and disorder in a variety of ways, including from community groups and residents' associations, in an **audit**. Information gathered about crime and disorder can then be passed on to the local police or youth offending team.

You can contact your councillor if you are concerned about activities in your area. Your local library or town website will tell you the names of your councillors and how to get in touch with them.

### Neighbourhood Watch and community messaging

Neighbourhood Watch schemes help prevent crime and protect a local area. They do this by the residents watching over their neighbourhood, which deters bogus callers and opportunistic burglars. They help reduce the fear of crime, particularly for the elderly and those living alone. They also provide a link with local councillors and the police. This is an example of partnership working.

Community messaging is a way of allowing the police to collect information and inform the public, by use of new technology. It works in this way. A person registers with the police their interest in fighting crime in their area. The police record a message, for instance about a spate of burglaries. The message is sent to individuals who have registered. A reference number is given for each message. If the person receiving the call has information relating to the enquiry, they can phone the police. In this way, the police can reach a large number of possible witnesses or informants without the need for individual interviews.

### CCTV cameras and security patrols

In Britain there is one CCTV camera for every 14 people. They have been useful in reducing crime in town centres and have been proven to reduce low-level disorder. After major crimes, films can be used to track the movements of suspects. Films can also be produced as evidence.

Security patrols are usually organised by local people, who pay a private firm of security officers to watch an area for incidents of crime and disorder. They tend to be used only in well-off areas because of the cost. They are an effective but expensive way of combating crime.

### Youth forums

Local councils run youth forums. They work like a school council. They are a chance for young people to give their opinions on issues that concern them. Young people's perception and experience of crime can be passed to the council, which can use the information when making decisions about crime and disorder reduction. This is another example of partnership working.

## Activity

Operation Mullion was an example of partnership working to reduce crime. It was based around Mayfield School in Portsmouth, which had suffered from serious antisocial behaviour and criminal activity.

1 Use the Internet to find out:
   * what the problems were that the school was experiencing
   * what was done to solve them
   * what the results were
   * who was involved in the scheme.

Use the Google search engine to start your search and remember that the first websites that it lists will probably provide you with the most information.

2 You could use some of these ideas when you are planning your assignment.

## Personal, learning and thinking skills

The activity should help towards PLTS: Independent enquirer.

## Just checking

* What is a crime and disorder reduction partnership?
* What is the role of the council in fighting crime?
* How is technology used in the fight against crime?

# Unit 6 Assessment guide

This unit is assessed by an assignment that is marked by your teacher. You will need to show your understanding of the people that make up the justice sector, for example the police, the Crown Prosecution Service, the probation service, the local authorities (your local council) and the prison service. You will also need to show the difference between antisocial behaviour and offending behaviour and the factors that cause people to offend and re-offend. There are many sanctions that can be imposed on people before they are sent to court and you will need to show that you know about some of these. You will need to carry out a survey in your school, college or area about how people feel about crime and behaviour in their area. You will also need to show how crime can be reduced and come up with some ideas of your own to reduce crime in your community. Finally, you should show that you understand how crime can affect victims and witnesses and how they should be protected and respected.

## Time management

* Manage your time well. You will have research to carry out on the people that make up the justice sector and the types of penalties that may be imposed, and do a survey looking at people's views on crime. Ensure that you keep any research and the results of your survey in a folder or file. This will help you when you are ready to produce your report on your findings.

* Be well organised. This is your chance to show that you are an independent enquirer and a self-manager and therefore will contribute towards achievement of your personal, learning and thinking skills, a key part of the Diploma in Society, Health and Development.

* Be prepared with a list of questions that you could ask if your teacher arranges for a speaker to come and talk to your class or if you visit a court or police station. These questions might include 'What is classed as antisocial behaviour?' and 'Who is likely to exhibit this behaviour?'

* Your survey should contain what is known as 'quantitative' and 'qualitative' data. This means that you should design your questionnaire with a mixture of questions for which you have yes/no answers and questions that require a longer answer.

## Useful links

* There are lots of useful websites that will help with your investigation of the justice sector. These include www.homeoffice.gov.uk, which looks at different aspects of crime and the role of the police. Another useful one is www.respect.gov.uk, which focuses on the causes and effects of antisocial behaviour.

* You may see your area being patrolled by PCSOs (police community support officers), who often deal with antisocial behaviour. You could talk to them about the job that they do and find out what is classed as antisocial behaviour.

* Local authorities also deal with antisocial behaviour. You could call at your local council office to collect information about the powers that they have.

* Victim Support is a charity that helps victims of crime. You could find out what they can do to help by looking at their website: www.victimsupport.org.uk.

## Things you might need

* Craft materials or ICT equipment to produce the questionnaire and the results of your survey. You could use ICT to put your quantitative results into graphs and charts.

* Good communication skills when questioning people on their opinion of crime and bad behaviour in the community. You should remember to keep the results of your survey confidential.

* Good observational and thinking skills when assessing how crime is, and could be, prevented in the community.

# How you will be assessed

| You must show that you *know*: | Guidance | To gain higher marks you must *explain*: |
|---|---|---|
| The role of the justice sector. This includes the police, the Crown Prosecution Service, probation and prison services, and the local authority.<br><br>What is antisocial and offending behaviour and why do people commit it?<br><br>Antisocial and offending behaviour can be different between men and women, young people, prolific offenders and people who live in different areas and may be because of substance misuse, unemployment, mental health issues and social exclusion.<br><br>What are the penalties imposed before people go to court? These may include: cautions, fines, eviction, injunctions and mediation. | ✳ You could produce your information about the justice sector in the form of a diagram. Think about the process that someone may go through from first committing a crime to the time they are sentenced. Who might be involved? How long might it take?<br><br>✳ Find out what is meant by antisocial and offending behaviour. What are some of the factors that lead to it? What can be done about it? What people might be involved? Is the use of antisocial behaviour orders (ASBOs) a good thing?<br><br>✳ Write this up in the form of a report – use headed paragraphs. | ✳ The role of four of the organisations that make up the justice sector.<br><br>✳ Three of the different patterns of antisocial and offending behaviour and three examples of why people offend.<br><br>✳ At least four of the sanctions that can be imposed. |
| The different attitudes to crime and bad behaviour in the community, and how it is tackled.<br><br>Carry out a survey of at least 20 people of different ages on their attitudes to crime and behaviour in the area.<br><br>How crime can be reduced in the area. Options might include the work of the PCSOs and special constables, community partnerships and meetings, local councillors, youth forums, CCTV and security patrols, Neighbourhood Watch.<br><br>Produce some ideas of your own on how crime could be reduced. | ✳ Crime and antisocial behaviour can include offences such as graffiti, drugs, under-age drinking, noise, and theft.<br><br>✳ Your 'community' does not have to be the area where you live. It could be your school or college. If you choose to carry out your survey in your area, take care of your own safety. Design a questionnaire that you could use to carry out your survey. Try it out on your friends or your teacher first to see if the questions work.<br><br>✳ Put all of your ideas and findings into a report. | ✳ How the results of your survey show how people feel about crime. For example, it may show that older people are more worried about being robbed than younger people but younger people are more worried about assault.<br><br>✳ What measures are in place in your area to tackle crime and look at their effectiveness.<br><br>✳ How some of your own ideas to reduce crime could be put into practice. Explain what the outcome of these ideas might be. |
| How crime can affect victims and witnesses. | ✳ Imagine how you would feel if you were the victim of a crime and you had to go to court to give evidence against the person who had committed the crime. How would you feel if this person knew where you lived or worked? What might happen if you refused to give evidence?<br><br>✳ People who do give evidence should be given recognition for what they are doing and should be treated with respect.<br><br>✳ Put your information into a report. | ✳ How crime can affect the health, self-esteem, safety and security of witnesses and victims. How might this happen? Give some examples.<br><br>✳ Why issues of confidentiality, protection, recognition and the need for respect and information are important. Confidentiality is important to stop people finding out where you live or work. If they did, they might threaten you or your family. This might prevent you from giving evidence, which could cause another person to be a victim of crime. |

## Introduction

In this unit, you will first look at the ways in which children develop and at how the development of children is monitored through the use of **milestones**. You will go on to examine the importance of play, change and learning in children's lives. What the government is doing to support children and the role of various professionals are topics that are also covered in this unit.

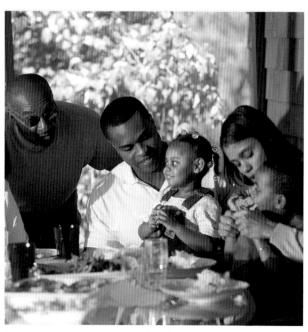

*Loving parents want to do their best for their children.*

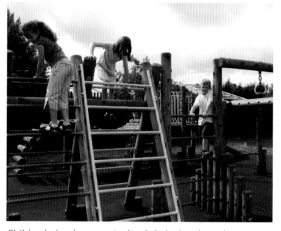

*Children's development is closely linked to their play.*

### Case study: Mark's story

Mark is 12 years old. He lives with his father and younger sister. Mark is an intelligent boy who has always done well at school. However, he has a medical condition that means he needs to use a wheelchair. He wants to be treated like any other boy of his age.

1 What problems will Mark have to overcome in his daily life if he is to achieve his desire to be treated like any other 12-year-old boy?

2 How can school help him to be treated like any other 12-year-old?

3 What help might his family need to help Mark?

These are the types of issues covered in this unit.

**Milestones** The different skills that a child should achieve by a specific age (e.g. children of six weeks should smile, showing that their visual and communications skills are developing).

## Play and change

Play is an essential part of learning. It is the way that children gain an understanding of the world around them. It is also how they learn to relate to others and to behave with others. You will be looking at how adults help children play and how different activities can be used to develop particular skills in a child.

Change happens to us all, such as moving house. Sometimes it is good; at other times it is less enjoyable. Children have to learn how to cope with change. In this unit you will look at the effects change may have on a child and how adults can help to make change something that the child is able cope with.

## The government's role

The government wants all children to have the best possible childhood. It consulted children to find out what they wanted. These became the aims of the government, which were set out in a Green Paper published in 2003 called *Every Child Matters*. You will find out how the government believes everybody who works with children and young people should put these aims into practice. These people are members of the 'children's workforce'. You will look at how important the Sure Start nurseries are in the government's plans for children. You will also find out how children who have problems can be identified so that they get the specialist help they need.

## How you will be assessed

To be assessed for this unit, you will need to produce one assignment. In the assignment you are to produce a resource pack that could be given to parents or carers to use to support their child or children as they grow and develop.

The assignment will contain two case studies. In the first case study you will look at the development of a child, as he or she grows older. You will also include information about experiences that improve their learning.

In the second case study, you will discuss an older child. Again, you will look at how their learning and development can be enhanced and the role of the children's workforce in this. You will need to plan activities that can help the children in both case studies develop.

You could use a real child or a child from a soap opera that you watch regularly.

## What you will learn in this unit

You will:

* Know the key stages in a child/young person's development
* Be able to recognise signs that could indicate that development might differ from agreed norms
* Understand how different experiences can enhance the learning and development of a child and a young person
* Understand how changes to, or in, a child or young person's life can affect their behaviour and development
* Know the purpose and broad overall structure of the children's workforce
* Understand how those working with children and young people can support their continuing development and well-being in conjunction with families and carers
* Be able to devise activities to support the development of children and young people

# 7.1 Remember the PIES?

In this topic you will first look again at the PIES and recall how they describe personal development throughout an individual's life. You will then look at some of the ways of finding out whether children are developing as they should.

## THINKING POINT

Look back to your own childhood. List the things you did (e.g. activities you took part in) that demonstrated your progress in terms of the PIES. For example, perhaps you can remember making something that would show your intellectual and physical development. Be prepared to share your memories with the rest of your group.

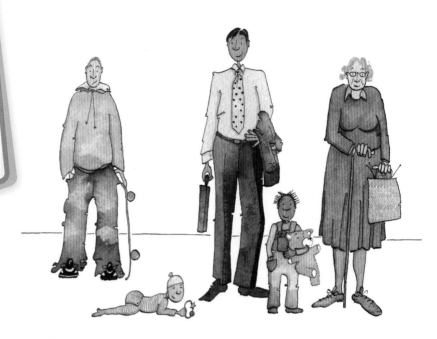

*The different stages of development.*

## What is normal development?

In Unit 4 you looked at the PIES – the physical, intellectual, emotional and social aspects of a person's life – and the ways in which people change and develop as they get older. You will have looked at different stages in a person's life and learned about the abilities that people acquire as they get older. However, you must remember that everybody is an individual. Each child will have different strengths and weaknesses. Some children may be ahead in their development in one aspect but not in others. For example, some walk at a very young age, while others have a larger vocabulary than most children of a similar age. This could be because of the environment that those children live in or because of the genes they have inherited.

Parents or carers of small children are always very concerned that their child is developing 'normally'. One way to reassure parents is to compare the child's progress against the 'developmental milestones'. Generally, the child will develop in all these aspects at the same time. That is, the different aspects of development are all linked; for example, as children gain fine motor skills (a physical development) they may use those skills to complete a jigsaw, which is an intellectual challenge. You can find out more information about developmental milestones on the Internet at www.babycentre.co.uk.

What is also important is to look at the *rate* of development. A child may follow a steady pattern of development but then fairly suddenly start to slow or even stop developing normally. For instance, if a child who has been developing normally does not try to walk at the expected age, this could be an indication of a physical disability. (On the other hand, the child may just be one who is at the far end of the normal range of development.) If there is concern, then parents can seek advice about what they can do to try to help the child; this may include finding out whether there is a medical cause for the child's lack of progress.

A **percentile chart** shows the normal way rate at which children should grow. There are different charts for boys and girls. They provide a guideline to assess whether physical development is occurring as it should. If a child is outside the normal boundaries, then medical help may be called on. For example, children who do not seem to be growing to a normal height may be given hormone treatment to assist the rate of growth.

Both parents and those who work with children need to be aware of the developmental milestones so they can recognise if development is not progressing as it should. At the same time, they must remember that every child is unique. No child will progress exactly along the lines set out in any textbook!

> **Percentile chart** A graph showing what percentage of all children will have reached a certain developmental stage (e.g. a particular height or weight) by their age.

## Case study: Ruth Lawrence's story

Ruth Lawrence was an exceptionally gifted child. Her father took great interest in her progress and she was described as being a maths genius. She gained a grade A in pure mathematics 'A' level at the age of nine and got a first-class honours degree in maths at the age of 13. She never went to school and was taught at home by her father, who went to university with her.

Ruth's intellectual development was obviously far outside the developmental norms.

1 How easy do you think it was for Ruth to make friends? Give reasons for your answer.

2 What do you think would be the effects of her unusual upbringing on her social and emotional development when she was a child?

3 Do you think it is a good idea to bring a child up in this way? Again, give reasons for your answer.

## Personal, learning and thinking skills

The activity should help towards PLTS: Reflective learner.

## Just checking

* What are developmental milestones?
* What are percentile charts?
* How can both of these be used to monitor a child's development?

# 7.2 What to look out for

In the last topic you looked at the idea of child development in terms of milestones. Now you will look at some of the most significant milestones in relation to the PIES.

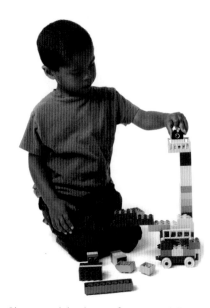

*Playing with bricks uses fine motor skills.*

## How development is monitored

Some milestones are of more significance than others. Some children may never crawl – instead they 'shuffle' on their bottom before learning to stand and walk. Crawling is therefore not a very significant milestone. However, if children do not start to walk before the age of about 18 months, then they may be investigated to see if there are medical reasons for this. A general practitioner will refer more serious cases to hospital, to see a **paediatrician**. The parent may ask for information or a concerned professional may do so. Health visitors are responsible for the care of children up to the age of five years. Children who attend nurseries will be monitored to ensure that they are achieving their significant milestones.

The table opposite sets out some of the significant milestones in a child's development. However, remember that these are merely guidelines for parents and carers, and that many children do not fit neatly into each category.

**Paediatrician** A doctor who specialises in the care of children.

## Self-concept

Our self-concept describes the way we think about ourselves. There are two aspects to this: self-esteem, which means how highly we think about our abilities and ourselves; and self-image, which we gain from other people's reactions to us. The development of self-concept begins in the first year of life.

## Moral development

This is our understanding of right and wrong. Young children believe they should not do something because of fear of punishment. As they get older, they begin to understand that something should not be done because it is wrong, not just because there may be unpleasant consequences. It is not easy to assess moral development. You may need to explain a story to the child or give the child a choice to make that will indicate to you how their moral development is progressing.

## Key milestones

| Age of child | Physical milestone | Intellectual milestone | Emotional milestone | Social milestone | Language development |
|---|---|---|---|---|---|
| 6 months | Sitting up without assistance | Recognises different tones in the carer's voice | Screams when annoyed | Tries to help (patting bottle) when being fed. Enjoys being played with | Recognises own name. Laughs and chuckles |
| 12 months | The child is mobile – crawling, shuffling or beginning to walk. Can pick things up with finger and thumb | Has a vocabulary of about three words | The attachment relationship should now be strongly formed. Looks for objects that have been removed (i.e. understands that things still exist even if they are not visible) | Is affectionate with family and familiar people | Understands simple words like 'bye bye'. Sounds become repetitive and are the beginning of word formation |
| 18 months | Can roll and throw a ball (hand–eye coordination) | Points to part of the body. Scribbles on paper | Can be clingy – doesn't like separation from main carer | Begins to be more curious about surroundings, so long as there is a familiar adult nearby | Words are becoming more understandable by others as well as carers |
| 2 years | Can walk up and down stairs confidently | Understands simple instructions. Points out objects | Shows strong emotions. Child knows own name and sex. Can recognise self in a mirror | Parallel play – the child plays alongside other children but does not interact with them | Can produce two-word sentences |
| 3–4 years | Can use crayons competently. Can walk on tiptoes | Can repeat a simple story. Knows primary colours and shapes | More comfortable with people the child does not know | Learns to take turns and share with others. Can play simple board games with adults. Imaginative play and role-playing | Talks well, asks questions and understands answers |
| 4–5 years | Can cut out a shape. Can catch a large ball | Can count up to 20. Drawings become more complicated. Can write own name | May begin to make strong friendships. Begins to mix more with own sex only | Cooperative play – the child can play and interact meaningfully with another child | Talks clearly, using basic grammar in speech |
| 6–8 years | Cuts out neatly and accurately. Can prepare simple food dishes (e.g. make toast) | Writing becomes clearer and letters are better shaped. Can tell a simple story | Can make and keep friends, because the child can understand another person's point of view | Plays with others without the need for parents to 'keep the peace' | Vocabulary reaches about 5,000 words. Can understand and tell complicated stories. Understands jokes |

### Just checking

* What will happen to a child who is not achieving particular milestones?
* Who is responsible for monitoring the development of a child?
* Using the table above, describe the abilities of a typical two-year-old.

Look at the photograph of the two children. List, in terms of PILES, the different ways in which a child changes between the ages of 9 and 16. For example, the child develops sexual characteristics. This is an example of a physical change. It may help you to try to remember how you thought and felt when you were aged about 9.

# 7.3 'Aren't you getting big!'

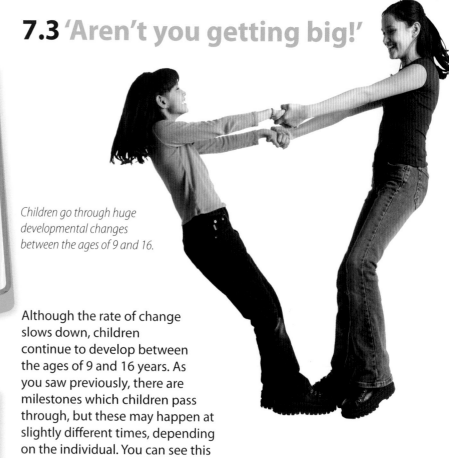

*Children go through huge developmental changes between the ages of 9 and 16.*

This task involves observing the social interaction between members of your group. First, decide how many people you want to observe and for how long. Choose an observation method to use (you could create an observation sheet to help you do this). Then carry out your observation.

1 Write a short report of your findings.

2 What was successful about your method? Was there anything that did not work well?

3 If you were not happy with your method, explain how you would do things differently next time.

**Baseline assessment** This is a clear picture of the individual child's level of development in all aspects of the PILES. This can be gained from reports from parents or carers at home, and childcare professionals that the child has come into contact with.

Although the rate of change slows down, children continue to develop between the ages of 9 and 16 years. As you saw previously, there are milestones which children pass through, but these may happen at slightly different times, depending on the individual. You can see this if you look at your year group in school; some Year 10 students look similar to an adult in their development, while others will look more like a child in Year 8. This is normal; however, by the time children reach the age of about 18, almost all healthy people will have reached their adult size and proportions.

Opposite is a table showing the major stages in development between the ages of 9 and 16 years.

## Observation and assessment

It is important that children are assessed regularly. This is to ensure that they are reaching their developmental milestones as they should. If a child is not reaching them, then steps can be taken to help him/her.

There are various different ways of observing a child, depending on what the person observing is trying to find out.

### Written accounts
The child is observed taking part in an activity. The observer writes down what the child is doing. It is important to decide at the start what type of activity is to be observed, as otherwise it can be easy for the observer to try to cover too many of the child's activities at once.

### Time sampling
The observer decides how often to monitor the child's activity, e.g. at 5-minute intervals. The observer then notes down what the child does at the specified time. The possible problem with this method is that even if the child does something interesting in between the time limit decided, the method does not allow it to be noted down.

| Age of child | Physical milestone | Intellectual milestone | Language milestone | Emotional milestone | Social milestone |
|---|---|---|---|---|---|
| 9–10 years old | Reaction times speed up. Can ride a 2-wheeler bike. Writing and drawing improves as they have better control over fingers. Writing becomes 'joined up'. | Begins to think and use reason. Reading and storytelling improves and gets more complex. | Sentences become longer and more complicated, in both speech and writing. | Makes friendships, usually with members of the same sex. Has an increasing awareness of the feelings of others. | May wish to join groups such as the Brownies or Beavers. |
| 11–12 years old | Girls may enter puberty e.g. the breasts may begin to develop. Boys will get taller, but sexual characteristics will develop later. In both sexes, body proportions will become more adult. | Concentration improves and lasts for longer on single tasks. Able to produce pieces of extended writing. Begins to have opinions on more abstract issues such as beliefs, morals, etc. | Continues to speak and write more competently, with increased use of vocabulary and description. | Friendships become longer-lasting and increase in intensity and importance. The opinions of the 'peer group' gain more importance. Begins to become more aware of the opposite sex. | Gradually, more leisure time is spent with friends than with parents or carers. |
| 13–16 years old | Both sexes progress through puberty. Body shape and size changes rapidly (for more detail, see childcare textbooks). | Gains the ability of abstract thought such as planning ahead, working out possibilities and thinking about one's own thoughts. Becomes more interested in adult issues such as poverty, morality, religion, etc. | Handwriting is clear and done quickly. Should be able to express views and ideas clearly and confidently to others. | Becomes very interested in the opposite sex. May form sexual relationships. Relationships with members of the opposite sex tend to be short-lived and intense. May become 'moody' and suffer mood swings. | The influence of the peer group becomes extremely important. Much time is spent with friends and their opinions and beliefs are significant to the individual. This can lead to conflict with parents or carers. |

*Key milestones 9–16 years old.*

## Tick charts

The observer decides what behaviour or skill to monitor, then sets up an activity to allow the child to demonstrate capability in the chosen skill. A prepared list is then used so that it can be ticked when the child demonstrates competence.

## Event sampling

This is used to monitor a child's behaviour during a particular event e.g. when the child is playing alongside others. The child's behaviour is watched and recorded throughout the event. It is a method often used if a child's behaviour is causing concern in specific situations.

Once the child has been observed in any of the ways above, assessment has to be made. This has to be done carefully, to ensure that the information is balanced and unbiased. The observer should have knowledge of what the child has already achieved, to see if the child is progressing. This is called the child's **baseline assessment**. The observer should also have a clear idea of what the child should be achieving at his/her age, i.e. a sound knowledge of the developmental milestones for a child of that age.

**Personal, learning and thinking skills**

English – thinking and listening, writing.

**Just checking**

* Why is it important that children are assessed?
* Use the table to describe how children change between the ages of 9 and 16.
* For each of the four methods of assessing children, give an example of an activity or aspect of development that can be observed. Explain why you think the method you have chosen is particularly suitable.

# 7.4 What shall we do today?

Children learn through the activities they take part in and the different experiences they have. In this topic you will look at how these experiences can help the development of the child and young person.

### Learning through routines

Children need routines in their lives. Partly because they have very little power, a routine helps children feel secure, as they will then know what will happen to them. Within the daily routine there will be many opportunities for learning. For example, getting dressed is good practice for **fine motor skills**, as doing up buttons is not easy for small fingers. (Tying shoelaces can be a major problem!) Brushing hair can be a chance to practise counting.

### Social interaction

Children learn how to react to others by mixing with people. This is how they come to know about facial reactions, responding to others and basic manners. Any **interaction** with people, either familiar people or strangers, can be a chance for the child to practise talking and behaving appropriately. For example, a visit to a café gives children an opportunity to make a choice and perhaps speak to a waitress or person at the next table. These simple interactions with others can be used to reinforce skills taught at home and at nursery.

As children get older, they should be encouraged to mix socially with adults. This improves social skills and teaches them how to communicate with older people. This can be useful for young adult life, when the individual enters the workplace for the first time and has to mix with a wide variety of people.

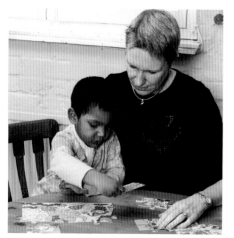

*Doing jigsaws uses intellectual and physical skills.*

### Developing curiosity and concentration

Children's intellectual abilities will be developed more if they are exposed to a wide variety of activities and experiences. Reading books together helps a child recognise letters and objects in the pictures. Owning a pet teaches a child the importance of caring for others and being consistent. Outings are especially useful to develop children's understanding of the world; for example, a trip to the beach could involve explaining about the tides or what sand is.

Board games are very important in teaching children social skills such as sharing, taking turns and learning how to win and lose graciously, as well as the importance of following rules. These can be difficult for small children and at all times it is important to choose toys or games that are appropriate to their age and not beyond their intellectual ability.

**Fine motor skills** Control of the smaller muscles, such as those in the fingers (e.g. holding a pencil). These skills are more difficult to acquire than gross motor skills.

**Interaction** All involvement with other people (anything from a simple act such as buying an ice cream from a shopkeeper to the deep conversation you may have with a close friend).

### Developing concentration and memory

Small children cannot concentrate for long. They gradually acquire the ability to do this as they get older. Both concentration and memory are vital for long-term educational success. Children can be helped to develop both of these skills by the use of counting games or by singing songs they have to learn the words to. The important thing is to try to make such activities fun, so that children are acquiring skills without seeing the process as hard work and without fear of failure.

## Challenging the child

While it is important to choose activities appropriate to the child's age, at the same time children need to be challenged so that they are continually progressing. This has to be done carefully, as demands that are unrealistic for a child can lead to failure, which is disheartening. All children need to be challenged in different ways, physically and intellectually. However, it must always be remembered that all children have their own dislikes and favourites.

Forcing a child to take part in activities that they seem to show no interest in serves little purpose. Some children do not enjoy ball games and forcing them to regularly play in this way will not increase their enjoyment of it. Instead, the adult needs to find another way by which these children can develop their skills and knowledge.

## Play opportunities

Play is crucial to a child's development. There is a belief that the recent explosion in the use of computer games and DVDs to occupy children is affecting their understanding of the world because they are not playing as they used to.

Concerns about health and safety mean that children's lives are more restricted than they used to be. Climbing trees and building dens away from the eyes of adults may result in scraped knees or bruises but they provide chances for risk assessment and excitement that make childhood special. Messing about in sand or with water provides an understanding of scientific concepts such as conservation of mass. Playing with others helps children learn about social interaction in a way that cannot be taught through a screen.

## The role of the adult

The role of the adult is to monitor, suggest, advise and provide overall control of the child's activity. Sometimes this may mean that the adult takes an active part in the child's play. At other times, they may stand back and let children make mistakes or sort out the problem for themselves.

At all times, the adult should have realistic expectations about what the child or young person can achieve. If too much is expected, then the child or young person will fail and this can affect confidence. However, if praise is given for little achievement, in the belief that children should be shielded from failure, then they will become unrealistic in their view of themselves. They will also expect praise when it is not earned. This is not helpful to the balanced development of the individual.

### Activity

1 Describe a day in the life of a small child you know (or think back to your childhood).

2 For each activity that the child takes part in, identify the opportunities for development in terms of the PIES.

### Just checking

* How does social interaction help the development of the individual?
* How should a child be challenged?
* What is the role of the adult in the development of the child and young person?

# 7.5 When things happen

No one's life turns out quite as they plan it. Some changes can be expected, such as leaving home. Other changes, like the early death of a parent, cannot. This topic looks at how such changes can affect the development of a child or young person.

## STARTING 'BIG SCHOOL'

Before you started at your secondary school, you probably visited it for a day. Think back to the activities you did on that day and describe how and why the day helped you adjust to the move to secondary school.

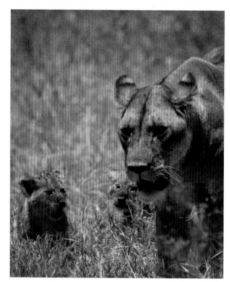

*All young animals need support from their parents.*

## Adapting to change

We all have to adapt to changes. Life would be very boring if every day was the same as the thousands that have already passed. Some changes that occur in our lives can be foreseen. We know that we will have to leave primary school, leave secondary school, leave our parents' home and so on. These changes can be planned and prepared for. Some may appear exciting, such as a move to a new house or the birth of a new baby, although even changes that appear exciting may be worrying or frightening at first. However, many things that happen to us cannot be planned for, such as the death of a parent, the loss of a job or illness in a family member.

As mentioned in the previous topic, children like a routine. Change tends to bring disruption to that routine. Naturally, children's understanding is rather limited. They are **self-centred**, which means that their view of a change in a family's fortunes may not be the view that adults would take. For example, the move to a foreign country may mean leaving a pet behind. This is probably not the biggest factor in the adults' mind when planning the move but may be the most significant to the child. The priorities of the child may be very different to the parents. Parents need to be aware that the child may be very concerned about something that the adult does not see as a problem at all.

**Self-centred** Tending to see things and events only from your own point of view.

Children may have feelings about events that seem to adults to be irrational. It is very common, for instance, for children to feel that a divorce between their parents could have been avoided if they had been 'good'. Even children who have lost a parent through illness sometimes feel guilt about their behaviour, because they believe that if they had been better behaved their parent would not have left them. Such irrational feelings need to be discussed with children to try to set their mind at ease and to help them come to terms with what has happened.

## Diploma Daily

Dear Dorothy

I am 13. My parents are getting divorced. It was not really a surprise as they have been rowing for a long time, but I still do not want it to happen. I am staying with my Mum and my Dad has bought a new flat. They say I will still be able to see my Dad but I am worried that I will not see him because that's what happened when my friend's parents split up. I am really unhappy about it all.

Love Eleanor

1 List all the concerns Eleanor may have about her future relationship with her divorced parents.

2 Write a reply to Eleanor giving suggestions for how she could come to terms with what is happening to her.

## Keeping everyone informed

Regardless of the type of change that is occurring, experts on child development agree on one thing: children will best manage change and any adverse effects if they are kept informed of what is about to happen. In times gone by, it was believed that it was better if children were not informed of what was going to happen, as they would be protected by not knowing what was going on. These days it is widely recognised that even small children should be given as much knowledge as possible of what is going to happen and how this will affect them. Of course, the language and degree of explanation given will depend upon the age and understanding of the child.

If children are struggling with unhappy feelings about what is happening to them, then this often has an effect on their schoolwork. They may be naughty to gain attention if they feel that nobody is paying them attention at home. Alternatively, they may become distracted and lose concentration; what is going on at home is of greater importance than lessons at school. If the child is experiencing some difficulty at home it is always useful to inform the school, so that allowance can be made for a loss in effort or concentration.

### Personal, learning and thinking skills

The activity should help towards PLTS: Reflective learner.

### Case study: Ben's story

Ben is two. He has been staying at his grandparents' house for a few days. He really enjoyed himself there, as he loves his grandparents very much. His dad has come to collect him and take him home. When they get home, there is a horrible shock. His mum shows him a baby. 'This is your new baby sister,' she says. Ben didn't want a sister! Nobody had asked him about this!

1 How might Ben react to his baby sister?

2 How will the arrival of the new baby affect Ben?

3 Describe how this situation could have been dealt with more satisfactorily.

### Just checking

* Why do children find change hard to manage?
* What is thought to be the best way to help a child manage change?
* How can change affect a child's performance in school?

Britain's future depends upon its children and young people. You will now find out how the government is determined that all children and young people will have the best possible start in life. You will also see how grown-ups sometimes have to help children and young people cope with change.

## Every Child Matters

In 2000, an eight-year-old girl called Victoria Climbié died in hospital in London. Her aunt and the aunt's boyfriend (her carers) had cruelly treated her. An investigation into her death found that several professional people, such as social workers and workers at the hospital, had come into contact with Victoria without realising what was happening to her. As a result, the government published a **Green Paper** called *Every Child Matters*. The idea was to ensure that services for children were organised to ensure that such a tragedy would never happen again.

The government decided that children's needs would be best met by linking together all the services that children come into contact with. Children were asked what they considered their most important needs to be and meeting these then became the aims of the government. There are five main aims. These are that children should:

* be healthy
* stay safe
* enjoy and achieve
* make a positive contribution
* achieve economic well-being.

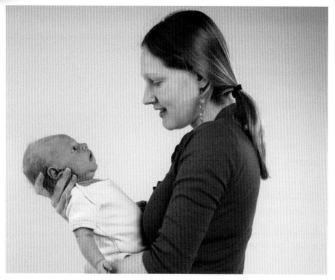

*Caring parents want the very best for their child. What would you want for a young child's future?*

**Green Paper** A document for discussion the government publishes that sets out its ideas regarding policy and proposals in a particular area.

### What this means

All the services that children come into contact with have to consider all the above aims as they make their policies. For instance, schools should no longer just be concerned about achievement. They should now consider the health of children, for example, by changing the school meal service so that the food is more nutritious. They should also try to ensure that students leave school with an understanding of how to become economically secure. Local authorities should ensure that the areas in which people live are safe for children as they play or go to school.

### How it works

The diagram on page 177 shows which groups of people are involved in working towards the aims of *Every Child Matters*. Representatives from each of the agencies in the spider diagram meet together so they can decide the best ways to meet each aim. For example, representatives from education, Connexions, the Learning Skills Council and the youth offending teams may work together to find ways of maximising the chances of all children to achieve. Connexions will work with employers and young people to ensure that there is a match between what the young person has to offer and what the employer is looking for. If the person eventually finds a job or training which is appropriate, then Connexions could be said to be meeting the aims of helping the individual in making a positive contribution and achieving economic well-being. In this way, the different skills and knowledge of each separate body can be combined to achieve the best possible outcome.

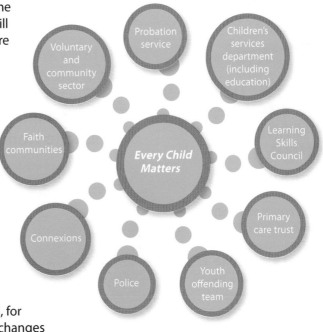

## Changes and transitions

As children grow, they will experience many changes or transitions. Some are expected, such as going to school. Some are unexpected, for example the death of a parent. Many of these changes will have an effect on the individual. Some may be very difficult for the individual to deal with. Changes such as dealing with family break-up, discovering that you have been adopted, or coping with physical or mental ill-health (either personal or that of a close family member) can have profound long-term effects on the person. Children and young people will need support from other family members or from other concerned adults (e.g. teachers) who can help guide and support the person as they come to terms with what is happening to them. As stressed in topic 7.5, giving information is vital. Coping with such changes can have a deep effect on the person and may change the way they view the world for the rest of their life.

### Activity

Read again the aims of *Every Child Matters*. They were written with someone like *you* in mind.

1 Give an example of what each aim means to you.

2 Can you think of any way in which you are achieving these aims?

3 Are there any that you feel you are not achieving? If there are, why are you not?

### For your project

You could investigate how a local organisation such as the local nursery or primary school has used the aims of *Every Child Matters* in its planning.

### Just checking

✳ What are the aims of *Every Child Matters*?

✳ How are the aims put into practice?

✳ How might the death of a parent affect the development of a child or young person?

# 7.7 All hands on deck

Everybody who works with children should have an awareness and understanding of the aims of *Every Child Matters*. Now you have looked at the thinking behind *Every Child Matters*, let's see how it is organised to work in practice.

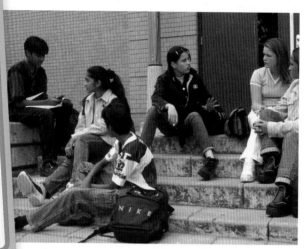

*The aims of* Every Child Matters *were drawn up by young people, for young people.*

## Sure Start

One of the most important ways in which the government is seeking to implement *Every Child Matters* is through the Sure Start nurseries. Research has shown that some children have already fallen significantly behind their peer group by the age of three years. In particular, if their language skills are not as good as they should be, this will affect their progress in many other ways. The government decided that the best way to tackle this was to offer high-quality childcare, especially for those children who are more likely to fall behind. These are often children from poorer families, or where the mother is very young.

As well as providing childcare, Sure Start nurseries are places where other agencies can become involved. The parents will be in the building each day, so it is the ideal place to offer help from Jobcentre Plus, social services, education and the local primary care trust (which deals with health matters). In this way, parents can speak to experts in the area they have concerns about. They can get help with problems and find out what to do to make themselves more employable. By 2008, there should be 2,500 children's centres providing this type of integrated help and support. This is an example of how services are being brought together so that agencies that are meant to help people are more easily available and accessible.

## Case study: The nursery worker's story

Jane is a nursery nurse. She chats almost every day with Sarah, who lives on benefits with her little boy, David. Sarah left school with no qualifications but now regrets this, as she wants to get a job when David goes to school and earn more money for them both. She asks Jane for help.

1 What help might Jane be able to offer?

2 Use the Internet to find out what the aims of Sure Start are.

# The Common Assessment Framework

Some children have more need of expert help than others. They may be disabled physically or mentally, or have an emotional problem that shows itself in **challenging behaviour**. These children require specialist help, often from more than one type of service provider.

For example, physically disabled children may need equipment to help with movement. They may need to attend a school that can cope with a wheelchair. The home may need adaptations to make wheelchair access simpler. The parents may require an adapted car so their child can be taken out in it.

The Common Assessment Framework is designed to identify all the child's needs through the use of one form, on which service providers can gather all the relevant information about the child. In the case above, the agencies involved could include the school, the primary care trust, the housing department of the local authority and the Benefits Agency. This information is then shared between all the people who can help, so that parents don't have to keep repeating their story to different people. This will also save time for the professionals, who will have one source of information to work from to assess all the needs of the individual child.

## Common Core of Skills and Knowledge

The 'Common Core of Skills and Knowledge' for the children's workforce, proposed within the framework of *Every Child Matters*, sets out the basic skills and knowledge needed by everybody whose work brings them into regular contact with children and young people. There are six main areas:

* effective communications and engagement with children, young people and families
* child and young person development
* safeguarding and promoting the welfare of the child
* supporting transitions
* multi-agency working
* sharing information.

The government is planning that soon, all the members of the children's workforce will have a basic understanding of the six areas of the Common Core. They will form part of the qualifications for anyone who works with children and young people.

**For your project**

You may want to investigate the Common Core of Skills and Knowledge and link its aims to the work of a childcare setting other than a school.

**Activity**

Take each of the skills and knowledge from the Common Core and give an example of how your school is achieving it. For example, your school may have a school council. This provides *communication* between the students and the teachers. When a school has a parents evening, this is an opportunity for your parents or carers to *communicate* with the school. If the school has a nursery, then it is providing *engagement* with younger children, who are below school age.

**Functional Skills**

The activity will help towards FS: English – literacy.

**Just checking**

* What is the Sure Start scheme?
* What are the benefits to (a) parents and (b) professional agencies of the Common Assessment Framework?
* What is the Common Core of Skills and Knowledge?

# 7.8 Helping children develop – in all ways

## WHAT IS HAPPINESS?

'We live in a very materialistic society but the things that bring happiness are not things.' What does this mean? How does it relate to the way that children and young people should be brought up?

The chief concern of parents – and the purpose of the children's workforce – is to ensure that children and young people develop satisfactorily in all aspects of their lives. This topic looks at some of the ways in which this can be done.

## The need for good communication

Good communication between a child and carers is essential. If children do not learn language in the first few years of life, they actually lose the ability to do so at all. This will affect all their future achievements in school, as success in the classroom depends upon a child's ability to understand what is going on.

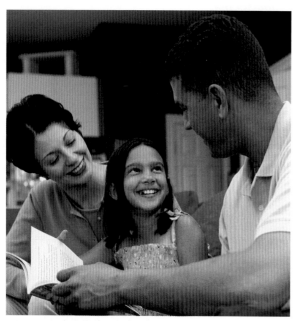

*What invaluable skill is the child learning here?*

Other, more subtle aspects of life are passed on through satisfactory communication. For example, the child learns *how* to speak to others – you know that it is not a good idea to speak to your teacher in the same way as you speak to your friends. Children become able to express feelings through speech, not actions – the tantrums associated with two-year-olds are caused by their inability to express their strong feelings in any other way. We all gain confidence through being able to state our thoughts and opinions clearly to others, and gain respect from others by doing so.

## Building relationships and providing support

Only if children are able to form a satisfactory first relationship, that with their parents or carers, will they be later able to make good relationships with other people, as children and adults. All adults who regularly come into contact with a child need to treat that child with respect and consistency. Children need to have boundaries, that is, to know what they can and cannot do. They may complain about this, but boundaries provide the security that children need to feel able to tackle new things.

Adults have to know when to take part and when to stand back if a child is playing. For example, children must learn to negotiate with their peer group; if adults constantly do this for them, social skills are not gained. Adults must be there to provide support, encouragement and reassurance, but be aware that, at times, children have to be left alone to sort out difficulties for themselves.

As children get older, their relationships with the peer group will become more important than the relationship with parents. In the teenage years the views and opinions of their friends will be vital for feelings of belonging and acceptance. Parents need to recognise the importance of the peer group and be ready to provide emotional support if there are disagreements between close friends.

## Managing transitions

As we saw in topic 7.5, leaving nursery and going to primary school are big changes for a child. Some will take this in their stride but others may find this very frightening. The best way to help children cope with change is to tell them as much as possible before the change occurs. This removes the fears the child may have and gives an opportunity for questions. A visit to the new building can help, just as you probably visited your secondary school during year 6.

Even at the age of 16, some teenagers will find the idea of starting college frightening. This is because, just like the four-year-old starting school, the young person is leaving the familiar and venturing into the unknown. There will be new people to meet and new systems to get used to. If the person has an inner confidence based on previous experiences, then such transitions can be managed satisfactorily.

## Challenging the child

Children need to be helped to move on, physically, intellectually, emotionally and socially. This is not easy. Some parents prefer not to see the child upset, or believe that failure would harm the child in some way. What is important is to choose activities that stretch children in a way that is realistic, so that they have the chance to succeed. If success is not immediate, then the adult needs to reassure the child so that they have the confidence to try again.

As children get older, if they have experienced success in tackling new challenges in the past, then they will be more likely to regard them as exciting rather than frightening. The young person will have the confidence to tackle new things and not to be put off by the occasional failure, if it happens.

## Managing behaviour

There are many different theories about how to manage a child's behaviour. However, most are in agreement that the way to ensure that a child behaves well is to act as a good **role model**. For example, parents should not swear in front of children, as children will copy adult behaviour. As the child gets older, then reason can be used to explain to the young person why behaving well is better for the individual and everyone they come into contact with.

### Activity

Parent 1: 'I think children should be able to run about and make a noise in public places. They are only young once.'

Parent 2: 'I think children should be taught to consider other people. They shouldn't be allowed to run and scream if it disturbs others.'

1 Who do you agree with?

2 Compose an argument to support your point of view.

### Functional Skills

The activity will help towards FS: English – literacy.

**Role model** Someone that others look up to and copy.

### Just checking

* Why is good communication between adult and child important?
* How should transitions be managed?
* How can a child be challenged?

# 7.9 Continuing to grow, continuing to learn

This topic looks at the different ways in which children learn. It also covers the ways in which adults can help and support children as they learn.

## The importance of play

Play is the way children learn about the world. During play, children learn both social and manipulative skills, and develop their understanding of the world. For example, board games teach children about following rules, something vital if they are to become a valuable member of society. Role-play stretches children's imaginations and shows how to recognise other people's position in the world around them. Physical games such as ball games develop fine and gross motor skills. Children should be encouraged to take part in different types of play, so that all aspects of development are encouraged.

## 'Are you playing out?'

Children need to be encouraged to play both indoors and outdoors, as the different environments lend themselves to different types of activities. Some types of play, such as that with balls or large items of equipment, are suitable for use only outdoors. At all times, the equipment used should be safe, able to withstand the use it will get and be suitable for the age of the children using it.

Sometimes children seem to get more fun from the box an expensive toy has come in than the toy itself. The box can be a boat, a cave or a suitcase; in other words, with the box the children can use their imagination in a way they can't do with the toy. There is no need to spend large sums of money on children's toys. What is important is that activities are varied and that they are suitable for the age of the child.

## Something special

Days out and trips enable the child to vary their experiences. Children need to develop an understanding of the world in which they live, outside of their immediate surroundings of home and nursery. They should visit the seaside, see cows in fields and go to a museum or children's show at the theatre. These are all opportunities for a child to learn. When they are young, they will learn about appropriate behaviour and the outside world on trips; as they get older their trips are more likely to have some specific educational content.

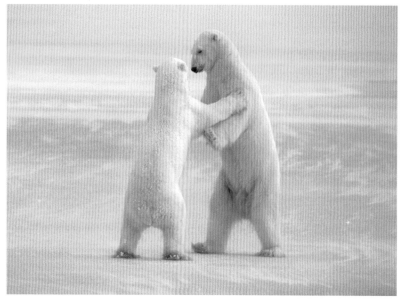

*Young animals learn through play.*

# What should the child learn?

Those people working with children and young people (e.g. in nurseries and playgroups) need to ensure that they are working towards clearly defined outcomes. These can be derived from the Early Years Foundation Stage, which is a set of guidelines developed by the government to help those working with children. It gives suggestions for how all those concerned with the development of children can help the child to make progress and achieve. You can find out more about the Early Years Foundation Stage on the Internet.

## Learning styles

Do you prefer to write notes or take part in a discussion to help you remember something? Which you prefer can give a clue to your 'learning style'. It is believed that we all learn best in one of three ways, and so can be classified as: **visual learners**, **auditory learners** or **kinaesthetic learners**. You may have done some work at school to identify your preferred style. We can all learn in each style, but it is now thought that a variety of activities, which cover all three, will enable more children to learn successfully. It is important to think about the three styles when planning activities. In this way, there is more chance of all children making progress.

## Supporting each child

Some children have particular needs that have to be addressed if they are to learn successfully. They may have physical, emotional or behavioural problems that will make learning more difficult for them. These children may need an 'individual education plan'. The plan is devised with the parents, child and teachers. It should include targets for the child, discussion of teaching and learning styles, methods that will suit the child best, and a later review to look at the child's progress.

Other children may need a mentor. These are adults, possibly not teachers, who are committed to showing an interest in the child over a period of time. They may discuss the child's problems and how to solve them, encourage the child when things seem difficult or provide advice and comfort. Some schools have a mentor scheme that children can join if they feel it would be of benefit to them.

## Learning to learn

Perhaps we now don't need to learn facts as people used to do, as the Internet has made so much information readily available. What we need to know is not facts, but how to learn new information successfully. This requires you to know how you learn best (your learning style), so that you can easily acquire new information as it becomes necessary. It also involves knowing how to use your memory successfully. Some schools have begun 'Learning to learn' programmes with younger children.

## Activity

You have been at school for at least nine years.

1 What do you find are the things that make it easier for you to learn? What makes learning difficult? Look at the definitions of learning styles below. Which do you think you are?

2 Give examples of things that you have done that made your learning easier.

**Visual learners** Those who prefer to use textbooks, mind maps and diagrams to learn.

**Auditory learners** Those who like debates, sound-bites and verse to remember information.

**Kinaesthetic learners** Those who prefer actions such as role-plays, visits and 'design and build' projects.

## For your project

As you have seen, play is very important in a child's development. You may want to look at how different activities, with children of different ages, aid their development in all aspects of the PIES.

## Just checking

* Why is play important in a child's development?
* How can individual children be supported to improve their educational chances?
* What is meant by 'learning to learn'?

# 7.10 Activity for a purpose

You have already looked at how important play is to a child's development and learning. You are now going to look at how different activities can be chosen to promote different aspects of development.

## What are activities for?

In this topic we will look at how different activities aid different aspects of children's development, based upon the PIES. However, don't forget that many activities will involve more than one aspect. For example, cutting and sticking activities will develop fine motor skills in a small child but will also involve the child in using imagination and being creative, which are aspects of intellectual development.

### Physical development

Physical activities develop fine motor skills (e.g. using the fingers) and gross motor skills (e.g. using the arms and legs) (see topic 4.1). When the child is under two years old, activities around everyday routines such as feeding and dressing are ways of improving both types of skills (e.g. using a cup or beginning to walk). Toys should be simple, such as building bricks, large crayons or playing with a large ball. As the child gets older, toys become more complicated.

By the time children reach about eight years of age, their physical skills will be quite well developed. Boys especially will take pride in their physical ability, often shown through their active participation in sport. Both sexes will develop physically and also socially through involvement with sports teams or some other regular sporting activity.

### Intellectual development

Our understanding of such things as time, length, temperature and number are all concepts that have to be acquired, through different activities. Intellectual development varies greatly between individuals, though the amount and quality of play and learning will have an effect on the rate.

Different types of toys will develop different aspects of the child's intellect. Toys such as Lego and Duplo will help with understanding size, shape and structure.

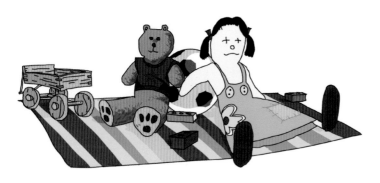

*Toys and games are used to help the child's development.*

Children also need to develop communication skills so that they are able to express their ideas and thoughts clearly. Young people should therefore be given the chance to exchange ideas, to get involved in debates or to give short presentations in lessons. All these allow young people to practise their communication skills. They are also activities that build confidence.

### Emotional and social development

Clearly, these two aspects of development are linked, as mixing with other children and adults (social development) can lead to emotional issues, both positive and negative. Children's ability to relate to others develops with age. By the age of three, they can begin to understand the idea of taking turns, sharing and making friends. This is the time to introduce simple board games, such as ludo, in which the children have to take turns. Playing games like football develops team spirit as well as an awareness of rules and winning and losing.

Reading stories with children, or encouraging them to tell stories (not lies!), helps develop their imagination and can give them opportunities to understand that other people have a different point of view from themselves. It can then help them to appreciate that other people's opinions and views are as important as their own. This helps encourage their emotional development. This is also a chance for children to come to an understanding of their own emotions, which can be very strong.

Young people will develop strong relationships with individuals outside the family. Girls tend to have one or two special friends, whereas boys will often form larger, looser groups of friends. At the age of about 13, they will start to have relationships with the opposite sex. Many of these relationships will be intense but short-lived. Through these relationships, young people learn how to relate in a deep, satisfying way with others.

## Case study: James's story

James is a four-year-old child who appears intelligent for his age. However, he does not seem to get on with members of his peer group.

1 What activities could you encourage James to take part in that would help his social and emotional development?

2 For each activity suggested, explain how it will help.

### Cultural development

Britain is now widely held to be a multicultural society. This means that there are many minority ethnic groups, who have different customs and beliefs from other groups. For example, in some cultures, women are likely to let all decisions in the home be made by the man. A child from an ethnic minority may have to come to an understanding of two cultures, first that of the home (whatever it may be) and then that of the mainly **secular**, white majority. The child from the white majority should be encouraged to have an understanding of other cultures. This can be done through the sampling of different foods, the celebration of different religious festivals and the display of pictures around the walls of a nursery or school to show different clothing or homes.

In this way, children gain an understanding that everybody's life and background is not exactly like their own. Schools provide an ideal way for children and young people to learn about other cultures. By mixing with others socially, we can gradually come to understand different cultures.

**Secular** Not religious.

## Just checking

* How does play help a child develop physically?

* Why is it important for all young people to have good communication skills?

* Explain how team games help young people develop in all aspects of the PIES.

# Unit 7 Assessment guide

This unit is assessed by an assignment that is marked by your teacher. You will need to show that you understand how children and young people develop not just physically, but intellectually, emotionally, socially and in their language skills. You will need to show that you know how development is measured and by whom and what might indicate that a child is not developing as expected. Changes to a child or young person's life, such as moving house, starting school or family breakdowns, can affect their behaviour and development in a negative way. You need to show in your assignment that you understand how these experiences can affect both a child and a teenager's development and well-being. The children's workforce might include teachers, nursery nurses, health workers, social workers and Connexions advisers. You will need to show that you have an understanding of the structure of the children's workforce, how these people work together and with families/carers, and what their job roles entail. As part of your assignment you will need to suggest activities that could help to support the development of a child and a teenager. These activities might focus on physical, intellectual, emotional, social or cultural development. Because of the importance of confidentiality, it is not advisable to use real children or young people as examples in your assignment. Instead you should use case studies; these may be designed by yourself or by your teacher, or may even be a character on a TV programme.

## Time management

* As this unit focuses on the development of children and young people, you may find it interesting to consider how your own development and well-being are promoted. Have there been any life changes that have affected you in some way? Who supports your development and well-being? Who could help you if you had a problem and weren't able to go to your family for help? How are classroom activities designed to help you learn? If you considered some of these questions it would help you to gather evidence required for this unit and save you some time!

## Useful links

* A useful website for researching the role of the different sectors is www.everychildmatters.gov.uk/strategy. This will give you information about how different groups of the children's workforce are supporting children and young people.

* Another useful website is www.need2know.co.uk. This gives information designed for teenagers on how to stay physically and mentally healthy and where they can get support from.

* Your teacher may organise a visit from someone who works with children or young people. You should make sure you ask plenty of questions. For example, you might want to know what they would need to do if they suspected that a child was not developing properly. Whom would they need to contact? Why would it be important to involve the parents or carers of the child at all times?

* You may undertake some work experience in a nursery or primary school. Although you should not use or identify any of the children you meet in your assignment, you may find it interesting to see what stages of development the children are at. Are all at the same stage and if not, why not? You could also identify the ways in which the children's activities help to promote their physical, intellectual, emotional, social and language development. This might give you some ideas for your assignment.

* Remember that the teachers and other staff members at your school or college are all part of the children's workforce. You could ask them questions about the ways in which they support young people and how they work with parents or carers.

## Things you might need

* You may be asked to produce a resource for parents or care workers to use to help them support their child's development. It should be appropriate for a child aged 3–7 years and a teenager. This could be produced in any format you like, including a CD Rom or a booklet using ICT or craft materials. You should use pictures and graphs or charts where appropriate but you should not use photographs of children that you know or information that could identify anyone.

* Copies of percentile charts might be useful to illustrate how growth is assessed.

# How you will be assessed

| You must show that you *know*: | Guidance | To gain higher marks you must *explain*: |
|---|---|---|
| The key stages of development for a child and young person. These will include 0–3 years, 3–7 years, 7–11 years, and 12–16 years.<br><br>How to recognise that a child or young person is not developing as expected | ✱ All children develop at different rates but development usually follows the same sequence (e.g. crawling before walking).<br><br>✱ Milestones may be measured against normal stages of development. These might include: physical (when a child starts walking); intellectual (when they start to read); emotional (when they develop self-awareness); social (when they can interact with others); language (when they say their first word).<br><br>✱ A way of measuring physical growth is percentile charts. This checks the height of a child against the average height of boys or girls of the same age. | ✱ What the key stages of physical, intellectual, emotional, social and language development are for a child aged 3–7 years and for a 12–16-year-old and give examples of what these might include.<br><br>✱ What signs might indicate that a child or a young person was not developing in the expected way. You might want to think about physical or learning difficulties and give examples. These may range from severe to moderate impairments. You may think about growth problems due to hormone imbalances or genetic problems when explaining the use of percentile charts. |
| How different experiences help learning and development of children and young people.<br><br>How changes in life can affect development. | ✱ These experiences might include the use of routines – for example, cleaning teeth twice a day. You could also include social interactions, the use of play, and other activities that stimulate development and the positive role of an adult.<br><br>✱ Serious illness of a lone parent can lead to a teenager needing temporary foster care while their parent recovers. | ✱ How at least three of these different experiences could affect both a younger child and a teenager in a positive way. For example, you may explain how an adult who teaches a child aged 7 how to ride a bike has a positive impact on the physical, intellectual, social and emotional development of the child.<br><br>✱ How life changes can affect both a teenager and a younger child and give at least three examples of these for each. |
| What is the structure and purpose of the children's sector. You could present this as a diagram with a written explanation.<br><br>How does the children's workforce support development and well-being of children and young people? How do they work with families and carers? | ✱ These might include teachers, nursery nurses, health workers, social workers, learning mentors, special needs workers, educational psychologists and Connexions advisers.<br><br>✱ People who work with children and young people can support them by: good communication, providing empathy, encouragement, and reassurance, by building good relationships with them, based on trust. | ✱ The different sectors that work with children. These include the statutory sector (NHS, social services, education services, youth justice), the voluntary sector (which may include play schemes, Scouts/Guides, youth clubs), and the private sector, where services need to be paid for.<br><br>✱ How the children's workforce can support a child or teenager. Give at least three examples for each and explain them. |
| What activities support the development of children and young people. You do not have to carry out the activities, just suggest what could be appropriate to help the development of a child and a teenager and why. | ✱ You could devise a creative activity that would help the development of physical fine motor skills, stimulate intellectual and emotional development and by working with other children in a cooperative way, also promote social development. | ✱ Suggest an activity for a child and a teenager and explain how it can help support development and well-being in at least three areas. This will include physical, intellectual, emotional, social and language development. |

# 8 PATIENT-CENTRED HEALTH

## Introduction

In this unit you will learn about the patient-centred approach to health care. The overall structure of the health sector is explored, in relation to the organisations and services that are in place to ensure care is individualised and holistic. You will look at common conditions and how they affect individuals, families and carers, as well as the normal baselines for health and their measurement.

**THINKING POINT**

Think of the last time you went to the doctor, or to hospital, or saw a nurse. Write about that experience of the health service. Were you pleased with the care you received? What do you think could have been done differently? Include some of the professionals you met and what their role was in your care. Did you feel at the centre of that care?

### The maze of health service provision

Health care services can often seem like a maze. There are lots of different departments, some with names we have never heard of or don't know what they mean. Working our way through these when we need treatment can often be frustrating. The health care organisations are making more effort to ensure the services are tailored around us and that our journey through the 'maze' is a smooth one.

### About this unit

In this unit we will look at the structure of health care and some of the services that are available for us to access. Some of the services are there not just when we are ill but also to ensure we don't become ill – they offer what is known as preventive health.

In other units you will have looked at what is meant by health and well-being. Health conditions affect us not only physically and mentally but also socially and emotionally. Organisations that provide health care aim to take all our needs into account and to provide **holistic care**. However, the focus of medical services will inevitably be on the treatment of physical and mental health problems. It tends to be support groups that assist with any emotional and social needs, sometimes with the involvement of local authority social services. This is an example of organisations across the sectors working together, in what is called joint working or **multi-agency working**.

When people become ill their families are affected as well. Imagine if your mum or dad became seriously ill. How this would make you feel? You would be worried and perhaps be unable to concentrate as well as you should on your studies. You might want to go with your parents to any hospital appointments. You might need to do much

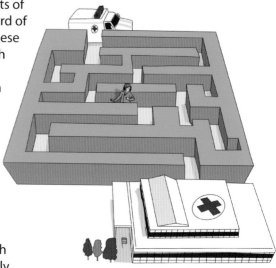

*Health care services can often seem like a maze.*

more in the way of helping out around the home. Health professionals and organisations need to be aware of the impact of illness not only on their patients but on the whole family network as well.

There are thousands of different types of conditions and diseases that can affect us. Some are short term – those people recover from or are cured of in a matter of days or weeks – while others affect people long term, even for the rest of their lives. Care services are now provided around the patient and the condition. To ensure patients' journeys through the health sector are smooth and effective, there are now what are known as **care pathways**. These are simply a 'map' of the journey a patient takes while accessing health care for their particular condition. This 'map' also shows the range of professionals the patient will meet on the way.

> **Holistic care**  Care that meets all the patient's needs – physical, emotional, social and mental health.
>
> **Care pathways**  The journeys patients with particular conditions take through the health service.
>
> **Multi-agency working**  Where different organisations work together to achieve an agreed outcome.

## Activity

Once you have completed this unit you may wish to attend a health care organisation for your work experience. There are many different places you can do this – not just hospitals, which are the first places most students think of when they want experience of the health service. Below is a short list of places you could try:

* dentists – there will be lots around your community
* pharmacies – try your local chemist and remember that some supermarkets also have chemist counters
* health clinics – contact your primary care trust for details and contacts or write to the manager of your local health clinic
* health and fitness gym clubs – these have physiotherapists and dieticians working in them
* St John Ambulance – you could join up as a cadet volunteer and learn vital first-aid skills as well.

1  Write a letter to your chosen employer for work experience. Remember to say what course you are doing and what you hope to gain from the placement.

2  Write a list of questions that you will ask the employer; one question could be 'How many people do you employ?'

3  In small groups write a list of all the different departments you know of within a hospital (e.g. surgery, paediatrics).

4  For each department, write a short description of what services it will offer (e.g. paediatric = care of children, including outpatients and on children's wards).

## How you will be assessed

For this unit you will be assessed by one assignment. You will need to investigate common conditions and their care and treatment, and produce an account of your investigation. You need to briefly investigate at least three conditions and then focus on one condition of interest to you. As part of the investigation you also need to explore the structure of the health sector. You should use the common condition that you are focusing on as the basis of this exploration. Parts of the investigation may be group activities, but your account should be your own work.

## What you will learn in this unit

You will:

* Know the basic structure of the health sector as it supports the patient-centred approach
* Know the normal baselines for health and how they are measured
* Be able to use simple measures for your own health baseline
* Know common conditions that can affect individuals throughout the life cycle and how they are treated
* Understand the potential impact of a range of common conditions on the well-being of individuals, their families and carers
* Be able to map a patient/care pathway for a common condition
* Understand the range of health care practitioners involved in a patient/care pathway for a common condition

# 8.1 Structure of the health sector

Most health care in the UK is provided by the National Health Service (NHS) and this topic looks at its structure and organisation. Important services are also provided by the voluntary and private sectors, and these are also looked at in this topic.

## The National Health Service

The NHS was created in 1948 by the Health Minister Aneurin Bevan. The idea was to offer free health care to the entire population. Since then, the NHS has changed many times and will continue to do so as our health needs change and technology advances. It is managed nationally by the **Department of Health**, which is responsible for setting targets such as reducing waiting lists for operations and appointments. It also funds the NHS – it holds all the money and gives this out to the NHS organisations across the country. Each region, for example the West Midlands, has its own **strategic health authority**. These authorities link to the Department of Health for their own areas but also have a responsibility for management of services to their regions.

Care provided by the NHS is referred to as 'statutory care'. Private care is provided by organisations that are run to make a profit; these include private hospitals and private residential care homes. Voluntary care is provided by charities or community groups that are not for profit.

### Modernisation

The NHS is currently going through what is called 'modernisation' – it is changing the way it offers services and provides care. It is basically updating its way of working, just as you would update your wardrobe! These changes are looked at in the next topic.

**Department of Health** The department of government that is responsible for health care and the National Health Service. It is headed by the Secretary of State for Health, a cabinet minister.

**Strategic health authority** Regional NHS body that is responsible for enacting Department of Health policy and for supervising the provision of health care in its area.

### Snapshot

More and more insurance companies are now offering various types of private medical and health insurance. Years ago there was only one type available and it was not affordable by many people. Today insurance companies offer various types of cover to suit different budgets and needs. Private health insurance offers people the opportunity to pay a set amount of money each month and in return be treated privately for any health conditions. Although the treatment will be the same as it is in the NHS, there will be no waiting times.

## The structure of the health service

The health sector is divided into three service areas: primary care, secondary care and tertiary care.

The frontline of the NHS is officially called primary care. The initial contact for many people when they develop a health problem is with a member of the primary care team, usually a general practitioner (GP). Primary care covers health services provided at your local health centre and within your local community.

Hospitals and outpatient services are referred to as secondary care. Access is often via referral from primary care services. An example of this is when a GP refers someone to the hospital for an X-ray.

Tertiary care is provided by specialised hospitals or departments. These are often linked to medical schools or teaching hospitals. They treat patients with complex conditions, who have usually been referred by hospital doctors. Hospices treating people with incurable cancers are examples of tertiary care.

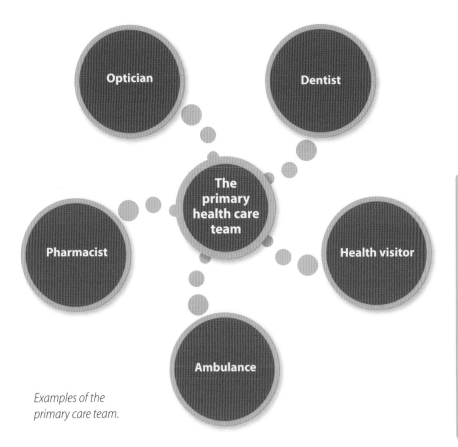

*Examples of the primary care team.*

## Voluntary and community services

Outside the NHS, there are around half a million voluntary and community organisations (VCOs) in the UK. These range from small, local community groups to large, established, national and international organisations. Some have no income at all and rely on the efforts of volunteers while others are, in effect, medium-sized businesses run by paid professional staff.

There are many charities that focus on health-related issues – some examples are given below. Do you know of any more? You could study some or one of these for your project.

* Cancer Research UK is a charity dedicated to cancer research.

* St John Ambulance provides first-aid services to community events, as well as first-aid training.

* MIND aims to create better lives for those with mental illnesses.

## THINKING POINT

If you felt ill, how long would it take for you to get to see your GP? Is that satisfactory? Have you ever heard of NHS Direct or used its services?

# 8.2 Getting to the heart of it

The government wants to reshape the NHS so that it is a personal health service for every patient. The NHS Improvement Plan shows how the NHS intends to do this. This topic looks at the plan and what the government aims to do.

## The vision

In 2004 the government published *The NHS Improvement Plan*. The document set out the priorities for the NHS up to 2008. The government's plan is that:

✱ patients will be treated in hospital within a maximum of 18 weeks from referral by their GP

✱ patients will be able to choose between a range of providers (hospitals, clinics)

✱ in every setting, the quality of care will continue to improve and patient safety will be a top priority

✱ people with long-term conditions such as diabetes will be supported locally by a new type of clinical specialist, to be known as community matrons, and services closer to home will ensure much better support, to minimise the impact of patients' conditions on their lives.

### Progress

The NHS has worked to change the way it provides services and is on track to achieve the targets.

✱ The maximum waiting time for an operation has fallen from 18 months to less than 9 months.

✱ The maximum waiting time for an outpatient appointment has fallen from 26 weeks to 17 weeks.

✱ Currently, 97 per cent of patients are able to see a GP within two days.

✱ Growing numbers of patients are taking advantage of new services such as **NHS Direct** and NHS **walk-in centres**.

✱ At accident and emergency departments, 94 per cent of patients are seen, diagnosed and treated within four hours of their arrival.

**NHS Direct** An NHS organisation that provides health advice by telephone, on the web and via interactive digital television.

**Walk-in centres** Clinics that give people fast access to treatment and health advice, without an appointment.

## Activity

Look at the progress made to date by the government.

1 For each one, list the benefits to patients and the health services involved.

2 How can we as individuals support the NHS in achieving its targets in reducing waiting lists for hospital care?

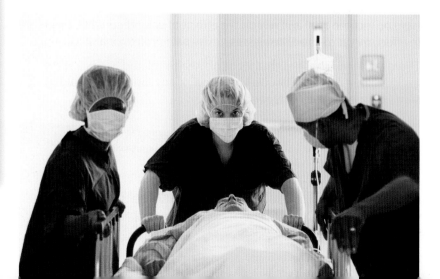

*Surgery waiting times are improving.*

## Innovation

'Choose and book' is a service that allows patients to choose the place, date and time for an appointment at a hospital or clinic. The aim currently is for them to be able choose from at least four or five different service providers (eventually people should be able to choose any provider). It has been in place since 2004. The benefits are that people can choose a time, date and clinic that suits them best and fits in with their various other commitments. It is a relatively new service and differs in each area. Visit www.chooseandbook.nhs.uk for more information and to see what's on offer in your area. Look too at the HealthSpace website (https://www.healthspace.nhs.uk); the plan is that we will all have access, via this NHS site, to our own health records; we will also be able to see appointment dates and note our personal preferences about our care and health.

### Case study: Mrs Fairhurst's story

Mrs Fairhurst went to see her GP, Dr Chand, again, as the varicose veins on her legs were getting worse. (Our veins have valves in them that ensure the blood flows in one direction only; in varicose veins these valves are weak or broken and blood collects in the veins, which become swollen and twisted.)

Over the last few months Mrs Fairhurst had tried the previous suggestions given by Dr Chand, which included wearing compression (tight) stockings and losing weight, but the varicose veins were getting a lot worse and she wanted now to look at further treatment options, including surgical removal.

Dr Chand informed Mrs Fairhurst that she needed to be referred to a specialist at the hospital for assessment, and told her about the 'choose and book' system. Mrs Fairhurst was offered the choice of three hospitals that she could attend and Mrs Fairhurst chose the one closest to her home, for convenience. She was then offered a selection of dates and times; she opted for a morning appointment on a Friday as her husband doesn't work Fridays and would be able to go with her to the hospital.

1 Look back at the section on the NHS Improvement Plan – does the 'choose and book' system support the NHS's targets? If so, which one?

2 Many health care appointments are wasted, as people do not turn up for them without letting the organisation know so that it could be assigned to another patient. Is Mrs Fairhurst more or less likely to turn up for her appointment? Give reasons for your answer.

3 How does the NHS Improvement Plan support and improve patient journeys and experiences of the NHS?

## NHS Direct

Since 1997, NHS Direct has been at the forefront of 24-hour health care – delivering telephone and e-health information services day and night direct to the public. It has a health website, and 2004 saw the addition of the NHS Direct digital TV service – one of the largest interactive services in the UK. Over two million people now access NHS Direct every month.

NHS Direct is staffed by nurses and allows you to access health advice straight away. You can call NHS Direct when you are not feeling well – you tell them your symptoms and they provide self-help advice and advise you whether you should seek further help from a medical professional.

### Just checking

✳ What is the maximum waiting time from referral by a GP to treatment in hospital as set out in *The NHS Improvement Plan*?

✳ What is 'choose and book'?

✳ List the benefits to patients of NHS Direct.

THINKING
POINT

Think about how you get goose pimples on your skin or shiver when you are cold. Do you know why this is?

*Blood pressure can be taken manually or digitally using a sphygmomanometer.*

Activity

1 Measure your temperature and record it; write down everyone else's in the class.

2 Work out the average body temperature of all the members of your class. Note also the range.

# 8.3 Measuring health

This topic covers some simple tests and measurements that can be done to assess a person's physical state of health. Once taken, the measurements can be compared against the normal baselines of health.

## What are baseline measurements?

There are measurements we can take that assess the body's health. We know what the normal measurements should be and therefore we can often diagnose illness and disease if they are abnormal. Sometimes there is no illness or disease when the measurements are abnormal – but they can then be a warning sign that the body is not coping and adjustments need to be made to our lifestyle. One example is high blood pressure. There is often no direct cause or reason for this but if we let it continue we are at risk of strokes and heart attacks. By cutting out salt in our diet and doing more exercise we can reduce our blood pressure.

The commonest measurements made are: temperature, pulse rate, blood pressure, peak flow, body mass index (BMI) and waist circumference. The last three are looked at in the next topic.

### Temperature

Body temperature normally varies over a very narrow range, of 36.5°C to 37°C. Our temperature is affected by having a warm drink, what clothes we are wearing and what the weather is like. This is why when we measure temperature we should do so at the same time each day and prior to eating and exercise. When females ovulate, the body temperature increases and this is used by some women to plan pregnancy.

**Hypothermia** is caused by prolonged exposure to the cold. Our bodies' internal survival mechanism is to start shivering when cold, to produce body heat, to produce goose pimples on the skin to prevent heat loss, and to reduce blood flow to the extremities to protect the internal organs. Those most at risk of hypothermia are the elderly and babies.

Fever is a condition where the body temperature increases and is a response to infection, surgery or illness. Bacteria and viruses die at high temperatures and therefore to protect us the body will raise its temperature to kill the bacteria. However, high temperatures can lead to fits and even death.

There are various ways to measure temperature but the most common used today is a tympanic thermometer (one which is inserted into the ear). Whatever method you use, follow the instructions carefully.

### Pulse rate

Your pulse rate is the rate at which your heart is beating. When measuring a pulse rate we count how many beats there are in a minute and the measurement is then expressed as 'bpm' (beats per minute). The average resting pulse rate for an adult is 60–100 bpm; it is faster in children. The 'predicted maximum pulse rate' (what you would expect it to be just after vigorous exercise) is 220 minus your age, and the target for a healthy pulse rate during, or just after, exercise, is 60–80 per cent of this. For example, for a 34-year-old the predicted maximum pulse rate is 220 – 34 = 186, and therefore the expected pulse rate during exercise is 112–149 beats per minute.

Pulse rate is a good indicator of health and can in some instances tell us that there are problems internally, such as heart disease, stress, infection or internal bleeding. A low pulse rate can also be a sign of heart disease. **Malnutrition** and hypothermia (extreme coldness) can cause a low pulse rate.

You can feel someone's pulse where an **artery** crosses a bone. The most common and easiest place is at the wrist, at the base of the thumb. The tips of the index and middle fingers should be placed on that spot, as the tips are very sensitive. It is best not to use your thumb, as you may feel your own pulse.

### Blood pressure

Blood pressure is measured in millimetres of mercury (expressed as mmHg). It is recorded as two numbers, for example 120/70 mmHg. The first or top one is the systolic and is the pressure of blood in your arteries as your heart contracts (pumps blood out); the second or bottom number is the diastolic, which is the pressure of blood when your heart relaxes or rests between beats.

We can have high blood pressure (**hypertension**) and not know about it, but it can lead to conditions such as stroke, heart attack and kidney disease. Approximately one in four adults in the UK has high blood pressure. Our blood pressure also temporarily increases with exercise, anxiety, pain and infection.

Blood pressure can be taken manually or digitally using a sphygmomanometer. The person should be sitting down and the machine should be at heart level. It is best to use the person's left arm, as this will achieve a more accurate reading.

**Malnutrition** A condition caused by lack of essential food, vitamins and nutrients.

**Artery** A blood vessel transporting oxygenated blood from the heart to the rest of the body.

**Hypothermia** A condition where the body temperature drops below 35°C.

**Hypertension** Blood pressure over 140/90 mmHg.

### Activity

The taking of a pulse rate has for long been associated with the medical profession. The Royal College of Physicians even has the image of a pulse being taken on its logo.

1 Take your resting pulse rate and make a note of it. Now jog on the spot for a few minutes. Take your pulse again immediately after this and every minute until your pulse rate is back to your resting pulse rate.

2 Plot a graph to display your findings.

### Case study: Travis's story

Travis is a 31-year-old man who has been admitted to a medical ward for the night at his local hospital after a road traffic accident. He had to have 38 stitches to a cut on his right leg. An X-ray confirmed he had broken his left leg and this has been set in plaster by the fracture team clinic. Before he settles for the night the nurse takes his baseline measurements and records them as: temperature, 36.5°C; blood pressure, 120/75 mmHg; pulse rate, 75 bpm. In the morning the health care support worker comes to see if Travis requires anything before the doctor and nursing team see him. She finds that his face is flushed, and he says that he feels weak and shaky. A nurse takes Travis's observations again and records them as: temperature, 37.4°C; blood pressure, 130/80 mmHg; pulse rate, 100 bpm. The doctor reviews Travis and suspects an infection and asks for blood tests. These confirm the doctor's suspicion. Travis is prescribed antibiotics and within a few days the infection is clear and his baseline measurements return to normal.

1 Which of Travis's baseline measurements had become abnormal?

2 List all the hospital staff who were involved in Travis's care. Note that they are not all explicitly mentioned in the case study.

### Functional Skills

The activity will help towards FS: Mathematics.

### Just checking

✱ What is the average resting pulse rate for an adult?

✱ At what body temperature is the condition hypothermia diagnosed?

✱ Name three diseases or conditions that high blood pressure can lead to.

# 8.4 Further measurements for health

There are other measurements as well as temperature, blood pressure and pulse rate that we can take to assess someone's health and well-being. These are body weight and 'peak flow' and in this topic we will look at these.

## Body weight

There are two common measures of body weight. Body mass index (BMI) allows for the fact that taller people will weigh more. Waist circumference is a simpler measure of body size that provides information about the distribution of body fat. Carrying too much fat increases the risks of conditions such as coronary heart disease and diabetes.

### Body mass index

Body mass index is an indication of whether you are underweight, overweight or the ideal weight for your height. It is a measurement tool that was developed in the 1980s, when **obesity** started to increase in Western society. It is used for adults only and should not be used for children, pregnant women or muscular athletes.

People who are obese are more likely to develop all sorts of health problems, including heart disease, stroke, diabetes and certain types of cancer. A simple measure such BMI can quickly indicate whether a person should think about losing weight.

**Obesity** A condition of being unhealthily overweight. It is defined as a BMI of over 30 kg/m².

**Respiratory** To do with respiration, that is, breathing.

*A height/weight chart.*

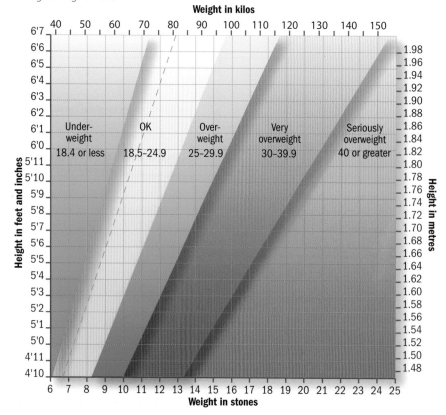

To determine your BMI, measure your height in metres and multiply this number by itself to give your height squared. Weigh yourself and record the result in kilograms. Now divide your weight by your height squared. Once you have done this, look at the chart to check your BMI status.

For example, Stanley is 1.6 metres tall and weighs 65 kg. His BMI calculation is as follows:

$$1.6 \times 1.6 = 2.56$$
$$65 \div 2.56 = 25.39$$

### Waist circumference

People who carry their fat around their waist and abdomen are more likely to suffer from the consequences of being overweight. The measurement at which there is an increased risk is defined as:

* over 94 cm for men
* over 80 cm for women.

To determine your waist circumference, locate the upper hip bone and place a measuring tape around the abdomen (ensuring that the tape measure is horizontal). The tape measure should be snug but should not cause compressions on the skin.

## Breathing

### Peak flow

Peak flow records how well a person can breathe. It is measured using a peak flow meter. A person blows out into it as hard as they can and it shows how fast the air flows out of the lungs (this is called the 'expiratory flow rate').

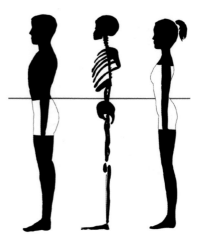

*Where to measure your waist circumference.*

This test is commonly performed for people who have asthma or other **respiratory** conditions. The better controlled the asthma, the harder the person will be able to blow out and the higher the peak flow score will be.

Peak flow readings are measured in litres per minute. As a guide, a 25-year-old male who is 6 foot (1.83 m) tall should have an average peak flow of 627 litres per minute, while a child aged between 6 and 15 years and who is 4 foot 7 inches (1.40 m) tall should have an average peak flow of 254 litres per minute.

The peak flow meter has a disposable mouthpiece; a clean mouthpiece should be used each time. The user takes a large breath and seals their lips around the mouthpiece. They then breathe out as quickly as they can. A scale at the side of the meter shows the reading. This is usually done three times, and the highest value is taken.

### Case study: Mike's story

Mike is eight years old and has had asthma since he was five. Now that he is older, his GP has asked that he starts to monitor his condition by using a peak flow meter. The peak flow meter is provided through a prescription and Mike's mum collects it from the local pharmacist. The **practice nurse** at the GP surgery explains to Mike how to use it and why it is used. He is told that the better controlled his asthma is, the higher will be his peak flow reading. Finally the practice nurse gives Mike an asthma diary with a section for recording his peak flow readings. At his next appointment the GP will use this information to decide whether the medication is working or not, or if it needs to be increased or possibly changed. If Mike's condition worsens and isn't being managed well with the medication, his GP will refer him to a **paediatrician**.

1 What sort of peak flow reading would you expect for a healthy boy of Mike's age?

2 What is the role of a practice nurse in asthma care?

**Practice nurse** A nurse who works within a GP's surgery or health centre.

**Paediatrician** A doctor who specialises in the care of children.

### Just checking

* What two conditions are you at risk of if you have a large waist circumference?
* What does BMI stand for?
* What is expiratory flow rate – air into or out of the lungs?

### THINKING POINT

Around one in seven children in the UK have asthma. It is estimated that one in three people will have cancer in their lifetime. Around two and a half million people in the UK have diabetes and a similar number have coronary heart disease. Do you know anyone with any of these conditions?

The terms 'disorder', 'disease' and 'medical condition' are often used interchangeably, although the term 'condition' can additionally cover injuries, disabilities, syndromes and infections. In this topic you will learn about some common conditions.

### Diabetes mellitus

Diabetes mellitus is a disease that affects how the body uses glucose, a sugar that acts as a fuel, for energy. When we eat, **glucose** from the food enters the bloodstream. The pancreas is a long flat organ in the body that aids digestion and produces insulin. Insulin is needed to let the glucose into the body cells, where it is used as fuel. Without insulin, glucose stays in the bloodstream, where it can reach dangerously high levels, damaging the kidneys and eyes. People with diabetes don't produce insulin, or the insulin they do produce doesn't work properly.

There are two types of diabetes: type 1 and type 2. In type 1 diabetes, the pancreas doesn't make any insulin at all and therefore the person needs to inject themselves with insulin throughout the day. This is the less common form and usually occurs before the age of 40. In type 2 diabetes the body produces insulin but it doesn't work properly. This is the more common form and occurs in adults over the age of 40. It is treated by lifestyle changes such as exercise and diet; insulin may be required.

The symptoms of both types are the same: tiredness, thirst, weight loss, blurred vision and slow healing of wounds and sores. At present there is no cure for diabetes and it is therefore a lifelong condition.

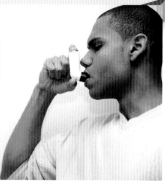

*Asthma affects the airways and lungs, such that sufferers find it difficult to breathe.*

### Case study: Brenda's story

Brenda is 65 and has had type 1 diabetes since she was 22. She injects herself with insulin throughout the day. Having had the condition for most of her life, Brenda is used to it and has learned to adapt her lifestyle around it. This includes what she eats and drinks and ensuring she always takes her medication with her wherever she goes.

**1.** Does the body produce insulin in Type 1 diabetes?

**2.** What type of diet changes do you think are required for people with diabetes?

**Glucose** A sugar used by the body as a fuel for energy.

**Nausea** Sensation or feeling of going to vomit or be sick.

**Radiotherapy** The use of radiation to treat cancer.

### Migraine

Migraine is characterised by a severe, throbbing, one-sided headache with **nausea** and/or vomiting. There are two types of migraine, common and classical. In common migraine, as with severe headaches, people may experience sensitivity to light, noise and smell. For example, bright light hurts their eyes and noises hurt their ears. This is why many people with migraine go to bed to lie down in a dark bedroom. In classical migraine, people experience the same symptoms as in common migraine but they have what is called an 'aura' before an attack starts, such as seeing flashes of light.

Migraine attacks can last for 4–72 hours and sufferers on average have 13 attacks a year. Migraine affects 15 per cent of the population and over two-thirds of sufferers are female. Both children and adults can experience it, although it is rare for someone over the age of 40 to start having migraines.

Migraines are treated with medication that can be taken at the start of an attack, but some people suffer so many attacks that they take medication every day to prevent them.

## Cancer

Cancer is the second leading cause of death in the UK. The cells in our bodies have a natural life cycle: they grow, divide and die. Cancer cells are abnormal body cells that do not die but keep on growing and dividing. They form a tumour, which can damage the surrounding body tissues. There are over 200 types of cancer. They all behave differently, grow at different rates and need different treatments. **Radiotherapy** is a cancer treatment that is administered by therapeutic radiographers.

## Some other common conditions

The table below presents some key points about three more common medical conditions.

### Asthma, stroke and epilepsy

| | Asthma | Stroke | Epilepsy |
|---|---|---|---|
| What is it? | A disease affecting the airways and lungs. Because the airways are narrowed, sufferers find it difficult to breathe | A brain injury that has occurred because blood flow to the brain has been interrupted, causing brain tissue to die | A condition whereby there are sudden bursts of excess electrical activity in the brain, causing a temporary disruption in the normal messaging activity between brain cells |
| What are the symptoms? | Wheezing, cough, tightness in chest, short of breath | Can include severe headache, blurred vision, difficulty swallowing or talking, weakness on one side of the body | Epileptic seizures and 'black-outs' |
| How is it diagnosed? | Chest X-ray; pulmonary function test; peak flow | X-rays and scans (CT and MRI) of the head | History of recurrent seizures and electroencephalography (EEG), which records brainwave patterns |
| How is it treated? | Inhalers; lifestyle changes | Lifestyle changes; rehabilitation; medication (drugs that keep the blood thin) | Medication (anti-epileptics) |

### Activity

1 Discuss with people in your class or at home whether or not they have had headaches. If they have, ask them to describe them to you. Was it throbbing, pulsating? How long did it last? What caused it? Have they ever had a day off because of a headache? Write up your findings in a short report.

2 Use the Internet to research headache clinics and write a magazine article on them. Include the role and title of the consultant who manages people with headaches and the different types of headaches.

### Functional skills

This activity supports FS: English; ICT.

### Just checking

❋ What are the symptoms of a migraine?

❋ What does a therapeutic radiographer do?

❋ What part of the body does a stroke affect?

# 8.6 Treatment of common conditions

When someone has been diagnosed with an illness, disease or condition, treatment needs to be planned, discussed and decided on by the patient. Some conditions do not require treatment, such as chicken pox, while others require medication or surgery. We need to treat both the cause of the condition and the symptoms. For some illnesses there is no treatment or cure and the care is then provided to minimise the symptoms.

## Pharmaceutical treatment

Some medicines are 'prescription only', which means they are available to you only if your GP or a hospital doctor has prescribed them. 'Over the counter' medicines are those that can be bought from a **pharmacist** without a prescription. The table below gives some examples.

### THINKING POINT

Have you ever taken any medication? Was this prescribed by your GP or was it bought from a pharmacy? Have you ever had an operation? If so, did you have a general anaesthetic or a local anaesthetic?

*Use of pharmaceuticals for common medical conditions*

| Type of medicine | Information | Examples of conditions it can be used for | Examples of medicine |
|---|---|---|---|
| Tablets and capsules | These vary on how to take them. Some are taken with food, without food or just with a drink | Infections<br>Pain relief<br>Migraine prevention | Antibiotics<br>Paracetamol |
| Creams and lotions | These are rubbed into the skin | Skin conditions such as eczema | E45 |
| Inhalers | These deliver medicines to the lungs | Asthma<br>Hay fever | Salbutamol |
| Liquids | Easy to take and so often used with children | Colds and coughs | Many different types available |
| Suppositories and pessaries | These medicines are inserted into the rectal passage | Constipation<br>Pain relief | Glycerine |

**Pharmacist** A health care professional (not a doctor) who specialises in drugs and medicines.

## Case study: Kathleen's story

Kathleen was 36 when she was diagnosed with cervical cancer. She had had an abnormal result from a smear test done in the NHS Cervical Cancer Screening Programme, which she attended every three years, and her doctor sent her for further tests. As soon as possible after the diagnosis was made, she had an operation to remove the cancer. The screening programme had allowed early intervention in her case, and she made a successful recovery.

1 What is early intervention?

2 Find out what other screening services the NHS offers.

## Lifestyle changes

Some conditions, especially the long-term or lifelong ones, require sufferers to change their lifestyle. Lifestyle includes things such as diet, exercising, and giving up smoking and reducing alcohol intake. A healthy lifestyle is not just required by people who already have medical conditions: it will benefit everyone, and help them to stop becoming ill. This is referred to as preventive care – preventing illness is always better than treating illness that has already occurred.

## Complementary medicine

Complementary medicine is becoming more and more popular and the NHS now offers it for some conditions. The NHS holds a directory of complementary practitioners and hospitals where such treatment is available (see www.nhsdirectory.org). Remember, however, that complementary therapy is to complement and not to replace medical treatment. Three popular types are acupuncture, aromatherapy and hydrotherapy:

* *Acupuncture* involves fine needles being inserted into the skin. It is used to treat pain, sports injuries, addictions and back problems.

* *Aromatherapy* has been shown to help in cases of stress, tension, headaches, migraine and pain, and its use in cancer care is increasing. Oils obtained from flowers, plants and trees are massaged into the body, added to baths or used in room vaporisers.

* *Hydrotherapy* has been proven to help in cases of stress, back pain and **arthritis**. A typical treatment involves a bath similar to a jacuzzi. Hydrotherapy was a common treatment in Roman times.

### Case study: Lavender's story

Lavender is 24 and has suffered from migraines since she was 14. She has generally had around three a month but last year decided to try aromatherapy, after reading in a magazine that it can help with migraines. Lavender has had a few aromatherapy massage sessions and when she feels a migraine coming on she uses peppermint oil. She reports that the migraines now come just once a month and are shorter in length. The peppermint oil also lessens her feeling of nausea.

1 Where else, other than in magazines, can you find information on treating conditions?.

2 Do you think the aromatherapy had a positive or negative effect on Lavender's migraines? Explain your answer.

## Exercise

A **physiotherapist** works with people who have physical symptoms or conditions due to illness or disability. One treatment offered by them is therapeutic exercise; that is, they teach patients some exercises suited to their condition. Some hospitals have specially designed gyms for this treatment.

### Activity

A new campaign by the Department of Health called 'Small Change, Big Difference' aims to persuade people to change their lifestyle before they become ill. Visit the campaign web pages on www.dh.gov.uk and read about it.

1 Plan a school or college campaign based on similar lines to 'Small Change, Big Difference'.

2 Produce a poster or leaflet that would form part of that campaign.

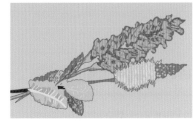

*Essential oils are obtained from plants like peppermint and lavender.*

**Arthritis** A condition where body joints are sore, swollen and painful.

**Physiotherapist** A health care professional (not a doctor) who treats the physical problems caused by accidents, illness and ageing, particularly those that affect the muscles, bones, heart, circulation and lungs.

### Just checking

* What is meant by a 'prescription only' medicine?
* What is the role of a pharmacist?
* What is the Department of Health's campaign to prevent illness called?

## THINKING POINT

Has a close member of your family ever been ill or admitted to hospital? Think about how this made you feel. Did it worry you? If the answer is no, imagine how you would feel if a loved one did become ill and require hospital treatment.

## Case study: Mike's story continued

Mike (from topic 8.4) now treats his asthma with inhalers. They help, but exercise still makes him very short of breath and wheezy. Once at school after playing football he had a very serious asthma attack and needed to go to hospital.

1 How is Mike's asthma likely to have further effects upon his physical health if he can't exercise properly?

2 Are there likely to be any effects on his emotional well-being?

**Occupational therapist** A health professional who assesses and treats physical and mental conditions using activities to promote independent living.

**Counselling** A process whereby patients are helped to deal with their problems by talking to a trained person.

**Depression** A mental health condition marked by feelings of sadness, despair, loss of energy and difficulty dealing with normal daily life.

# 8.7 How medical conditions can affect individuals, families and carers

Medical conditions can affect not only on the individual sufferer but also family members and carers. This topic covers the PIES – physical, intellectual, emotional, social aspects looked at in Unit 4 – as well the possible financial consequences of ill-health.

## Physical effects of ill-health

Most health conditions affect us physically in some way. Some change how we look or act, while others may prevent us doing physical activities we enjoy doing. These changes may be short term, for example breaking a leg, or lifelong, as in the case of a limb amputation. Health and social care organisations offer rehabilitation services that aim to help people to live independently following conditions that have affected their physical function. An example of a professional involved in such care is an **occupational therapist.**

When patients are affected physically by an illness, families and carers need to help them with things like personal hygiene, as well as shopping and cleaning.

## Emotional and intellectual effects of ill-health

Medical conditions can affect us psychologically, both directly in the case of mental health problems but also indirectly in the case of physical conditions. Many people with long-term conditions suffer from **depression** and require **counselling** and support. If people can no longer work because of ill-health, they may worry about paying bills. Families and carers will also suffer emotionally (with stress and anxiety), as it is very worrying when a loved one is ill.

## Social effects of ill-health

Some illnesses can affect us socially. Stroke is one example of this, as some stroke patients have difficulty in walking and talking, which obviously will limit their social lives. Some activities they could do before the stroke they will no longer be able to do and this can cut them off from some of their social circles.

## Economic effects of ill-health

There are more than one million people in the UK who have been unable to work for at least six months because of illness. Diseases and illness cost the country a lot of money, and not only in terms of the health care costs. When people are unable to work through illness the government has to provide financial support through benefits.

For some people who have worked all their life, suddenly not being able to work causes great stress and worry. There are still bills and mortgages to pay. Some people may have to sell their house or car and luxuries such as holidays cease.

## Case study: Tony and Natalie's story

Tony and Natalie have been married for 10 years and live in a five-bedroom detached house. Tony used to play football at the weekends and Natalie enjoys painting. Tony was a 42-year-old managing director but recently he suffered a stroke, probably caused by his high blood pressure. The stroke affected his left side and he now has mobility problems. As a result, he has had to give up his job. Natalie has been a housewife for the last seven years; she hasn't worked in that time and does not drive a car. They have two children – Robert aged six and Andrew four.

1 What effects will the stroke have on Tony? Consider the physical, intellectual, emotional and social impact.

2 What impact will Tony's stroke have on his wife and his two children? Again, consider the physical, intellectual, emotional and social impact.

## Young carers

Young carers are children who help look after a family member who is ill, disabled or has a mental health illness. Their responsibilities may include cooking, cleaning, shopping and assisting with personal care. There are over 175,000 young carers in the UK and their average age is 12. Many young carers miss out on opportunities that other children have to play and learn.

Whatever their background, young carers have lots to deal with. Many struggle educationally because of their caring responsibilities. They are more likely to suffer emotional and psychological difficulties, when young or in later life. Caring for a physically disabled adult is hard work, and young carers suffer in particular from back problems. In terms of their personal identity, they may have difficulty seeing themselves as an individual in their own right with a future, and not just someone who looks after other people.

### Activity

1 Visit www.patient.co.uk and make a list of at least 10 charities and support groups.

2 Design a leaflet describing two of the charities and support groups.

## Case study: Olivia's story

Olivia is 14 years old. Her main loves are badminton and hanging out with her friends. When Olivia comes home from school she takes on the role of sole carer for her mum, who has depression. Since last year, Olivia has joined the young carers club in her home town. She attends every two weeks and has the opportunity to meet other young carers and get advice and support from the young carer workers. She says, 'Gill is my support worker and she is great. The young carers club takes the young carers out to places, to give us a break. All the staff are really friendly and they try to ensure we get the support from other agencies too, like GP, social workers and teachers.'

1 What effect on Olivia has her mum's illness had?

2 What professionals and organisations support Olivia in her caring role?

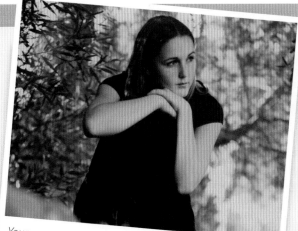
Young carers need support in their roles.

### Just checking

＊ Name a condition that affects us physically.

＊ What is the name of the professional who can help us cope with illness and live more independently?

＊ How can illness affect us economically?

## 8.8 Care pathways and professionals

**THINKING POINT**

Imagine you are planning a long car journey that will take at least five hours. What planning will you do beforehand? Will you use a map to plan the quickest way there? Will you plan rest breaks? Anything else? Why would you plan all of this?

In this topic we will look more closely at the term 'care pathway' and what it means. We will also look at the range of health care professionals and organisations that could be involved in a care pathway.

### What is a care pathway?

A care pathway is an outline of the care that a patient may require for a certain condition, including tests and examinations. Pathways originally were made for patients with complex conditions, but they are now used for a wide range of conditions, including obesity.

A care pathway is presented from the patient's point of view. This helps to ensure that the care they receive is individually tailored to them and meets their needs. The pathway is planned for the whole journey and not just one visit to a hospital. It generally includes the different departments and organisations that the patient will encounter in the whole episode of care for their condition. Care pathways are an important way to develop and keep partnerships between different health professionals and organisations and they also 'empower' patients.

Care pathways are primarily documents that are designed by health care managers when planning services in partnership with patients. If you were to look at one you would see it is very difficult to interpret, as they use language or terminology that is unfamiliar. However, some NHS trusts do provide simple diagrams for patients that explain the care pathway.

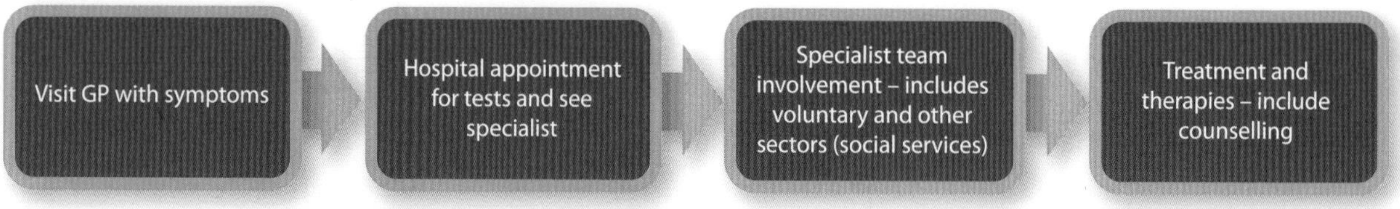

Visit GP with symptoms → Hospital appointment for tests and see specialist → Specialist team involvement – includes voluntary and other sectors (social services) → Treatment and therapies – include counselling

*The process of a care pathway.*

### Case study: Jane's story

Jane is 27 years old and for the last two months has had symptoms of extreme thirst, tiredness and loss of weight. She visited her GP, who ordered some blood tests that were sent to the hospital's **pathology department** for analysis. One test measured Jane's blood glucose levels. At her next appointment, Jane's GP informed her that her glucose level was abnormal and possibly indicative of diabetes; a referral to a hospital **specialist diabetic team** and **consultant** was necessary. The hospital team advised Jane she would need insulin therapy as she had type 1 diabetes and educated her on how to administer it; they also recommended dietary changes and gave her

contact numbers for **Diabetes UK** local support group. At the support group Jane will be able to meet other people who have diabetes, such as Brenda, who we met in topic 8.5. The hospital team drew up an individual plan of care for Jane. Her GP and primary care team would monitor her condition but she would need to return to the hospital in a year for tests to ensure the diabetes was not affecting her health too much.

1 Make a list of all the professionals and services Jane came into contact with during her care pathway.

2 Map out Jane's care pathway as illustrated in the diagram above.

## Case study: Tony's story – the stroke

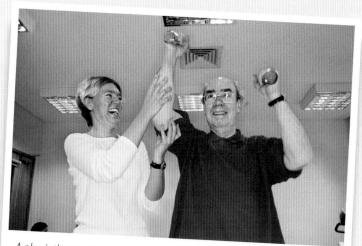

*A physiotherapist is one part of a stroke rehabilitation team.*

**Diabetes UK** A charity that funds research into diabetes and helps those who live with the condition.

**Specialist diabetic team** A health care team specialising in diabetes and consisting of doctors, nurses, dieticians, podiatrists and administration staff.

**Pathology department** A hospital department that offers diagnostic laboratory services.

**Consultant** The most senior rank of hospital doctor.

Following his stroke, Tony (from topic 8.7) was driven by ambulance to hospital, where he was seen in the accident and emergency department. After a doctor there had seen him and made a diagnosis, he was transferred to the neurology ward, where he was under the care of a consultant neurologist. Scans were performed by diagnostic radiographers to assess the severity of the stroke and plan further care. A range of scientists were involved in examining Tony's blood samples. Dieticians assessed his ability to swallow and eat; they then planned a diet for him. While on the ward the stroke rehabilitation team assessed Tony. The team's occupational therapists and physiotherapists advised him on the physical activities that would aid his rehabilitation. After discharge from the hospital, Tony was supported in the community by his GP, as well as the local authority's social services department. Tony continues to visit the hospital for follow-up care and rehabilitation therapy.

1 List all the professionals who have been involved in Tony's care.

2 Draw a map of his route through the health service.

## Just checking

✳ What is a pathology department?

✳ Is diabetes a long-term or a short-term condition?

✳ What do care pathways aim to provide?

# 8.9 Supporting the care pathway approach

In this topic you will learn what organisations and services support the concept of patient-centred care and care pathways.

## National Service Frameworks

National Service Frameworks (NSFs) are long-term plans to improve the care given by the NHS for certain conditions. They outline what is expected and they set standards. At present, there are NSFs for the following areas:

* cancer
* paediatric intensive care
* diabetes
* coronary heart disease
* mental health
* **renal** services
* long-term conditions
* children
* older people
* chronic obstructive pulmonary disease.

However, new NSFs are always being developed.

The NSFs have a number of aims and objectives. For example, the diabetes NSF has strategies to reduce the risk of developing diabetes, to identify diabetes in people who are not aware that they have the condition, and to improve overall diabetes care. The NSF for older people has strategies to tackle **ageism** and discrimination and to address conditions commonly related to older people, such as stroke. The mental health NSF focuses on the safety of people with mental health problems, their carers and the public. Key objectives include ensuring that mental health services are accessible to those who need them, are non-discriminatory, and offer choices that promote independence.

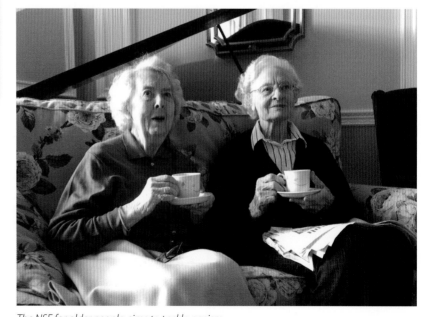

*The NSF for older people aims to tackle ageism.*

## PALS

Since the year 2000, NHS trusts around the country have been asked to provide a patient advice and liaison service (PALS). It is a confidential service created to help patients, their families and carers find the answers to questions or concerns regarding the care and treatment they receive. Patients, relatives and carers may all sometimes need to turn to someone for help, advice and support. The PALS is there to help sort out any problems and guide people through the different services available.

## NICE

NICE is the abbreviation used for the independent organisation called the National Institute for Health and Clinical Excellence. It is responsible for providing national guidance on promoting good health and preventing and treating ill-health.

NICE produces guidance in three areas of health:

* *public health* – guidance on the promotion of good health and the prevention of ill-health for those working in the NHS, local authorities and the wider public and voluntary sector

* *health technologies* – guidance on the use of new and existing medicines, treatments and procedures within the NHS

* *clinical practice* – guidance on the appropriate treatment and care of people with specific diseases and conditions within the NHS.

**Renal** To do with the kidneys.

**Ageism** Discrimination against someone due to their age.

### Activity

Most hospitals and primary care trusts have a PALS.

1 If you are on work experience in a health care setting, ask your placement supervisor about the local PALS. You may see posters on walls advertising the service or leaflets in patient waiting areas. Collect examples of these for your portfolio.

2 If you are in a hospital on placement, there may be a PALS office. Ask if it can be arranged for you to visit the PALS team to find out more about them.

### Diploma Daily

#### World's Biggest Coffee Morning!

September saw the 'World's Biggest Coffee Morning' take place. It is one of the biggest fundraising events in the UK, with an estimated 2million people raising their mugs for Macmillan. The event has helped the cancer charity to raise over £7 million for people affected by cancer. Every year 270,000 people are diagnosed with cancer in the UK. Macmillan aim to support every one of those people and their friends and families too.

1 Visit Macmillan's website, www.macmillan.org.uk. Find out about the sorts of information they can offer.

2 In what ways can they support people with cancer?

### Just checking

* What are NSFs and what are they intended to improve?
* What are the key objectives of the mental health NSF?
* What does NICE stand for? Describe in detail which three areas of health it produces guidance for.

# Unit 8 Assessment guide

This unit is assessed by an assignment which is marked by your teacher. You will need to show that you understand how health can be measured – for example, measuring temperature, pulse, blood pressure, peak flow, waist circumference, and body mass index. You will need to explain what the normal measurements (values) are. You will need to carry out some health measurements yourself and interpret them to assess health. You will need to investigate some common health problems and their signs, symptoms and treatment. You will need to show that you understand how illness affects the physical, intellectual, emotional, social and financial well-being of everyone involved. When a person is diagnosed with a health problem, they will experience treatment by a range of health care workers in different organisations, such as the GP's surgery or the local hospital. You will need to investigate this for one common health problem, and you will also need to show the structures of the different organisations that provide this health care.

## Time management

* Keep any class work safely in a folder, for example charts containing results of measurements. Keep any research that you do, for example when investigating diabetes or asthma, in a folder, so that you know where to find it when you write up your report. By being well organised, you will show your teacher that you are an independent enquirer and a self-manager.

* Carry out as many activities in class as you can. These will include health measurements of temperature, pulse, blood pressure, peak flow, waist circumference, and body mass index. By carrying out these measurements, you will gather evidence for your assignment.

* Be prepared with a list of questions that you could ask if your teacher arranges for a speaker to come and talk to your class. These could contribute towards your primary research.

## Useful links

* There are lots of useful websites that will help with your investigation of three illnesses. For example, www.patient.co.uk is a website used by lots of GPs to give their patients information about their health.

* Another useful website is www.nhs.uk where you will find information on diseases and also the structure of the National Health Service, the largest provider of health care in the UK.

* You may also be able to get leaflets from your local GP's surgery or clinic about common health problems and how to recognise them.

* Work experience will also be useful, as you may meet health care workers who can explain how illnesses can affect patients and their families.

* You could talk to a family member or friend if they have a health problem and ask them how it affects them physically, intellectually, emotionally, socially and financially.

## Things you might need

* The relevant charts on which to record measurements; these will help you to compare your own health measurements against the normal values.

* Evidence from health care workers or people suffering from illnesses, to confirm that you spoke to them about an illness and its treatment. This will contribute to your primary research that you need to undertake to gain higher assessment marks.

* Craft materials or ICT equipment to produce your booklet containing information on one common illness, its treatment and who provides it.

* ICT equipment to help you carry out your investigation of three common health problems. Your teacher may advise you which ones you should investigate.

* A reference list will be needed to show where you got your secondary research information from. You should make a note of every book and website that you have used in your investigation and put this list in your assignment.

# How you will be assessed

| You must show that you *know*: | Guidance | To gain higher marks you must *explain*: |
|---|---|---|
| What measurements are needed to check whether someone is healthy. These will include: pulse rate, blood pressure, peak flow, waist circumference, body mass index and temperature. You also need to show that you can use them correctly. | ✳ Watch closely when your teacher or a health worker shows you how to carry out these measurements. Ask for help if you are still not sure so that you don't get an incorrect result.<br>✳ Find out what the normal result (or value) is.<br>✳ Record three of your own measurements. If you work with a friend you can check each other's blood pressure and compare this and your other results with each other.<br>✳ Put this information on to a chart and keep it safely in a folder. | ✳ What the normal values are for each measurement.<br>✳ How each one is measured.<br>✳ Your own results and compare the results to the normal values. |
| The signs, symptoms and treatment of three common illnesses, such as diabetes, cancer, coronary heart disease or asthma. How any of these illnesses can affect the patient, the family and their carers. Think about the physical, intellectual, social, emotional and financial well-being of all concerned. | ✳ Present this information as a report. Try not to copy from textbooks as this will not be your own work. You should use a variety of information, including leaflets.<br>✳ You could ask a health care worker about the treatment of these illnesses. You might consider the well-being of a relative caring for an ill spouse or partner. They may be unable to spend time relaxing through hobbies (physical impact). They may be unable to go out with friends if the patient needs 24-hour care, leading to isolation; they may be worried about their partner's condition (emotional impact). The patient may need medicines, special foods or have to pay parking charges when visiting hospital (financial impact). To achieve a higher mark you need to show that you have used primary research, so speak to a health care worker or a patient. Make sure you are sensitive when asking questions and remember the information is confidential. | ✳ The signs, symptoms and the treatment required by three patients suffering from different common conditions.<br>✳ At which stage of life it may affect them. You could add information about the measurements of health where relevant.<br>✳ The impact of ill-health on the patient, family and their carers. |
| What happens to the person who is ill and what the role is of the health care workers who will come into contact with them. Think about how the patient will first seek a diagnosis – where will they need to get treatment from? Who will provide the treatment? What is their job role? | ✳ Choose just one of the conditions that you have investigated.<br>✳ Find out what the roles of three health care workers are and how their care supports the patient. For example, you might investigate the role of the doctor, nurse and physiotherapist if you are investigating the journey of a patient with asthma. Present this information in the form of a booklet, which can be produced using ICT or craft materials.<br>✳ Talk to health care workers if you can, to show you have carried out primary research. | ✳ What happens to the patient throughout their treatment and what support, care and treatment may be offered from start to finish.<br>✳ The roles of three health care staff that the patient would come into contact with. |
| The structure of health care organisations. The largest provider of health care is the NHS but people may use health care from private or charitable organisations. | ✳ You could present this as a diagram, with a written explanation, showing how the primary care services and the secondary care services are organised in the NHS. You could link this to your detailed investigation of one illness.<br>✳ Private organisations may include hospitals, care homes and complementary therapists. Charitable organisations may include those that provide day care, e.g. Age Concern, or care for the terminally ill, e.g. hospices. | ✳ How health services within the health sector are organised and how they support patients. |

## Introduction

This unit will show you how society has looked on people with disabilities in the past. Earlier attitudes have shaped the way today's society looks at people with disabilities. You will learn about the many self-help groups that have grown out of the need of people with disabilities to feel valued and to have their independence. You will begin to understand how the various movements and campaigns over the years have helped develop a different attitude towards people with disabilities, and how they have encouraged positive acceptance and inclusion. You may have experienced this in your own school, through anti-bullying policies and the inclusion of students with physical and learning disabilities.

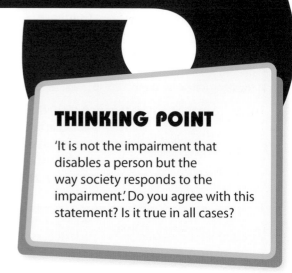

**THINKING POINT**

'It is not the impairment that disables a person but the way society responds to the impairment.' Do you agree with this statement? Is it true in all cases?

### Models of disability

We are all different! Because we are all different, it is easy sometimes to see people as better or worse, right or wrong. When you walk through your town or shopping centre, how many times do you make a judgement about someone you see? What do you base that judgement on – their style of dress, their age, their colour, their behaviour? Do you automatically feel sorry for anyone who has a physical disability?

Prejudices come from many areas and we **stereotype** people. These prejudices and stereotypes are based on historical **attitudes**, on how the media portray a certain group, and on what parents or peers think. Do you use your own judgements based on what you see and know, or do you follow others?

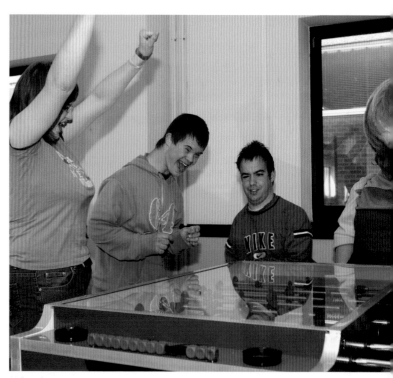

*Value diversity.*

In this unit you will learn what the social model of disability is and how it compares with the medical model. You will begin to understand how the social model challenges society and how it has helped to change our attitudes towards people with any kind of disability.

# Barriers

You will realise that, as a service provider, you may get on better with some clients than with others. Think about why that might be. Could it be that you feel more awkward with someone you don't understand? But if you find out about the person's culture or interests, that might help you to get on. You may then learn to value the many different people who make up the society we live in.

There are many barriers that people with disabilities face every day. There are physical barriers, such as not being able to get into buildings. There are language barriers that might stop them getting the right information. Other barriers stop people accessing certain services, including health services. People with learning disabilities have to overcome barriers to access the curriculum. There are also barriers that come from people's attitudes towards others. You will look at these and develop your own opinions and values.

## How you will be assessed

For this unit you will be assessed by one assignment. For this assignment you need to investigate the social model of disability and produce a report. You will also need to identify and reflect upon your own attitudes and those of society, enabling you to develop further as a reflective learner. As part of your report, you should assess at least one piece of legislation and a resulting policy that supports the social model of disability. You will also need to investigate how the social model of disability helps to promote independence and choice, appropriate support and service provision, employment and the removal of barriers that promote disability. You will need to carry out a survey in order to investigate this. Some of the research for this unit could be carried out in small groups, with sharing of information. However, your report should be entirely your own work.

## What you will learn in this unit

You will:

* Know about the development of the social model of disability, its aims and objectives
* Understand what is meant by the social model of disability, why it is important in addressing discrimination, how it supports independence and choice, and how it differs from the medical model
* Understand how the social model of disability shapes and is continuing to influence the development of support, service provision and the environment
* Understand how potential barriers in society and the environment might be overcome
* Know about the role of ethics, key legislation and policies which support the social model of disability
* Be able to recognise your own values and attitudes, and your own personal and social responsibility to others

---

**Attitudes** Personal views or feelings about a person or thing.

**Stereotype** A generalised and oversimplified opinion or image of someone else, such as 'Football players aren't very intelligent'.

---

## Activity

1 What type of disabilities do you know of? Make a list. Discuss these as a group or with your friends to see if anyone has come up with anything different. Make a master list.

2 Now look around your classroom. What problems do you think each of these groups might have if they had to use the room? What changes could be made so that as many groups as possible could use it?

# WHAT DO YOU THINK OF THIS?

'On the towpath we met and had to pass a long line of imbeciles… It was perfectly horrible. They should certainly be killed.'

This diary entry by the novelist Virginia Woolf was written in January 1915.

**Disability** A condition that restricts someone's ability to perform particular activities.

**Impairments** Reductions in strength, quality or ability, possibly because of an injury or disease.

# 9.1 Then and now: from Bedlam to…

In order to recognise where your own and society's values and attitudes come from, it is useful to look at some historical attitudes towards disability, and compare them with attitudes more prevalent today.

## The influence of the past

It is important to see where society's thinking about **disability** has come from. The statement in the starter stimulus (left) is typical of the times and the way people thought about disability. Past attitudes can be seen in myths, literature, theatre and folklore. Some of our current negative attitudes and stereotypes have been reinforced by society and religion over many centuries. You will still come across these negative attitudes in individuals and you may notice how certain parts of our society and environment are not helpful or inclusive of people with various disabilities. For centuries people have worked to change these views but, as you will see, it is only within the last 30 years that real changes have been made. The social model of disability has developed as a result of these negative attitudes and values.

Historical attitudes to disabilities have shaped how society thinks about people with disabilities today. But such attitudes can still be seen in many cultures around the world.

In medieval times, witchcraft became linked with people with disabilities. During the 'great witch hunts' of 1480–1680, people were told how to identify witches by their **impairments**; people thought these 'witches' also created disability in others. A woman who gave birth to a disabled child was often accused of being a witch. Between 8 and 20 million people, mainly women, were put to death as witches across Europe. Many had disabilities.

### Fairy tales

We are bound to be affected in later years by the images and stories that are shown to us early in our lives, and many of these relate to people with disabilities. For example, disability has been linked with evil throughout the folklore of Britain and Europe. The fairy tales by the Brothers Grimm, such as Hansel and Gretel, often portray the witch as deformed, blind and ugly, with a stick. Look at the way everyone who is evil is shown in the tales we are told when we are young, such as 'the ugly sisters' in Cinderella. Pirates have similarly often been portrayed as both evil and disabled, for example, R. L. Stevenson's Long John Silver and J. M. Barrie's Captain Hook.

### Entertainment

Throughout history, people with disabilities have been used as entertainment. Games were held at the Coliseum in Ancient Rome where disabled children were thrown under horses' hooves; the Romans also staged fights between dwarfs and women, and blind gladiators were made to fight each other. In medieval times, court jesters were often disabled.

You will have probably heard of people with disabilities being used in more recent times as entertainment in circuses and freak shows. For many people with disabilities, however, working in a circus was a career at which they could at least make a living. Some people's disabilities prevented them from doing physical work, so at least being in a circus helped stop the idea that they were a drain on society, worthless and objects of pity.

## Present attitudes

Society has come a long way from when people were put into places like Bedlam. Now, because of much campaigning and the development of the social model, people with disabilities can live as a group while keeping their independence.

The majority of children and adults with disabilities now live at home with their families. There are some who live in residential schools or establishments, some in health service establishments and some children are in substitute family placements. Unfortunately, though, there are still cases where disabled children lose all contact with their families.

Residential care may still be the best solution for some people with disabilities. The most important thing is that they and their families have a choice, that they are empowered to make the decision based on the many different factors that affect them.

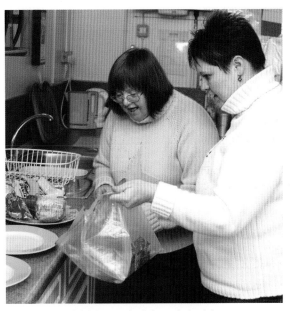

*The majority of children and adults with disabilities can now live at home with their families.*

## Activity

Look at the passage below from the *Pictorial Handbook of London*, published in 1854. It describes the conditions of the Hospital of St Mary of Bethlehem ('Bedlam'):

'*Bethlem Hospital* was founded in 1547, and the early treatment of the miserable creatures committed to its brutal rulers, appears to have been characterised by utter indifference to the feelings and comforts of the patients, and a studied aggravation of their miseries. Indeed, to our shame be it recorded, these miseries were made the materials for actual *profit* to the hospital; a sum of about 400*l.* being annually collected by exhibiting the poor maniacs, chiefly naked, and uniformly chained to the walls of their dungeons, and by exciting them to the most violent manifestations of their maladies. This practice of showing the patients, like wild beasts, was abolished in 1770, but the abolition was unaccompanied by any other improvement in their treatment. Recently, however, the unfortunate lunatics have been more humanely treated.'

1 In the passage above, find five things that happened in the past to people with a mental disability that would not happen today.

2 Produce a diagram or collage to show historical attitudes and stereotyping.

## Just checking

* Think back over your childhood: can you name three stories in which disabled people were the bad guys?

* Can you see three words written in the description of Bethlem Hospital that would cause offence today?

* Make a list of what you think may have influenced your attitudes.

# 9.2 Ethics, equality and you

## CHALLENGING VIEWS

Many people have minor impairments, such as those who use hearing aids, or glasses or contact lenses. They are not usually discriminated against. People who are deaf or blind, however, are often discriminated against, perhaps because there are more barriers to communication. Would you be prepared to challenge attitudes and practices that prejudice and exclude people with disabilities?

This topic looks at how various groups of people have fought for equality and how this has had an impact on key legislation and provision. It also takes into account the role of charities in promoting the rights of people with disabilities.

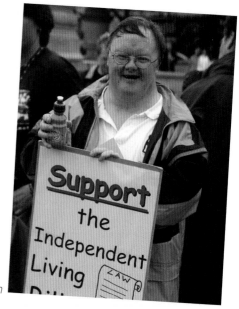

*The fight for equality goes on in many aspects of society.*

## People with disabilities fight for equality

The struggles of people with disabilities to gain civil rights have led to legislation in the USA (e.g. the Americans with Disabilities Act 1990) and the UK (e.g. the Disability Discrimination Act 1995), as well as many other countries, including South Africa, India and Australia. The United Nations adopted the UN Standard Rules on Equalisation in 1992. Examples of UK legislation are presented in the table below.

*Key UK legislation on disability*

| Key legislation | Aims and provisions |
| --- | --- |
| Mental Health Act 1983 | Aims to protect the public as well as the patient. People with a mental illness are sometimes compulsorily detained in psychiatric hospitals, and the Act regulates how and when this can happen |
| Disability Discrimination Act 1995 (DDA) | Gave rights to people with disabilities in employment, access to education, transport and housing, and obtaining goods and services |
| Discrimination Act 2005 | Goes further than the DDA and actively promotes the rights of people with disabilities to equal opportunities. It also promotes positive attitudes towards people with disabilities and encourages their participation in public life |
| Human Rights Act 1998 | Aims to ensure that your and everyone else's rights in all areas of our lives are respected |
| Care Standards Act 2000 (CSA) | Ensures that services, including residential care, nursing homes, children's homes and many others, are regulated and national standards are applied |
| Children Act 2004 | Aims to improve the lives of children and covers all the services that children might access, including schools, day care and children's homes. It also encourages services to work more closely together for the benefit of the child and supports the *Every Child Matters* programme |
| Equality Act 2006 | Created a single Commission – the Commission for Equality and Human Rights (CEHR) – to replace the Equal Opportunities Commission (EOC), the Commission for Racial Equality (CRE) and the Disability Rights Commission (DRC). It also made **discrimination** on the grounds of religion or belief, sexual orientation or disability unlawful. The CEHR promotes understanding of the importance of equality and diversity in our society |

The government makes laws and then local authorities (and others) have a duty to carry out those laws. Legislation is based on the idea that adjustments need to be made to services to allow people with disabilities to have access to buildings, transport, workplaces, environments, education, communications and equipment.

Schools and colleges have to take into account the needs of disabled students and to make reasonable adjustments to their policies, practices and procedures so that disabled students are not placed at a disadvantage in comparison with other students. Can you think of any adjustments your school has had to make to accommodate a student with any impairment?

Schools should also include in the curriculum the study of how society has portrayed and treated people with disabilities in the past and today. This may have been taught in your PHSE lessons.

## Charities for people with disabilities

To give to charity or be charitable has traditionally been seen to be a good thing in many religions, including Christianity, Islam and Judaism. Unfortunately, charities centuries ago led to pitying or patronising attitudes towards people with disabilities. While charities attempted to care for people with disabilities, the views of the time led to institutions being built to care for the 'less fortunate'. People with disabilities in this way were kept away from society, which developed into a policy of **segregation**.

Today, however, the role of charities has changed dramatically. Numerous campaigns have been run by disabled people alongside charities – such as Scope, Mencap, the Royal National Institute of Blind People (RNIB) and the British Institute for Learning Disability (BILD) – and together they have fought for the rights of disabled people to have independence and choice in their lives. These charities have had a big impact on the development of the social model of disability, which is the subject of the next topic.

**Discrimination** Treating a person or group unfairly or differently from other persons or groups of people (e.g. on the basis of prejudice).

**Segregation** Keeping particular groups of people apart from one another.

### Personal, learning and thinking skills

The activity should help towards PLTS: Independent enquirer; Self-manager.

### Functional skills

It will also help towards FS: ICT – find and select information.

### Activity

1 Look up the following on the Internet and see the work these charities do today. Their main aim is to promote equality for disabled people and to support them.

　＊ Cystic Fibrosis Trust

　＊ Epilepsy Action

　＊ Mencap

　＊ National Autistic Society

　＊ National Deaf Children's Society

　＊ RNIB

　＊ Scope

2 Choose one that particularly interests you, and prepare a short talk on it, describing how it is working to empower people with the specific disability.

### Just checking

＊ Give two examples of a physical impairment.

＊ Name two pieces of legislation that promote positive attitudes towards people with disabilities.

＊ There have been many others but which four charities have been named in this topic as having had an impact on the development of the social model of disability?

**Model** A simplified or idealised version or idea of how something ought to work.

# 9.3 Social and medical models of disability

In this topic the two key models of disability – the social and medical models – are looked at and compared. You will learn about the differences between the two. You will look at why the social model developed and why it is preferred by people with disabilities.

## The problem

Based on the medical **model** of disability, the World Health Organization (WHO) in 1980 gave the following definitions:

* *impairment* is 'any loss or abnormality of psychological, physiological, anatomical structure or function'
* *disability* is 'any restriction or lack (resulting from impairment) of ability to perform an activity in the manner or within the range considered normal for a human being'
* *handicap* is 'a disadvantage for a given individual, resulting from impairment or a disability that limits or prevents the fulfilment of a role that is normal (depending on age, sex, social and cultural factors) for that individual'.

Can you see why these definitions might offend and hurt people who are disabled? The above definitions disempower people with disabilities. Why? Do you think people with disabilities were consulted about these definitions?

## The medical model

The 'medical model' of disability sees the disabled person as the problem. People with disabilities are seen to be dependent on others for their basic needs and not able to do much for themselves. The thought is that the world will stay as it is and people with disabilities must fit into it. That might mean being isolated at home or being put into a specialised institution.

This model, together with historical views, has led us to have pity for people with disabilities or in some cases fear.

Usually the focus is on the impairment rather than the needs of the person. It gives the impression that people with disabilities are sick, helpless, useless, unfortunate and incapable of controlling their lives. It has often been non-disabled professionals who say where these people go to school, what support they should get, where they should live and what type of work they should do, if any.

The medical model creates a cycle of dependency and exclusion. Both disabled and non-disabled people have accepted this model, which has made this cycle difficult to break.

*The nature of the medical model of disability.*

Child development team

Specialists

Social workers

Doctors

Surgeons

GPs

Special transport

Speech therapists

**The impairment is the problem**

Educational psychologists

Occupational therapists

Special schools

Benefits agency

Sheltered workshops

Training centre

This approach has been and still is used by most agencies that deliver services for people with disabilities, including education, health and rehabilitation, and by employers. It involves certain assumptions about impairment, disability and handicap. It has led to people being excluded and segregated from society.

## The social model

The term 'social model' was first used in 1975. It has been developed as an alternative to the medical model and, most importantly, this was done by people with disabilities and their supporters.

The social model of disability challenges the way people who do not have disabilities think about people with them. It begins with the view that society in general takes little or no account of people who have impairments, which means they are often excluded from participating in education, work and social activities.

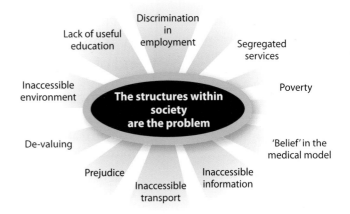

The problems people with disabilities have in society.

In the last 30 years, people with disabilities have campaigned for an approach to disability based on human rights. It is beginning to be accepted that disability discrimination, prejudice, negative attitudes and stereotypes are not acceptable. The disability movement has advocated a different way of looking at disability.

The social model defines 'impairment' and 'disability' very differently to the medical model:

* *impairment* means that some part, or parts, of your body, senses or mind are limited in their functioning, in the long term or permanently

* *disability* is the loss or limitation of opportunities to take part in the normal life of the community on an equal level with others due to physical and social barriers.

Compare these definitions with those given by the WHO at the start of this topic. What are the differences?

Impairment and chronic illness exist and sometimes pose real difficulties, but supporters of the disability movement believe that the discrimination against people with disabilities is socially created and has little to do with their impairments.

## Activity

1 In pairs, discuss the differences between the medical and social models of disability. What has changed? Why do you think people with disabilities wanted and needed a change in the way society viewed them?

2 Write your own definition of the social model. Your definition should indicate how the social model supports independence and choice for people with disabilities.

## Just checking

* Which model suggests that a person with a learning disability needs to be 'cured'?
* Which model suggests that people with disabilities can and should be supported to be independent?
* When was the term 'social model' first used and who helped develop it?

# 9.4 What is the social model?

This topic looks more closely at the social model of disability. It shows how it differs from the medical model and why. The social model challenges society's ideas about people with disabilities and presents another way of looking at disability, to get rid of discrimination and to value diversity.

## The message of the social model

The message of the social model could be summarised as follows: 'If you want to make a difference to the lives of people with disabilities, you must change your society and the way it treats people with impairments.'

That is, if people would reconsider their attitudes towards people with disabilities, that would probably change the way solutions are found to issues that affect them.

The social model starts with the idea that all disabled adults and children have a right to belong to and be valued in their local community. With this model, you start by looking at the strengths of the person with the impairment and at the physical and social barriers that obstruct them, whether in the environment, at school, college, home or work.

## Some differences between the models

The social model of disability has made us all look at how we can prevent prejudice and stereotyping. It has also made us look at how people with disabilities can be included in society and how we can **empower** those with disabilities.

For example, look at these different attitudes to the same issues:

* The medical model will say a person is not able to use existing structures such as buildings and public transport because their disability limits what they can achieve.
* The social model will criticise the designers, manufacturers and contractors who did not consider how people with disabilities could access those structures when they were designing, manufacturing or constructing them.

The disability movement has said that, 'put simply, it is not that someone can't walk which disables them but that they have to climb steps to get into a building. It is not that someone can't speak that creates disability, but the fact that society fails to communicate with such a person.'

## Challenging prejudice

This way of seeing things opens up opportunities to get rid of prejudice and discrimination against people with disabilities. To ensure that the needs and rights of people with impairments are met, society must adjust the social and physical environment. Rather than attempting to change people with disabilities to fit the existing environment, the disability can be reduced by changing the environment.

The table below compares the attitudes underpinning the medical model and the social model.

*Comparison of the medical and social models of disability*

| Medical model | Social model |
|---|---|
| The child is 'faulty' | The child is valued |
| Person is labelled depending on their diagnosis | A person's strengths and needs are defined by themselves and others |
| The impairment becomes the focus of attention | Barriers are identified and solutions developed |
| Assessment, monitoring and therapy programmes are imposed | A programme is designed based on the outcome to be achieved |
| The person is segregated and alternative services provided | Necessary resources are made available to ordinary services; appropriate training is made available for parents and professionals |
| Ordinary needs are put on hold | Relationships are nurtured |
| Re-entry into mainstream if normal enough or permanent exclusion | Diversity welcomed and the child is included |
| Society remains unchanged | Society evolves |

## Case study: Anisa's story

Anisa is an 11-year-old student with **Asperger's syndrome**. She is an intelligent girl but finds it difficult to make friends. She has just started attending the local secondary school and is afraid she may be bullied. She has a support worker who sits with her during lessons so that she doesn't need to talk to anyone else. She always answers questions in the lesson but is aware that some of the students are laughing at her. The teachers are concerned they may not be able to meet her needs adequately.

1 What are the problems that Anisa is going to face at her new school? Discuss with a friend how these problems could be resolved.

2 Using the social model, how do you think the school should be tackling the issues of Anisa attending? How can Anisa be empowered?

3 What could be done to help Anisa have more confidence to interact with other students? How could the other students help with this?

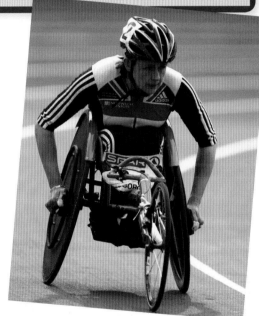

*A role model. Born with spina bifida, Tanni Grey-Thompson, pictured, is a highly successful athlete. She has won 11 Paralympic gold medals and has held over 30 world records. In 2005 she was made Dame Commander of the Order of the British Empire, for her services to disabled sport.*

## Role models

The social model of disability has helped change attitudes to and perceptions of people with disabilities. There are many examples of people who, through their own determination and support from a society that cares, have achieved success in many fields.

## Just checking

* Who does the medical model blame for the problems the disabled have?
* The social model starts with what idea?
* Give two examples of how the social model differs from the medical model.

# 9.5 Looking at things differently

In this topic you will look at two case studies. They show the impact the two models of disability can have on a person. You will look at how people with disabilities can and want to be equal and some of the attitudes that can prevent them from fully integrating in our society.

## Coping, cures and fears

As you have seen in the previous topics, the medical model focuses on how a person copes with their impairment. Disabled people have historically been 'treated' by the medical profession, who look for cures to enable the 'unfortunate' person overcome the tragedy of their disability. This is in sharp contrast to the social model of disability, which looks at ways society can adjust to accommodate a person with a disability.

**Down's syndrome** A genetic condition that features learning disability, which may range from moderate to severe, as well as some physical anomalies.

**Special school** A school that has pupils with statements of special educational needs (SEN), and often with one particular type of disability, such as deafness, whose needs cannot be fully met from within mainstream provision.

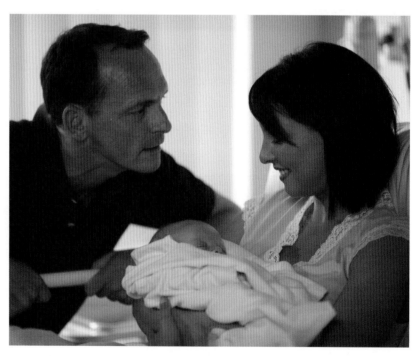
*Honey, Billy and their baby, Janet, from* EastEnders.

If you watch *EastEnders* you will probably be aware of the storyline of Honey and Billy's baby, Janet. It showed very clearly the anxiety and fear that some parents feel when they have a baby with **Down's syndrome**. It has also shown how those fears can be overcome.

## Case study: Michele's story

Michele gave birth to a girl but it seemed to her that not all was right with her daughter. Over the next few months she felt as if the doctors and nurses were dismissing her, that they had expert knowledge that they wouldn't share with her. After many months and numerous consultations, the diagnosis was finally made: her daughter had Down's syndrome. The doctors told her not to worry, and that there were special homes that would look after her child if she couldn't cope.

Michele's feelings were mixed. She felt relieved that someone had finally told her what was wrong with her child but she also felt a despair creep in. Michele's hopes for 'normality' and for a bright future for her daughter were dashed by the diagnosis. She now felt that life for her child was hopeless. She would have to go to a 'special' school and she wouldn't be able to mix with 'normal' children. She was afraid to go out, not knowing what people's reactions would be. As she herself said:

'I wanted to take my baby out and show her off to everyone. But she's got problems and she's not normal. I feel very conscious about the way she is and that people will stare at her. Some people aren't bothered about disability but some will think 'What's wrong with her?' I used to be scared of children with disabilities, when they were on those special buses going to school. So I know people will think like that, because I think like that myself.'

1 What does Michele think the future holds for her daughter?

2 Which model of disability is being used here by the doctors? Give examples to support your answer.

3 How could the social model of disability be applied to support Michele and her daughter?

## Case study: John's story

My name is John Edwards. I am 17½. I've been studying at college for one year. Before I came to this college I was in a **special school** with other disabled people like me and I really liked it there.

I am studying AS Applied ICT. I have support in taking my notes; I dictate to my support worker and I have support with my personal care. All staff and students have been really helpful and supportive. From day one I felt really welcome and they sorted out all my needs to help me to study well and get my grades.

When I'm not studying, I really enjoy watching rugby and meeting with friends. I like going to the pub, and I enjoy meeting new people.

It was a real challenge coming to a mainstream college, because I had to learn how to mix with non-disabled people. I felt I had to show them that just because I was in a wheelchair didn't mean I didn't have a brain.

I had to go on work experience. I needed to tell them what I needed and I looked around the building to see if it was accessible. I got a message the next day to say they were very sorry but they didn't have the right access into the building or facilities for me, so I wouldn't be able to go there. I felt annoyed and upset at this because I was really looking forward to it.

1 Which aspects of John's experiences described here are influenced by the medical model and which by the social model of disability? Give reasons for your decisions.

2 Where has the social model been applied to support John's education?

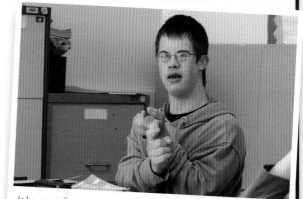

*John at college.*

## Just checking

* How does a person get Down's syndrome?
* What is a 'special school'?
* Give an example of stereotyping from John's story.

## HOW WILL HE COPE?

James is 19 years old. He wants to go on work experience to a laboratory. James is in a wheelchair and his parents are very concerned that the lab won't have the facilities to support a person with a disability. How will he gain access to the building and move around the labs? What will happen about his lunch? How might other people react to him? Do you think the laboratory would and could **enable** James to access the work placement?

**Independence** Freedom from the control, influence, support or help of others; the ability to make your own decisions.

**Enable** Give people the means and the ability to do things for themselves.

## Snapshot

The Disability Rights Commission (DRC) was an independent body set up by the British Parliament to end discrimination towards people with disabilities. The passing of the Equality Act 2006 meant that in October 2007 the DRC was replaced by the new Commission for Equality and Human Rights, which has powers across all equality law (race, sex, disability, religion and belief, sexual orientation and age).

# 9.6 Enable, not disable

This topic looks at how the social model of disability has influenced attitudes and affected provision. You will learn how this model has enabled and supported disabled people to be independent and have a choice in how they live and work.

## Positive acceptance

There has been a growing culture of acceptance of the differences between people. This is where the social model of disability has developed from. It aims to promote the rights of people with disabilities to **independence** and inclusion in our society.

The social model of disability has changed many people's outlook on life – and it could change yours. The social model of disability seeks to **enable** people with disabilities to look at themselves in a more positive way. This increases their self-esteem and independence.

## Choice and control

Many people believe that independence is about doing everything for yourself. People with disabilities often need assistance in their everyday lives, so people have thought they cannot be independent. People with disabilities have challenged this assumption.

How many times a day do you ask for help to do something? It may be as simple as 'Could you hold my bag please while I put my jumper on?' We all live in a society and depend upon each other. Being independent is not about doing everything for yourself.

Choice and control are two of the most important things commonly denied to people with disabilities. One way of overcoming this is to give them the finance and support they need to employ their own care workers to assist them with their everyday lives. This would in turn give them independence. Direct Payments are cash sums which may be paid by local authorities to people to enable them to buy the social care services and support which they have been assessed as needing. This could include home-care support for personal care needs, alternatives to day care and residential provisions provided by their local authority. Can you think of the advantages that this method offers?

## The health needs of people with disabilities

People with physical and/or learning disabilities often have other health needs as well. Some disabilities are in fact associated with particular health problems; for example, people with Down's syndrome often have thyroid disorders, and people with cerebral palsy may also have epilepsy, blindness, or deafness.

Find out about other health needs related to a particular physical or learning disability or impairment.

People with disabilities are more likely to experience a dissatisfying service. As well as the obvious issues that may cause a problem, such as wheelchair access, there are many other issues that can prevent a person with a disability accessing appropriate health care. It may be that someone with a visual impairment, for example, cannot access information in an easy-to-understand format. People with learning difficulties may have problems with accessing services by themselves, but such difficulties are easily overcome by the provision of a support worker.

If you need to go to the doctor, do you make your own appointment or does one of your parents make it for you? Think of all the skills involved with making an appointment. You need to be able to use the telephone, tell the time, explain to a stranger what you need, organise how to get to the health centre, remember to attend at the right time, and make the journey. This can create a lot of anxiety – and that is before you even get to the doctor! Then you have to be able to explain what is wrong. All this on top of feeling poorly!

It is very important that some people with physical and learning disabilities have a support worker to help them access services.

Specific strategies that services should use to improve the health of people with learning disabilities have been recommended in a 2001 White Paper entitled *Valuing People*. These include health action plans (HAPs), training and regular health checks.

## The educational needs of people with disabilities

Universities and colleges are legally required to offer 'reasonable adjustments' and ensure that disabled students are treated fairly. The number of disabled students going on to higher education has increased in recent years; this is because universities and colleges now have to have policies and practices in place to ensure that each student has an equal chance to participate fully in the educational environment.

Because of the social model of disability, students can now access education more easily. As well as access to the environment, there are two areas that have developed to enable this to happen:

* *Alternative format.* Many disabled students have problems accessing text-based documents, so alternative versions are used, such as Braille or sometimes tapes with spoken versions of the text. Students with **dyslexia** can also use tapes. Other formats include using large fonts in documents.
* *Assistive technology.* As well as wheelchairs and hearing aids, this usually refers to devices that use computer technology, such as spell-checkers, and computers running specialist software.

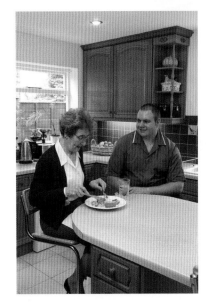

*Look at the photograph. What support is being given and why is this important to the disabled person?*

**Activity**

1 Look at the policies your school or college has on inclusion and anti-bullying.

2 Write a report showing how your school or work placement environment supports independence and inclusion.

**Dyslexia** A language-based disability in which a person has trouble understanding written words.

**Just checking**

* What are Direct Payments?
* What happened to the Disability Rights Commission?
* Give two examples of assistive technology.

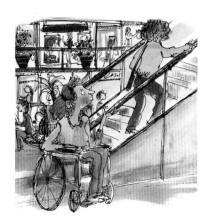

# 9.7 Breaking down barriers

This topic looks at the barriers in society and the environment that create problems for people with disabilities and how those barriers can be overcome.

## Barriers

The opportunities available to people with disabilities are limited by a multitude of barriers (see also topic 1.8). Heavy doors and inaccessible public transport are just two examples of what makes travelling such a hassle – not the fact that someone is disabled. Every disabled person can make their own list of the barriers that limit their inclusion in society. One huge but invisible barrier is other people's negative attitudes.

The social model of disability empowers people with disabilities to challenge society to remove those barriers.

In work, school, leisure and entertainment facilities, transport, training and higher education, housing or in personal, family and social life, it is practices and attitudes that disable people and create the barriers.

## Twelve basic needs

People with disabilities have identified 12 basic needs which, if met, would enable them to participate fully in society:

* full access to the environment
* accessible transport system
* technical aids/equipment
* accessible and adapted housing
* personal assistance
* inclusive education and training
* an adequate income
* equal opportunities for employment
* appropriate and accessible information
* advocacy
* counselling
* appropriate and accessible health care provision.

People with disabilities say that if the barriers were removed, gradually they could play a full part in community life, working and paying taxes like everyone else. In the long run it is cheaper and more economical to support people with disabilities to be independent than providing services in such a way that a disabled person will be dependent on society for the rest of their lives.

What are your views on this?

## Environmental barriers

The disability movement has said that it is the way the environment is designed that presents many barriers. New buildings now have to have ramps or lifts so that they do not present environmental barriers.

---

*How do you think people feel if they come across barriers such as these?*

Inclusive Involving as wide a range of people as possible. One of the government's aims set out in *Every Child Matters* is that all disabled children will be fully included in society (see topic 7.6).

Advocate Someone who is employed to speak for the person with the disability.

Shop managers are becoming more aware that they can arrange their floor space better, so that there is adequate space to get around. Public transport is also being adapted so it can be more easily used by people with disabilities. Most families take play and leisure activities for granted, but barriers here may include the physical environment, the nature and type of public play equipment, and family resources.

## Education

For many years children with disabilities, both physical and learning, had segregated provision in 'special schools'. This has sometimes meant children being in residential institutions for most of the time. The thinking now is that, as far as possible, children should be included in mainstream schools, with the right level of support. There are, however, cases when it is appropriate for children to be in a school that can cater for their specific needs.

## Attitudes and emotions

You have seen in previous topics how people with disabilities have been viewed. If we have a more **inclusive** society, maybe this would help attitudes to change. Do you know anyone who has a disability? Have you talked to them about how they feel other people treat them?

## Language

People with learning disabilities may struggle to understand what is said to them at times, so care workers will use diagrams or make a special effort to speak clearly and simply. An **advocate** or a translator may be employed to help with communication.

Language barriers can also include a lack of accessible information. Someone who has a visual disability may need information written in Braille; someone who is hearing impaired may want the help of someone who can use sign language.

### Diploma Daily

Dear Dorothy

I really fancy this girl in my class. She's gorgeous! The problem is she is deaf and I don't know how to talk to her. When I try she doesn't understand what I am saying or maybe she doesn't want to hear it. We are in our last term at school. I might not see her again after we have left. She seems to be able to communicate with her mates but I'm not sure what to do.

Shaquille from Surrey

Dear Dorothy

I've just started secondary school and am worried about how I will cope. I have cerebral palsy and struggle to get up the stairs so I am often late to my lessons. It takes me a while to say what I want to say, so the other children just stare at me. I don't think I am going to make any friends. The teachers are very kind but don't ask me any questions because they think I might take too long in answering. I want to join in with the others and be able to get to my lessons on time. What can I do?

Coryn from Corby

1 In pairs, discuss what Dorothy's answers should be to these two letters in the *Diploma Daily*. How can Shaquille and Coryn overcome the barriers they are facing?

2 Produce a questionnaire to gauge the attitude of people in your school or work placement to potential barriers. Assess the information. How can the barriers be overcome?

### Just checking

* Can you think of three environmental barriers that a person in a wheelchair might come across on their way to and in the supermarket?
* If you use the social model, what type of education are children with disabilities entitled to?
* Name two language barriers and how they can be overcome.

## WHAT DO YOU THINK?

Do you have an impairment or disability, or do you know anyone who has? What is your experience of disability? Think about your own values and attitudes. Where do they come from? Is it from stories you have heard or read? Is it from the opinions of your family or friends?

In this topic you will be asked to begin questioning your own attitudes and values. It also looks at the changing role of the media and how it has influenced our thinking of people with disabilities.

### Your own attitudes

Everyone has some sort of experience of people with disabilities or some knowledge of disability issues. The attitudes of society are reinforced by the portrayal of people with disabilities in the media, books, films, comics, art and language. Many people with disabilities can be greatly hurt by negative views of themselves; these views create feelings of low **self-esteem**.

### The role of the media

Media professionals have grown up with the same common biases, stereotypes and negative images as the rest of society. This is bound to affect the way people with disabilities are reported and portrayed. This in turn will reinforce public stereotypes.

#### When the media stereotype people with disabilities

Have you ever, when you thought about 'disability', felt pity and conjured up a picture of someone who is dependent and imperfect? Those images are perpetuated by the media. Television and the press are perhaps the two most influential sources of information in the UK, providing us with both opinions and a view into many different areas. The media reflects and influences our norms, beliefs and **values**.

How do representations of disability in the media impact upon the life of a disabled person? Would you notice if a story, publication or television news programme presented biased, negative images of people with disabilities? Look at the table at the top of the next page. Can you see why this reporting might upset people with disabilities?

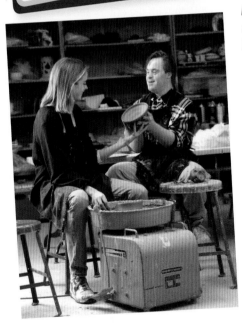

*What is your experience of disability?*

Should we challenge traditional views, opinions, perceptions and prejudices about people with impairments and disabilities and their place in society?

While reporters no longer use terms such as 'cripple', they may still use the word 'handicapped'. Often people with disabilities will be referred to as 'brave', 'courageous victims' or 'unfortunates'. Why do you think this might perpetuate the medical model of disability rather than the social model?

People with disabilities on television are often shown in either hospitals or nursing homes. This reinforces the view that they are dependent and need help; if the disabled person is cute, this works even better.

However, these images are changing. Many actors and television presenters have a physical or learning disability. Do you remember

## Examples of biased reporting

| Story line | Critical evaluation |
|---|---|
| 'For years the state's retarded have been warehoused, but now with the state school closure, many will have new choices and opportunities in the community.' | This article does promote choice, opportunities and inclusion, but look at the word 'retarded' – doesn't such labelling stereotype and devalue people with learning and mental disabilities? Even if the overall tone, subject matter, approach and issue are otherwise handled well, this one word gives a negative image |
| 'Mentally ill person goes on rampage.' | What image do you have when you read this? The implication seems to be that the person went on a rampage because they were mentally ill |
| 'Until stricter paediatric standards are in place, nursing homes won't be safe for children.' | This sounds at first glance as if it is caring, but why are children living in nursing homes at all? |

Paul Henshall, the trainee doctor in *Holby City*, or Julie Fernandez, the secretary in *The Office*? Both were in wheelchairs. The subject of disability is being handled openly, with respect and sensitivity.

There have been many campaigns over recent years that have had a huge impact on the way people with impairments and disabilities are treated and thought of. These campaigns have highlighted issues of access, inclusion and portrayal.

### Case study: Holly's story

Holly is 13 years old and has cerebral palsy. She attends the local secondary school, where some of her lessons are on the first floor. She has one friend who helps her to get to her lessons but generally she doesn't make friends easily. She is very aware of the stares she gets from other pupils in the school.

1 Holly often arrives late to a lesson when she has to struggle to climb the stairs to the first floor. How do you think this might affect her?

2 Holly doesn't find it easy to make friends. What do you think will have contributed to her feeling that people don't want to talk to her?

3 How will her experiences at school affect her self-esteem?

4 What would you do to include Holly and make her feel ordinary?

### Personal, learning and thinking skills

The activity should help towards PLTS: Creative thinker; Reflective learner; Effective participator.

### Activity

1 As a group, discuss the role of the media and how it influences our opinions.

2 Produce a collage of pictures from magazines and newspapers showing how people are portrayed. Use positive and negative images.

3 Present this to your group and give your opinions on how people are portrayed.

### Functional skills

It will also help towards FS: English – speaking and listening.

You have been asked many questions on this page. Now *you* need to keep asking the questions and challenging yourself and others.

### Just checking

* What kind of language might be used by the media and others to describe someone with an impairment?
* Give four words that the media has sometimes used to describe a person with a disability.
* Give two examples of people on TV who have a disability.

# 9.9 Our personal and social responsibility

Our society is made up of many different people. We are different because of our physical appearance, our race, colour, language, and our gifts and talents. In this topic you will reflect on your own personal and social responsibility towards others.

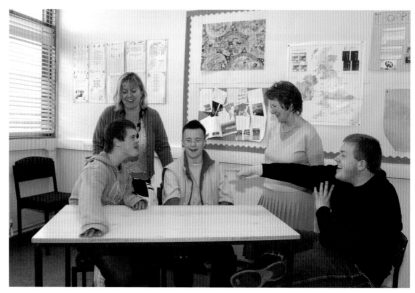

*Our society.*

### Social inclusion – working together

Social inclusion is about helping to ensure that everyone feels able and confident to contribute and to be involved in their community. **Diversity** should be valued.

People and organisations are becoming more aware and recognising the barriers that people with disabilities face, and this in its own right is a huge step to removing them.

Inclusion for people with disabilities within our society needs to be looked at in a **holistic** way. There are many charities, organisations, agencies and people with disabilities that are working together to promote the rights of children and adults to be part of a fully inclusive society.

The government's Department for Work and Pensions has asked employers to acknowledge their role in helping social inclusion for disabled people. Employers have to provide disabled employees with the assistance they require. This means not only making physical changes but also developing a positive and supportive culture at work among other employees, and trying to eradicate prejudice and stereotypical views.

Can you think of ways that this approach could also be used at school, in your class even?

# The National Social Inclusion Programme (NSIP)

Government departments and other organisations have worked together to challenge attitudes, to enable people to fulfil their potential and to greatly improve opportunities and outcomes for people with mental health problems. Some of this work is underpinned by the National Social Inclusion Programme (see www. socialinclusion.org.uk).

As you have seen in Unit 2, it is very important that there is coordination and communication between agencies. Developing a multi-agency approach to respond to the needs of children and adults with disabilities and their families means that our society can move from:

* children being cared for in institutions to being cared for at home
* children going to special schools to them going to mainstream schools
* separate child protection processes to integrated approaches to child welfare, which give support to the whole family.

The National Health Service National Service Framework for Children, *Every Child Matters* and the Children Act 2004, as well the extension of Direct Payments (see topic 9.6), have all helped with this approach.

The health, social care, children and young people and the community justice services work together to improve outcomes for disabled children, young people and their families, to give everyone equal opportunities in life.

## What does a socially inclusive society mean to you?

What can you do individually to help this process of developing an inclusive society and why should you? We all have a responsibility to the community we live in. We have to decide what we want that community to be like.

The following statements have been adapted from *Creating Accepting Communities*, a report produced in 1999 by MIND (the National Association for Mental Health, which campaigns for people with mental health problems).

* 'A healthy society is one that gets the best out of everyone regardless of their circumstances.'
* 'A healthy society is one that embraces **diversity** and is not threatened by cultures, beliefs or behaviours outside society's norms.'
* 'Everyone is part of society and nobody should be seen as a "burden".'
* 'If you socially exclude any group of people this damages not only the mental health of the excluded individuals but the mental health of society as a whole.'

If we as individuals are going to promote inclusion, it means leading public opinion. What can you do to help lead people's opinions?

## Activity

Either design a poster to affect and challenge the attitudes of others towards disability, or produce a leaflet and a display on how to combat discrimination and celebrate diversity. Provide contact details of relevant organisations for people who want to find out more about certain issues.

## For your project

Explain what you think is your personal and social responsibility towards people with disabilities and how you can help influence the opinion of others.

## Just checking

* What is meant by valuing diversity?
* Give two examples of organisations working towards an inclusive society.
* What do you believe makes a healthy society?

# Unit 9 Assessment guide

This unit is assessed by an assignment, which is marked by your teacher. You will need to show your understanding of what the social model of disability is, and how society treats people who have disabilities now and how they were treated in the past in asylums and institutions. You will need to show your understanding of how the social model of disability aims to help people become independent and how it feels that it is society that disables people rather than their impairments. You will need to compare this against the medical model, which focuses on people's medical conditions and what people can't do, rather than what they can. You will need to show that you understand how people with disabilities may be stereotyped or discriminated against and how changes in health and social care services, education, employment and the environment have helped them become independent. You will need to carry out a survey of an organisation, to identify any potential barriers that discriminate against people with disabilities. These might include the environment, stereotypical attitudes or language that is used. Legislation (laws) has helped people with disabilities to be treated equally and all organisations have their own policies based on these laws. You will need to investigate one piece of legislation and one organisation's policy. You will also need to examine your own views and feelings towards people with disabilities and consider how society feels about them.

## Time management

* Keep any class work in a folder; this will help when you need to write your report.

* Be prepared to listen to other people's points of view in discussion: their views may enhance your report. It will also help you become a reflective learner.

* If your teacher allows you to carry out the survey in class time, use the time wisely.

## Useful links

* Work experience may provide an opportunity to carry out the survey to assess how independence and choice can be promoted, and how potential barriers that prevent independence can be overcome. For example, you may visit an organisation that provides care and support for people with physical disabilities, where you will see how the environment is adapted to allow wheelchair access and therefore help to prevent discrimination. You could carry your survey out in your school or college, where you could assess the environment for any barriers to access.

* You may be able to talk to people who either have a disability themselves or represent a group of people who have disabilities. You could ask them whether they feel they are discriminated against or treated differently to other people. Remember to treat any information that you are given sensitively and maintain confidentiality.

* Useful websites to help you with your research on the social model of disability and associated legislation are: www.drc.org.uk and www.mencap.org.uk.

## Things you might need

* ICT equipment to investigate at least one piece of legislation relevant to the social model of disability. For example, you could research the Discrimination Act 2005 and assess whether it has been put into practice in your school or college.

* A copy of an organisation's policy that is based upon the piece of legislation that you have chosen.

* Permission from an organisation to investigate how they support people with disabilities and if there are any potential barriers. For example, if you went to visit a day centre for people with learning difficulties, it would be good practice to ask your supervisor if you could carry out your survey.

* People with whom to discuss society's attitudes towards people with disabilities. Talk to your family and friends about their feelings.

* To be honest about your own views and values. You are asked to reflect on your attitudes towards people with disabilities; do you call people names or feel sorry for them? Or do you treat them as equals who need a bit of extra help to do the things that you do? By being honest, you will be able to really think about your attitudes towards disability and those of society.

# How you will be assessed

| You must show that you *know*: | Guidance | To gain higher marks you must *explain*: |
|---|---|---|
| What the social model of disability is, how it developed and how it is different from the medical model. | Produce a report that shows how you have investigated how people with disabilities were treated in the past and how society treats them today. Remember that the social model of disability focuses on helping people to become independent while the medical model focuses on people's medical conditions and what they can't do, rather than what they can. | What the aims and objectives of the social model are. You will need to discuss how society needs to change its attitudes towards people who are less able and you should consider the labels that people are given, e.g. handicapped. How it empowers people and changes attitudes in society. |
| How the social model of disability affects support, service provision and the environment for people with disabilities. | Carry out a survey of an organisation (this may be your school, college or work experience placement) and identify how people with disabilities are supported. Service provision means the type of care a person with disabilities might receive. Do they have a care worker who allows them to be as independent as possible or do they receive a service that sees them as a medical problem? | How independence and choice are promoted and how improvements in the environment, education and employment can support people with disabilities in an organisation. |
| How potential barriers in society and the environment can be overcome. | In your survey, assess at least three potential barriers that may disable rather than enable people. This might include stairs, and a lack of a lift, toilet facilities that have no room for a wheelchair, canteen facilities where the counter is too high for a wheelchair user. Other barriers will include people's attitudes towards people with disabilities, language that negatively stereotypes people and a lack of educational support. | How these potential barriers (e.g. access, education, attitudes and language) might be overcome. For example, you could suggest how the environment could be improved and how people's attitudes could be changed to be more positive towards people with disabilities. |
| How legislation, related policies and ethical issues support the social model of disability. | Produce a report showing how your chosen organisation uses one piece of legislation and a policy to support the rights of people with disabilities. You could use the Discrimination Act 2005 or the Equality Act 2006. Ask your teacher or your work placement supervisor for a copy of a policy that an organisation uses to promote the social model of disability and equal opportunities. | How ethical implications affect policies in an organisation. Organisations need to show that they are acting ethically when supporting people with disabilities. This means respecting other people's rights, choices and independence. Legislation helps to protect people's rights and ensures they are treated correctly. |
| What your own values, attitudes and social responsibility to others are. | In your report, you should reflect on (think about) your own feelings and attitudes towards people with disabilities and give four examples of these. You should also consider what other people in society think. You should also reflect upon your social responsibility to others, for example when you act as an advocate. | In much more detail, why you have these feelings and attitudes. Where do your values and attitudes come from? Could you change them? How easy or difficult would it be to change society's views? Have you ever acted as an advocate – that is, spoken on behalf of someone else? |

# YOUR PROJECT

## Introduction

In this unit you will find information and advice on how to complete the project for your diploma qualification. Your project is unique to you. You will have ideas and interests of your own. Here the aim is to offer you guidance on how to meet your aims and objectives.

### What is the project?

The project is an important part of your diploma qualification. It enables you to undertake study of a topic that you can select. It allows you to explore a topic of interest in much greater depth and you can also decide what type of work it is. You may, for example, choose to do a report or an investigation. You will have a teacher project support link, who will advise and guide you through your project. You must complete your project within either one or two years. When completing it, you can work either alone or in a group – but check this with your tutor first.

### What exactly do I need to do to complete the project?

For your project, you are required:

* to select, either individually or as part of a group, an appropriate sector-relevant topic – that is, the topic must be relevant to the sectors covered by the diploma

* to identify a question, task or brief which specifies an intended outcome – that is, say what you are going to do and what you hope to achieve (these are your aims and objectives)

* to produce a plan for how you will deliver your intended outcome – that is, plan how you will achieve your aims and objectives

* to conduct research into the project area using appropriate techniques – this will form your project design, for example, using questionnaires or interviewing people

* to develop the intended outcome using selected tools and techniques safely – take into account health and safety and any professional codes of ethics

* to demonstrate the capacity to see a project through to completion – that is, complete your project on time and hand it in

* to share the outcome of the project and an evaluation of the project, including a review of your own learning and performance, with others, using appropriate communication methods – that is, present your project in various formats (written and orally) and reflect on what you think went well and what you would do differently if you had to do it again.

## Materials and resources

It is a good idea to keep a project notebook. This can be an ordinary notebook but it is important that you use it solely for the purpose of your project.

Inside you can make notes on:

* ideas for your project
* websites you have visited
* lists of things to do
* ideas you have
* reflections on what you think is going well and what is not.

As well as a notebook you will need other materials:

* an A4 lever arch file
* A4 paper – lined and plain
* USB storage (or floppy discs or similar)
* pens and pencils

* ruler
* eraser and pencil sharpener
* plastic wallets
* highlighters.

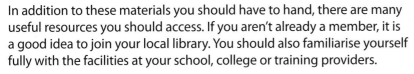

*A project notebook will help to keep you organised.*

In addition to these materials you should have to hand, there are many useful resources you should access. If you aren't already a member, it is a good idea to join your local library. You should also familiarise yourself fully with the facilities at your school, college or training providers.

Ensure you have an email address so that you can make enquiries via this method of communication.

Finally, become a readaholic! Read local newspapers, magazines and leaflets – it will increase your knowledge as well as giving you ideas for your project.

*Become a readaholic!*

## How your project will be assessed

The assessment evidence for all Projects may be presented in a format most appropriate to the type of Project – for example, journals, slides, CDs, videos/DVDs, audio tapes, photographs, artefacts, etc. The projects are marked by generalists and the Extended Projects are marked by specialists.

## What is covered in the rest of this unit?

* Choosing your project topic – how to choose your project subject and some ideas for topics
* Planning your project – developing your project aims and objectives and managing your time
* Information sources – finding and using information sources
* Ethics, confidentiality and health and safety – ensuring you complete your project with these in mind
* Research methods – how you will obtain information and data for your project
* Presenting your project – how to present your project in written and oral formats
* Bibliographies – how to reference and record what resources you have used

# Choosing your project topic

**THINKING POINT**

Has there been a particular subject in the course that has interested you? Is there something you have heard about that you would like to know more about?

Your first task is to choose a topic or subject for your project. Think of some ideas and write these down in your project notebook to discuss with your project mentor/tutor. Don't worry if you can't think of a topic straight away and feel confused. Work through the following pages and write some notes in your project notebook – take time to think of your topic and don't rush.

## The diploma areas

Below is a list of the main areas the diploma has covered. Look these over and write down in your notebook the ones that you have really enjoyed and would like to know more about. If you have a certain career in mind, for example as a social worker, it may be a good idea to choose an area that is related to this.

| Level 1 | Level 2 |
|---|---|
| Exploring the sectors | Principles, values and personal development |
| Exploring principles and values | Working together and communicating |
| Working together | Safeguarding and protecting individuals |
| Are we communicating? | Growth, development and healthy living |
| Is it safe? | Needs and preferences |
| Health, well-being and lifestyles | Antisocial and offending behaviour |
| Meetings needs | Supporting children and young people |
| Growth and development | Patient-centred health |
| | The social model of disability |

## Some ideas

Ideas 'For your project' are presented throughout the units of this book. Some more are suggested in the diagram on the next page.

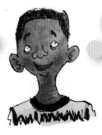

**Social care**

The development of social services

An investigation into care home provision in your local community

**Health care**

How the treatment of diseases has changed through history

The history of a role such as a midwife

Hospital infections – causes, symptoms and treatment

**Community justice**

Aims of parenting programmes

Explore the Neighbourhood Watch scheme and what its aims are

An investigation into what the Youth Taskforce is

A report on how antisocial behaviour is being managed in your community

**Children and young people**

The role of play in child development, including types of play

The role of Sure Start – case study on your local Sure Start centre

Early-years education – importance of play, assessment and development, including the workforce

*Some ideas for your project. These suggestions could be adapted to your own particular interests.*

## Some 'do's and 'don't's

Do:

✔ choose a topic you are interested in

✔ choose a topic that is related to the diploma

✔ discuss your topic with your tutor.

Don't:

✘ choose a topic just because your friend is doing the same

✘ choose a topic that is very personal to you as it can affect you emotionally

✘ choose a topic that you have strong moral feelings about – such as euthanasia – because your own personal feelings may affect how you approach and write up the project.

## Think it through

Talk through possible topics and any potential problems with your class colleagues. It's important that you choose a topic that there is lots of information on for you to find and read.

**Activity**

Once you have a topic in mind, explore the area in more detail by drawing up a spider graph or mind map. This will help you to see what you could cover within your project.

# Planning your project

Once you have chosen what area you want to look at in your project, the next step is to plan what you need to do and how you are going to do it. Planning will incorporate some deadlines, so that you know you can deliver it on time.

## Aims and objectives

Once you have chosen your topic, you will need to sit down and think about your aims and objectives.

### Aims

An *aim* is a statement of intent. So, in broad terms, you would say what you are going to do.

For example, a level 2 project aim may be:

* *In this project I aim to describe the importance of nutrition across the human life span.*

You may have further aims, in support of the primary aim of the project:

* *I aim to include examples of diet plans.*

### Objectives

Your *objectives* are what you are going to do or study to achieve your aims, broken down into tasks. For example, for the project above on nutrition, your objectives could be:

* *Describe what the human life span is*
* *Describe what is meant by nutrition*
* *Identify the nutritional requirements at the various life stages*
* *Design a diet plan for each stage of the life span*

## The main body of the project

You will also need to plan the content of your project – what you will put into it. It may be useful to map this out early on, by thinking of the headings you will use in your final report. You would normally start with an introduction and end with your conclusions. What comes in between will depend on what it is you researched for your project. See the example of Beth's project, opposite.

## Plan and manage your time

It's important that you plan your time and set yourself small tasks to ensure that you complete and hand your project in on time. You will need to plan and work around other commitments you have. If you can, put aside an evening a week to work on your project. Write yourself an action plan saying what you are going to do each week and review this regularly to make sure you are not getting behind. Write your action plan in your notebook.

## How well do you manage your time?

| | Yes | No |
|---|---|---|
| Do I usually turn up to class on time? | | |
| Do I keep most appointments and arrangements that I have made? | | |
| Do I leave things to the last minute and end up rushing them or not completing them? | | |
| Do I hand in my assignments on time? | | |
| Do I use my time effectively? | | |
| Do I make time to rest and relax? | | |

If you have answered mainly 'no' to these questions, then you need to address how you manage your time.

### Beth's project

For her project, Beth decided to look at MRSA, the hospital-acquired 'super bug'. In planning the content of her project, she broke it down into sections, as follows:

* Introduction
* What is MRSA?
* How is it spread?
* How is it treated?
* What are the symptoms?
* What effects does it have on health
* Prevention
* Hospital policies and practices on MRSA
* Conclusions

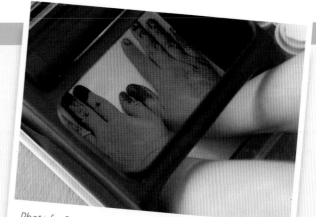

*Photo for Beth's project. Remember that you can include pictures in your project report.*

Beth had nine months in which to complete her project. To manage her time effectively and to ensure she could hand it in when she needed to, she drew up the following plan:

| | |
|---|---|
| Months 1 and 2 | Visit school and public library. Speak to librarian about resources and facilities. Do literature search (books and journals) |
| Month 3 | Internet searches |
| Month 4 | Write letter to infection control department at the local hospital for any information. Visit local health promotion department to locate materials on how to prevent infection spreading |
| Months 5, 6 and 7 | Draft writing of project report |
| Month 8 | Finalising project. Oral presentation to class |
| Month 9 | Hand in project |

# Information sources

There are thousands of books, articles and websites available for students to access and use for projects and research. However, you need to be able to find and locate these. It is important to make sure they are relevant before you use them.

## Types of information

There are many different types of information you can access and use for your project. To some extent which you use will depend on your chosen topic.

| Types of source | Examples |
|---|---|
| Books | Textbooks, dictionaries, encyclopaedias |
| Journals | Articles in professional journals such as *Health Service Journal*<br>Journals are similar to the magazines you read but their content is based on the area they cover. For example, nursing journals contain articles relating to nursing care. |
| Audiovisual | DVDs, CDs, media packages, including television programmes and films |
| Statistics | The Office for National Statistics has a website (www.statistics.gov.uk) where you can view various types of statistics |
| Internet | Access to websites |
| Newspapers | Newspapers cover many topics and you can search past newspapers on computers in public libraries |

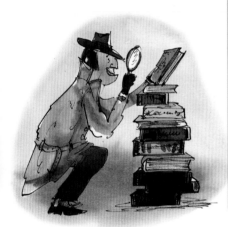

*Searching for relevant information is a skill you need to develop.*

To ensure the information you are reading is up to date, you should access books and journals written within the last 5 years and no longer than 10 years ago, unless of course you are doing a 'historical' investigation.

## Using the Internet

The Internet can be a valuable tool for your project. It contains millions of pages of information. However, unlike a library, the content of the Internet isn't catalogued, so you have to find the information for yourself. This is known as 'surfing the web'. Anyone can design and publish a web page and therefore some websites may contain information that is wrong, outdated or unreliable.

### Search engines

Use a 'search' engine and type in keywords relevant to your topic. When using search engines there is usually an option to just search British/UK websites, and you should click on this option if appropriate.

For example, if your project topic is on child development, type in 'child development' in the search engine box. Tens of thousands of websites will come up. You therefore need to try to reduce these, by typing in after 'child development' some keywords relevant to your project. So, if you are covering child development but want to know specifically about *assessing* child development, type in 'assessment' after 'child development'. You will find that some websites have been written for professionals, who may use language and terminology you don't understand. Try typing in 'key stage 4' or 'KS4' after your keywords. The engine should then search for websites relevant to 14- to 16-year-olds. If this doesn't help, ask your tutor to assist you. Remember, you can always ask for help!

Once you have found a page that you think may be helpful, make a note of its 'address' (e.g. www.nhs.uk).

Use search engines to locate various websites that are relevant to your project subject. Write down their 'address' in your project notebook. Show these to your project tutor, who will check their content and authenticity before you start to extract information from them.

### Gateways

An Internet gateway is a website dedicated to a subject and provides access through it to a number of other relevant websites. For example, www.intute.ac.uk is a free online service that provides access to websites on education.

### Providers of information

The following public bodies all produce information relevant to the diploma:

* The government produces information in many formats and you can visit its website at www.direct.gov.uk.
* The Department of Health also produces lots of information and its website is www.dh.gov.uk.
* The National Health Service's website is www.nhs.uk.
* Community Justice's website is www.communityjustice.gov.uk.

## Using public libraries

Almost all towns and cities have public libraries and it's free to join them. In addition to a wide range of books, most libraries have audiovisual aids and offer access to the Internet. The librarian will be someone who is experienced in locating information and may be able to point you in the right direction.

### Activity

Answer the following questions in your project notebook.

* How far back will you look for information? Two years? Five years?
* Will you use material published in the UK or does your project topic mean you will have to look at material published in other countries?
* What type of information will you use? Books, journals, the Internet? Consider how easily accessible and available these are.
* Will you be visiting your local library?
* How much time will you spend on your resource research?

# Ethics, confidentiality and health and safety

**THINKING POINT**

Has anyone ever copied your homework off you? How did this make you feel? Have you ever been told something, then found out that what you were told wasn't true? Have you ever told anyone a secret but only to find out that they have told many other people? How did this make you feel?

When completing your project or the research for it, there are key principles you must follow: protect people's rights and protect people from harm.

## Ethics and confidentiality

Ethics and confidentiality are covered in Unit 1 of this book. Read back over this section to remind you of these principles.

Ethics is concerned with standards of behaviour and is driven by a desire to protect people. Think of ethics and morals as the rules for distinguishing between right and wrong. We learn ethical norms at home, at school, in church and in other social settings. Although most people acquire their sense of right and wrong during childhood, moral development proceeds throughout life and human beings pass through different stages of growth as they mature.

There are several ethical principles you need to consider when completing your project. You could see these as a 'code of practice' for diploma students, much as the caring professions have their own codes of practice.

### Code of practice for the diploma student

* I will honestly report data, results, methods and procedures.
* I will not copy or plagiarise other people's work. When I do use information from a book or website, I will write the author down in my bibliography.
* I will adhere to confidentiality principles.
* I will respect fellow students and colleagues and treat them fairly.
* I will avoid discrimination against colleagues and students.
* I will obey school/college rules.

### Protection

When completing your project you must also ensure that you protect the rights of others. As humans, we have rights of protection from harm and protection of our privacy.

In completing your project, no harm should be done to others – either physical or psychological.

Ask permission when including any participants – tell them what you are doing and why. State in your project report that you have done so.

When writing up your project you must maintain confidentiality and not use any names.

# Safety first

It is essential that whatever methods you use in your project are safe and will not cause harm to you or others.

Below are examples of project topics that could cause health and safety issues.

* *Exercise.* If your topic involves any form of exercise, then participants must be used to exercising and not have any health-related conditions that could be affected by sudden exertion.

* *Chemicals.* Do not use any chemicals or substances (e.g. alcohol) in your project.

* *Interviews.* Ensure your safety by interviewing people you know. Do not, for example, go knocking on the door of people you do not know, asking if you can interview them.

*Remember* – always discuss with your project mentor what you intend to do and they will advise you regarding any health and safety implications.

# Research methods

Research can be defined briefly as the study to discover correct information. There are different ways to discover and obtain this information and these are called research methods.

## Questionnaires

Questionnaires are a valuable way to collect information. It is a good idea to ask people in your school or college to complete them. There are two main types of information you can get from using questionnaires: facts and opinions. Examples of facts are age, gender, religion and weight. Opinions include people's views and feelings about certain things. An example might be 'What do you think of school meal provision?'

To get the best out of this method in your project, you need to ensure a lot of people complete the questionnaire. You also need to allow time for them to complete the questionnaire and return to it you. So, if you are using this method, you need to plan early.

Below is a checklist of points you need to consider if using questionnaires:

* *Time.* Allow plenty of time for you to design the questionnaire and to circulate it to people.
* *Costs.* These will include postage costs if people need to return the questionnaire to you. It is often best either to email the questionnaire out or to ask people to leave it in a box left somewhere easily accessible to everyone, like a canteen.
* *Production.* The design of the questionnaire can take time, so plan for this early in your project action plan. You will also need access to a photocopier or printer to make copies of the questionnaire.
* *Permission.* Discuss permissions with your project tutor, as you may need permission to distribute the questionnaire, and the content and questions will need to be checked by your project tutor.
* *Confidentiality.* Don't ask people to put down their names on the questionnaire, to ensure their confidentiality.
* *Data extraction.* How will you use the information gained? Will you need support or assistance? Who will give this to you?

There are many different types of questionnaires you can design and your project tutor will support you and show you some examples.

## Interviews

There are two main ways for you to conduct interviews: face to face or by telephone. Equipment you will need includes a notebook and pencils and a voice recorder if you have one. This is so you can tape the interview and play it back again at a later date.

Safety tip! Never arrange to meet someone you do not know to conduct an interview. If you are doing interviews, discuss this with your project mentor. It is important to say whom you are interviewing. A good idea is to invite interviewees into your school or college and interview them there.

## Andrew's questionnaire

Andrew's topic for his level 2 project was the diet of people aged 14–16 years. Within his project, he included childhood obesity and diabetes, and the fact that many people do not eat enough fruit and vegetables. Within his project he wanted to know what sort of foods people of this age typically consumed. He designed a questionnaire which he asked his whole year-11 group to complete. It consisted of the following five questions:

✳ How many pieces of fruit do you eat each day?

✳ Do you eat nuts on a regular basis?

✳ Do you take vitamin supplements?

✳ Do you eat fish regularly?

✳ Do you eat chips more than 4 times a week?

He sent out 200 questionnaires, and 120 were completed and returned to him. He asked his functional maths and numeracy teacher to assist him in extracting and analysing the data. Andrew found that only 60 out of the 120 people ate at least two pieces of fruit each day – that's 50 per cent.

**1** What other questions could Andrew have had on his questionnaire?

**2** If 80 people out of 120 in Andrew's study ate two pieces of fruit instead of 60 out of 120, what percentage would this be?

### Top tips for interviewing

✳ Develop a list of the questions to be asked during the interview. Run these by your project mentor. Try them out first on some friends. You can then change any that you felt didn't go too well.

✳ Express clearly the purpose of the interview. It is important that you tell the person being interviewed why you are interviewing them. Remember to keep the things they tell you confidential.

✳ Try to have only a few questions that give responses of 'yes' or 'no', because they give limited information. These are called closed questions. Use open questions, as these require a full answer and encourage the interviewee to talk.

✳ If you have not understood the response or answer, ask the person to repeat and clarify.

✳ Do not assume answers.

✳ Avoid irrelevant discussions.

✳ Remember your own non-verbal and body language when interviewing. Keep good eye contact and nod encouragingly when your person is giving answers. This will put them at ease and encourage them to relax.

✳ Keep the interview short.

✳ At the end of the interview, summarise the answers given by the person, to check you have written them down and interpreted them correctly.

✳ Thank the person for their time.

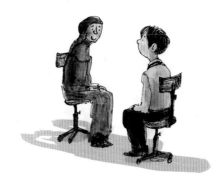

*It is important you are aware of non-verbal signs and body language when conducting interviews.*

### Activity

In preparation for your project interviews, practise the scenario and test your questions with your class colleagues.

**1** Ask them to tell you what they feel went well and what aspects you should change or what things you should do differently. This is peer review.

**2** Write their comments down in your project notebook, as you will need to write these up as part of your assessment.

# Presenting your project

Once you have all your information and you have made notes, you then need to put it altogether and set it out for presentation and assessment. Good presentation is critical, as you need to make sure other people can read and understand it.

## Written presentation

When putting your project report together, it's a good idea to divide it into sections:

* Title page. This should have your project topic title on it, together with your name and details.

* Contents page. This will list each section and give page numbers.

* Introduction. This briefly introduces your project topic, and sets out what your aims and objectives were.

* Main text. This is the largest part of your project. It describes your project work as a whole. You can include any graphs or diagrams within your main text.

* Conclusion. This is the final section of your report, in which you tie together what was presented in the project and sum up the main points.

* Bibliography. This is a list of all the books and other sources of information that you have used for your project.

Within each section, use further headings to set out the work.

Don't forget to number your pages and label any diagrams.

Once you have completed your report, you need to proofread it and it is also a good idea to get a friend or relative to do this as well. Proofreading is where you read the whole document to check for errors, spelling mistakes and sentences that don't make sense.

## Oral presentations

When presenting your project orally, you need to take the following into consideration.

### How long have you got to present?

You may have 5, 10 or 20 minutes, say. Plan your presentation accordingly. For example, if you are presenting on what an antisocial behaviour order (ASBO) is and you have 5 minutes, then you could present it as follows:

* Introduction (30 seconds).

* What an ASBO is, with examples (3 minutes 30 seconds).

* Ask whether the audience has any questions and circulate any handouts (1 minute).

### How many people will be in the audience?

You will need this information to ensure you have enough handouts, for example, if you are using them.

## What equipment can I use?

Will you use an overhead projector (OHP) or the computer and use Microsoft PowerPoint?

## Confident delivery

Remember when doing an oral presentation to speak clearly, slowly and loud enough for people at the back of the room to hear.

Many people are nervous about presenting in front of audiences. This is normal. After giving a few presentations, you will develop confidence and the skills to deliver a great presentation.

## Checklist for oral presentations

* Have I allowed myself enough time to prepare?
* Am I familiar with the topic?
* What is the purpose of the presentation?
* Who is the audience, and how many people will be in it?
* Have I got some examples, where appropriate, to help illustrate any points of my presentation?
* Do I need to consider audience participation?
* Do I want/need handouts?
* Do I want/need audiovisual materials?
* If so, will the audience be able to see them?
* Do I need to book equipment?
* Does all the equipment work and do I know how to use it?
* Have I practised my timing?
* Have I checked my tone and the projection of my voice?
* Have I practised not using fillers such as 'um' and 'ah'?
* Am I going to keep eye contact with the audience?
* During delivery, will I take notice of immediate audience feedback, such as yawns, wandering eyes, nods of agreement, smiles?
* How will I handle criticism?
* What will I do if I think the criticism is unfair?
* What will I do if the audience misunderstands some of what I say?
* What are my plans to overcome my admitted shortcomings?

Write notes on the above in your project notebook.

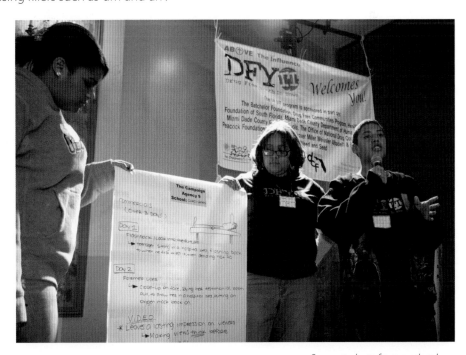

*Some students from a school in North Staffordshire giving a presentation on palliative care.*

# Bibliographies

The bibliography is an important part of your final project report. It should not be neglected.

## What is a bibliography?

A bibliography is an alphabetical list of the sources of information you have used within your project report or other assignment. Within it you will list: books, articles, newspapers, Internet sites, magazines and interviews.

## Why do I have to include a bibliography?

You should always include bibliographies in assignments, to acknowledge your sources and to show where you got your information from. It also shows that you have researched around the topic properly, and used different sources – not just one book. It also allows people reading your work to know where they can get further information. For example, when using a book you will probably use information from just a few pages, but the person could then go and find this book and read the whole of it, gaining further knowledge about the subject, if they so wish. If you use text from a book but do not acknowledge it, then this is known as plagiarism, which is stealing other people's work.

## The parts of the bibliography and the entry styles

### Books

When referencing books you need to note:

* the name of author (who wrote it) – put the surname first, then the initial
* the year of publication – what year the book was written, usually found on the first few pages of the book
* the title of the book – usually in italic type, or underlined
* the publisher – what company has published the book
* the place of publication.

For example, if you were referencing this book you would note it down as follows:

○ Allen, B., Forshaw, C., Haworth, L., Nicol, D. and Vollbracht, A. (2008) *Diploma in Society, Health and Development Level 2*. Heinemann, Oxford.

### Newspaper articles

When referencing newspaper articles you need to note the following;

* the name of the author (who wrote the article – put the surname first then their initials)
* the year of publication
* the title of the article
* the name of the newspaper – usually in italic type, or underlined
* the day and month the newspaper was printed
* the page number of the article.

For example, for the *Diploma Daily* article shown:

○ McIver, S. (2008) 'Residential care home to close down', *Diploma Daily*, 3 May, p. 12.

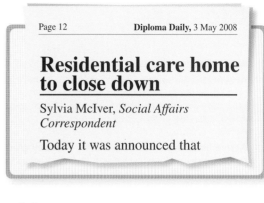

### Internet

**When referencing sources that appear on the Internet, you need to note the following;**

✳ the name of author

✳ the year of publication (this isn't always stated, but do look)

✳ the title of the web page

✳ date accessed – that is, the date on which you looked at the website

✳ the URL – the web address.

For example:

○ NHS Direct, Common health questions (accessed 7 July 2008), www.nhsdirect.nhs.uk

## Top tips

✳ Book and magazine titles are always in italic or underlined in a bibliography.

✳ Put the bibliography in alphabetical order, by the authors' last names.

✳ When there is more than one author, list the authors in the order they are listed on the title page.

✳ Be in the habit of writing down the bibliographic details of a source as soon as you decide to use it – use your project notebook.

✳ Email addresses should not be used without the permission of the owner of the address.

✳ Double-space your bibliography list (ask your ICT tutor to help you do this).

## Summary

✳ Plan your topic carefully

✳ Keep a project notebook

✳ Become familiar with your local library

✳ Ensure you have an email address

✳ Take time to choose your project aims and objectives

✳ Plan your time carefully – develop an action plan

✳ Use as many resources as you can

✳ Remember ethics and confidentiality and to be safe

✳ Decide early if you are going to use a questionnaire

✳ Plan your project presentation carefully

✳ Don't forget your bibliography

✳ Ask for help if you need it

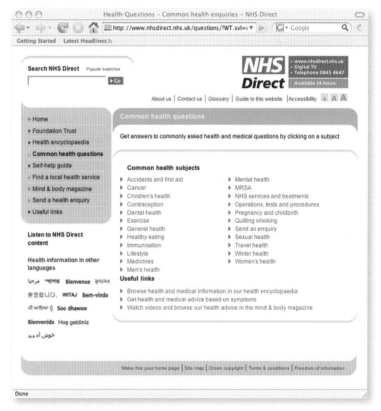

*The NHS Direct website.*

# Glossary

**Abuse** To treat wrongly, harmfully or inappropriately.

**Acceptable behaviour contract (ABC)** An informal procedure aimed at stopping antisocial behaviour; it is a voluntary contract and so has greater flexibility than an ASBO. Breaking an ABC may be a reason for serving an ASBO.

**Active listening** A structured form of listening and responding in which the listener attends fully to the speaker, and then repeats, in their own words, what they think the speaker has said, to check on understanding.

**Acute** Sharp or severe in effect; intense.

**Advocate** Someone who is employed to speak for the person with the disability.

**Ageism** Discrimination against someone due to their age.

**Agencies** Organisations that provide a government or local authority service.

**Alzheimer's disease** A degenerative disease marked by a loss of memory and decreasing ability to communicate, understand and function normally.

**Amniocentesis** A test where a little fluid is taken from the amniotic sac that surrounds the baby, and analysed. It can detect foetal conditions such as spina bifida (a defect of the spinal cord).

**Antibodies** Proteins in the body that help to kill microbes.

**Antisocial behaviour** A wide range of selfish and unacceptable activity that spoils the quality of community life. Repeatedly acting in a way that is likely to cause alarm, harassment or distress to people who do not live in the same house as the person carrying out the behaviour.

**Antisocial behaviour order (ASBO)** A court order given for general antisocial behaviour (see topic 6.2) or as part of a sentence if a person has been involved in criminal behaviour. It states exactly what the person can and cannot do, depending on the reasons why it was given. For example, an offender who has been harassing someone may be forbidden to visit the street the person lives in.

**Appendicitis** Inflammation of the appendix, which is a small tube of tissue attached to the lower end of the large intestine.

**Artery** A blood vessel transporting oxygenated blood from the heart to the rest of the body.

**Arthritis** A condition where body joints are sore, swollen and painful.

**Asperger's syndrome** A form of autism. People with this condition often want to be sociable but find it difficult to understand non-verbal signals. They often have good language skills and are intelligent.

**Assessment** The gathering and evaluation of information in order to be able to understand a particular situation.

**Assistive technology** Any product or service designed to enable independence for disabled and older people. Examples include a Zimmer frame, grab rails, shower stool, pendant and sensor alerts in case of falls.

**Attitude** A personal view or feeling about a person or thing.

**Audit** Systematic check and assessment on a situation. Councils are required to conduct regular audits of crime in their localities.

**Auditory learners** Those who like debates, sound-bites and verse to remember information.

**Authorised users** People with official permission to use something, such as a computer database.

**Bail** A sum of money paid by or for a defendant so that they can await trial in the community, rather than in prison.

**Barristers** Lawyers who defend or prosecute suspects in court.

**Borough** An area run by a council or local authority.

**Braille** A written language of raised dots, used by some blind people.

**British Sign Language** This is the language many deaf people prefer. The language makes use of space and involves movement of the hands, body, face and head.

**Care package** A collection of services to be provided to help an individual to maintain their independence, living in their own home.

**Care pathways** The journey patients with particular conditions take through the health service.

**Cerebral palsy** A condition caused by brain damage before or at birth which causes difficulty in controlling or moving muscles.

**Challenging behaviour** Behaviour that is dangerous (to the self or others) or very disruptive.

**Chronic** Having had a disease, habit, weakness for a long time.

**Clients** People who use the services or professional advice of the health, social care, community justice and children and young people sectors.

**Codes of practice** Sets of standards of conduct for workers and employers across the four care sectors.

**Co-habitation** An emotional and physical intimate relationship which includes a common living place and which exists without legal or religious sanction.

**Collaboration** Working together.

**Colleagues** The fellow professionals you work with.

**Communication** The giving or exchange of thoughts, opinions or information by speech, writing or signs.

**Community support officer** A uniformed member of the police service but without the powers of a full police officer.

**Concise** Brief and to the point.

**Confidential** Private and secret.

**Confidentiality** Keeping sensitive information secret.

**Consultant** The most senior of rank of hospital doctor.

**Contagious** Spread very easily.

**Counselling** A process whereby patients are helped to deal with their problems by talking to a trained person.

**CRB** The Criminal Records Bureau. The Bureau will search its files to identify job applicants who may be unsuitable for certain work, especially work involving children or vulnerable adults.

**Criminal record** A police file of someone's history as an offender. The record is deleted after a period of time, depending on the seriousness of the offence.

**Culture** A set of beliefs, language, styles of dress, ways of cooking, religion, ways of behaving and so on shared by a particular group of people.

**Custodial sentence** A sentence given by the court where the criminal is locked up in a prison or, for young offenders, a secure training centre, a secure children's home or a young offender institution.

**Custom** A practice or way of living that is traditional, or a habit.

**Data** A collection of facts about a person or organisation.

**Data protection** Legal safeguards to prevent misuse of information about an individual that is stored on a computer.

**Department of Health** The department of government that is responsible for health care and the National Health Service. It is headed by the Secretary of State for Health, a cabinet minister.

**Depression** A mental health condition marked by feelings of sadness, despair, loss of energy and difficulty dealing with normal daily life.

**Diabetes UK** A charity that funds research into diabetes and helps those who live with the condition.

**Dialysis** The purifying of blood, as a substitute for the normal function of the kidney.

**Disability** A condition that restricts someone's ability to perform particular activities.

**Discriminate** Treat a person or group unfairly or differently from other persons or groups of people (e.g. on the basis of prejudice).

**Diversity** A wide range of people, differing in terms of race, views, cultures and abilities, among other things.

**Down's syndrome** A genetic condition that features learning disability, which may range from moderate to severe, as well as some physical anomalies.

**Duplicating** Doing something more than once.

**Dyslexia** A language-based disability in which a person has trouble understanding written words.

**Effective** When something produces the intended or expected result.

**Eligibility criteria** A set of conditions which, if met, means someone can receive a service.

**Emergency** A sudden unforeseen crisis (usually involving danger) that requires immediate action.

**Emotional** To do with the emotions.

**Empathise** To understand another person's feelings.

**Empower** Allow someone to make decisions for themselves.

**Enable** Give people the means and the ability to do things for themselves.

**Enabling** Supplying with the means, knowledge or opportunity to do something; giving a person the ability to do a certain task.

**Environmentalist** Someone who is concerned with the protection of the environment.

**Epilepsy** A disorder of the nervous system that causes convulsions and/or periodic loss of consciousness.

**Ethnicity** The fact that someone belongs to a particular ethnic group. An ethnic group means people who share the same way of life and culture.

**Factors** Things that contribute to, or affect, something else.

**Fine motor skills** Control of the smaller muscles, such as those in the fingers (e.g. holding a pencil). These skills are more difficult to acquire than gross motor skills.

**Glucose** A sugar used by the body as a fuel for energy.

**Green Paper** A document for discussion the government publishes that sets out its ideas regarding policy and proposals in a particular area.

**Gross motor skills** Control of the larger muscles, typically those in the arms and legs (e.g. kicking a ball).

**Hazard** Anything that has the potential to harm someone in some way.

**Health** The state of being sound or whole, in body, mind and soul.

**Hierarchy** A system of persons or things arranged in a graded order.

**Holistic** Looking at a person or issue as a whole, rather than as a sum of parts. Looking at all the different needs of the client, including medical, social and emotional needs.

**Holistic care** Care that meets all the patient's needs – physical, emotional, social and mental health.

**Home-Start** A charity that provides informal and friendly support for families with young children.

**Hospice** A home or service providing care and support for people who are sick or terminally ill.

**Hypertension** Blood pressure over 140/90 mmHg.

**Hypothermia** A condition where the body temperature drops below 35°C.

**Immunisation** The administration of a substance (usually by injection) to help the body fight infectious disease.

**Immunity** Resistance to a particular disease caused by infection.

**Impairments** Reductions in strength, quality or ability, possibly because of an injury or disease.

**Implement** To carry out something, follow it through.

**Implementation** Putting a decision or plan into action.

**Inappropriate behaviour** Behaviour that is not suitable or proper.

**Inclusive** Involving as wide a range of people as possible. One of the government's aims set out in *Every Child Matters* is that all disabled children will be fully included in society.

**Income** The amount of money that goes into a household, generally from earnings from work but also from sources such as welfare benefits, pensions and investments.

**Independence** Freedom from the control and influence of others and from the need for their support; the ability to make your own decisions.

**Independent** Not having to rely on someone else to do things for you.

**Infections** Illnesses that are spread by the passing of microorganisms between people.

**Integrated** When all the different elements are combined as one.

**Intellectual** To do with the brain.

**Interaction** All involvement with other people (anything from a simple act such as buying an ice cream from a shopkeeper to the deep conversation you may have with a close friend).

**Interests** Those things that draw your attention, that you want to get involved with and spend time on.

**Interpersonal skills** Skills that allow us to interact successfully with others.

**Intervention** Any specific action a service provider takes on becoming involved in a case. Doing something to prevent or improve or control a situation; getting involved.

**Jargon** Specialist words and expressions when used inappropriately, with people who won't understand them.

**Joint working** Agencies working together.

**Judgemental** Making decisions or forming opinions on the basis of something such as appearance, without proper evidence, and being too critical.

**Justice sector** All the people and services involved in dealing with crime.

**Kinaesthetic learners** Those who prefer actions such as role-plays, visits and 'design and build' projects.

**Labelling** Identifying or describing someone with a label rather than as an individual. Labelling is linked to stereotyping, as people are expected to conform to the behaviour associated with the stereotype with which they have been labelled.

**Legislation** A law or group of laws as passed by Parliament.

**Life events** Any particularly important things which take place or happen during the life span.

**Life stage** A distinct period of growth or development in the life span.

**Makaton** A system of communication designed for people with learning disability that uses speech together with signs (gestures) and symbols (pictures).

**Malnutrition** A condition caused by lack of essential food, vitamins and nutrients.

**Medical history** A complete description of a patient's physical and mental condition, past and present.

**Menopause** The natural and permanent stopping of menstruation, occurring usually between the ages of 45 and 55.

**Microorganism** Organisms ('germs') so small they are not visible to the naked eye, but can be seen only with a powerful microscope.

**Milestones** The different skills that a child should achieve by a specific age (e.g. children of six weeks should smile, showing that their visual and communications skills are developing).

**Minutes** A record of what is said and decided at a meeting, made at the time.

**Model** A simplified or idealised version or idea of how something ought to work.

**Modelling** The demonstration of a type of behaviour in order for it to be copied.

**Monitoring** Making (and recording) regular checks on something.

**Motor neurone disease** A progressive, incurable, degenerative disease that leads to weakness and wasting of muscles.

**Multi-agency working** Where different organisations work together to achieve an agreed outcome.

**Multidisciplinary** Made up of professionals of different types (often from different agencies) working together to deliver services.

**Nausea** Sensation or feeling of going to vomit or be sick.

**'Need to know' basis** Giving only that information which is needed, and only to those who need to know.

**Needs** Requirements or things felt to be necessary.

**NHS Direct** An NHS organisation that provides health advice by telephone, on the web and via interactive digital television.

**Non-verbal cues** Methods of communicating other than talking, mainly body language and facial expressions.

**Nursing home** A place where adults can live with medical care provided under the supervision of nursing staff.

**Obesity** A condition of being unhealthily overweight. It is defined as a BMI of over 30 kg/m$^2$.

**Occupational therapist** A health professional who assesses and treats physical and mental conditions using activities to promote independent living.

**Paediatrician** A doctor who specialises in the care of children.

**Paramount** More important than anything else.

**Partnership** Care workers, professionals, the service user and families working together. People or organisations working together towards a common goal.

**Pathology department** A hospital department that offers diagnostic laboratory services.

**Peer group** A group of people of the same age who are important to the individual. The peer group will influence the behaviour and attitude of the individual because they value their opinion.

**Percentile chart** A graph showing what percentage of all children will have reached a certain developmental stage (e.g. a particular height or weight) by their age.

**Perception** Understanding of the issues.

**Person-centred planning** A process of helping people (usually with some form of disability) to find out what is most important to them and what they want from their lives.

**Perspective** A way of looking at things.

**Pharmacist** A health care professional (not a doctor) who specialises in drugs and medicines.

**Philosophy** An attitude that guides a person's behaviour.

**Physical** To do with the body.

**Physical reflexes** Automatic, uncontrollable responses to a physical change, such as moving away from something sharp that causes pain.

**Physiotherapist** A health care professional (not a doctor) who treats the physical problems caused by accidents, illness and ageing, particularly those that affect the muscles, bones, heart, circulation and lungs.

**Planning** Setting out detailed proposals for doing or achieving something.

**Police community support officers (PCSOs)** Uniformed police support staff. They do some of the tasks that do not require the experience or powers held by regular police officers.

**Policy** A document that tells service providers how to deal with particular situations in the workplace.

**Practice nurse** A nurse who works within a GP's surgery or health centre.

**Prejudice** An unreasonable feeling against a person or group of people, especially not liking a particular group of people.

**Preventive** Working to stop problems arising.

**Primary information** Information obtained by asking a person directly.

**Principle** A basic guide to the right way to behave, for example that you should try to treat everyone fairly.

**Procedure** A list of steps to follow to complete a particular task in the correct way.

**Professional bodies** Organisations that set standards for and look after the interests of their members, who all do one type of job. An example in the health sector is the Royal College of Nursing.

**Psychologist** Someone who studies the human mind and its functions.

**Puberty** The life stage when a person becomes capable of sexual reproduction.

**Radiotherapy** The use of radiation to treat cancer.

**Record** A written account of what has happened or been achieved, for example, in a meeting, or by a student.

**Reflection** Looking at yourself or back on something you have done, deciding whether you like what you see or have done well (or not) and using that to improve yourself.

**Regulations** Government orders (rules) which have the force of law, made to control conduct.

**Remedial** Working with existing problems to lessen them.

**Renal** To do with the kidneys.

**Report** A structured account of a particular subject matter, or of something that has happened.

**Residential home** A place where people (adults or children) live and are cared for and supported by staff with social care (not health) training.

**Respect** A feeling or attitude of admiration and regard for somebody or something.

**Respiratory** To do with respiration, that is, breathing.

**Response rate** The proportion (percentage) of questionnaires that are returned to you completed.

**Review** To look at something again with a view to improving it.

**Risk** The chance of suffering harm, loss, injury, danger or some other bad consequence.

**Rituals** Prescribed or set ways of behaving in certain circumstances or of conducting a ceremony, proceeding or service.

**Role model** Someone that others look up to and copy.

**SCOPE** A disability organisation in England and Wales whose focus is people with cerebral palsy.

**Secondary information** Information gained at second-hand, such as from books.

**Sector** The care industry is divided into sectors that are responsible for different aspects of the care of people, such as the social care sector and the health sector.

**Secular** Not religious.

**Segregation** Keeping particular groups of people apart from one another.

**Self-centred** Tending to see things and events only from your own point of view.

**Self-concept** This is a combination of our self-esteem, which is how highly we think about ourselves, and our self-image, which is how we think others think of us.

**Self-esteem** How highly you think of your abilities and yourself.

**Shared care** Professionals and others sharing in the care of an individual.

**Single assessment process** Sharing information about an individual and their needs, with the aim of having a good all-round understanding of the individual's needs.

**Skills** Abilities you have when you become expert at something.

**Social** To do with life with other people.

**Social isolation** Living without regular contact with other people, especially friends and family.

**Socio-economic** To do with a mix of social/class considerations and money.

**Solicitors** Lawyers who give legal advice and draft documents. Some appear in court for defendants.

**Special constables** Uniformed volunteers who give a few hours each week to support the police in enforcing the law.

**Special school** A school that has pupils with statements of special educational needs (SEN), and often with one particular type of disability, such as deafness, whose needs cannot be fully met from within mainstream provision.

**Specialist diabetic team** A health care team specialising in diabetes and consisting of doctors, nurses, dieticians, podiatrists and administration staff.

**Stakeholder** Someone who has a share in or an interest in an organisation.

**Stamina** The heart's ability to work under strain.

**Statutory** Required by law. The statutory services have been set up by Acts of Parliament and are funded by public money.

**Stereotype** A generalised and oversimplified opinion or image of someone else, such as 'Football players aren't very intelligent'.

**Stereotyping** Thinking a group of people will all have the same attributes, for example that all older people will be deaf and have memory problems.

**Stopcock** The main tap or valve on the pipe bringing water from the mains into the building.

**Strategic health authority** Regional NHS body that is responsible for enacting Department of Health policy and for supervising the provision of health care in its areas.

**Strategy** A plan or a method of getting results.

**Strength** The body's physical power.

**Summons** Written orders to attend court at a stated time.

**Suppleness** The body's ability to bend without damage.

**Support** Sustained help, emotional as well as physical, for a person in a state of pain, illness, distress or grief.

**Supported living** An arrangement whereby people with a disability can live within the community, with carefully tailored assistance.

**Terminology** Specialised words or expressions that are used by people in a particular work setting.

**Transmitted** Passed on.

**Ultrasound examination** A harmless, non-invasive and painless technique that generates images ('scans', produced by high-frequency sound waves) of the baby and its organs.

**Values** Beliefs about what is important and worthwhile in life and what is morally right.

**Victim Support** An independent charitable organisation which helps people cope with the effects of crime. It provides free and confidential support and information, and works to advance the rights of victims and witnesses.

**Visual learners** Those who prefer to use textbooks, mind maps and diagrams to learn.

**Vulnerable** A state in which being physically or emotionally hurt is more likely.

**Walk-in centres** Clinics that give people fast access to treatment and health advice, without an appointment.

**Welfare** Health, happiness, well-being.

**Well-being** People feeling good about themselves.

**Wisdom** The ability to discern or judge what is true, right, or lasting; insight.

# Temperature and blood pressure chart

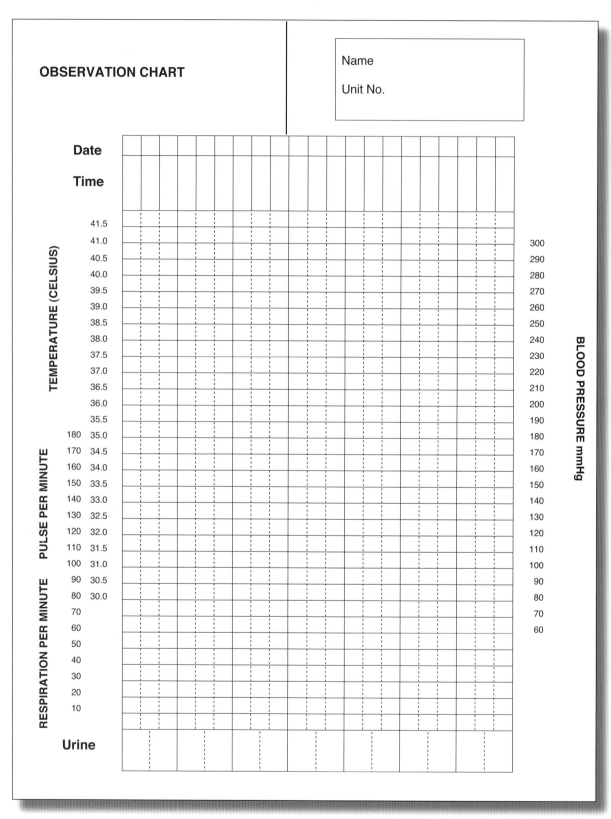

# Peak flow chart

**Peak Flow Diary**

To take a peak flow reading: put the marker to zero, take a deep breath, seal your lips around the mouthpiece, then blow as hard and as fast as you can into the device. Note the reading. Repeat three times. The 'best of the three' is the reading to record. Mark this with a cross on the chart.

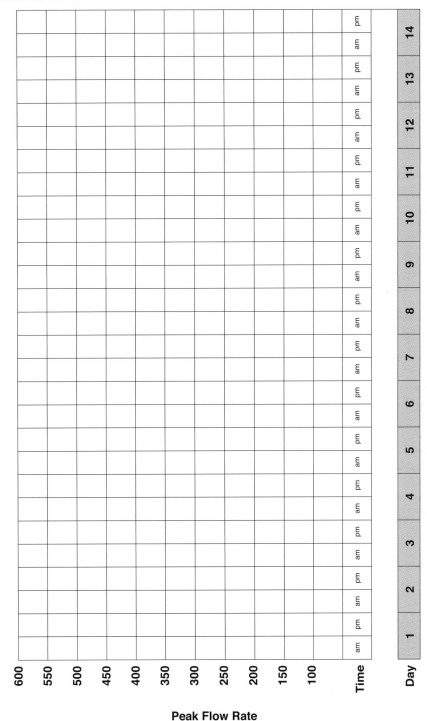

Date.......................

Name ......................

**Peak Flow Rate**

# Index

Pages in *italics* indicate pictures and diagrams; pages in **bold** indicate definitions of terms in the text, but more definitions may be found in the glossary on pages 248–51.